# Office and Operative Hysteroscopy

Springer-Verlag France S.A.R.L

Bernard BLANC, René MARTY, Rémy de MONTGOLFIER

# Office and Operative Hysteroscopy

Prefaced by John SCIARRA

and by Claude SUREAU

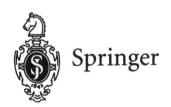 Springer

**Professeur Bernard Blanc**
Hôpital de la Conception
147, boulevard Baille
13385 Marseille cedex 5
FRANCE

**Docteur René Marty**
26, boulevard d'Argenson
92200 Neuilly-sur-Seine
FRANCE

**Docteur Rémy de Montgolfier**
Maternité
Hôpital de Salon-de-Provence
13300 Salon-de-Provence
FRANCE

ISBN 978-2-287-59652-0      ISBN 978-2-8178-0841-3 (eBook)
DOI 10.1007/978-2-8178-0841-3

© Springer-Verlag France 2002
Originally published by Springer-Verlag France, Berlin, Heidelberg, New York in 2002

SPIN : 10687993

# Foreword

Hysteroscopy is now an essential part of contemporary gynecologic practice. This is true in both the office setting as well as in the hospital operating room. Office hysteroscopy gives the practitioner the ability to obtain direct information of uterine pathology, with minimal discomfort, minimal risk and minimal cost to the patient. Furthermore, with modern small diameter instruments, hysteroscopy performed on an ambulatory basis provides immediate visual diagnosis in a true minimally invasive fashion. Similarly, operative hysteroscopy using newer endoscopes allows the surgeon to perform both simple and advanced uterine surgery with uterine preservation and fertility preservation. Evidence now clearly indicates that operative hysteroscopy gives excellent results, and is the minimally invasive surgical procedure of choice for the treatment of the septate uterus, intrauterine adhesions, endometrial polyps, intracavitary uterine fibroids and for the treatment of abnormal uterine bleeding by endometrial ablation. This volume of office and operative hysteroscopy written and assembled by Drs. B. Blanc and R. Marty is a comprehensive, practical text by experts in the field that covers all of the above aspects of diagnostic hysteroscopy and hysteroscopic surgery.

The possibility of visualizing the interior of the uterus has interested physicians and intrigued gynecologists for over a century. Hysteroscopy, however, did not become an important clinical procedure until the advent of fiber optic instrumentation, the development of modern lens systems and small telescopes, and the evolution of safe techniques to distend the uterine cavity with either fluids administered under pressure or with of carefully regulated carbon dioxide inflation. The hysteroscopic instrumentation available today, as presented in this text, allows the practitioner the ability to perform both diagnostic and surgical procedures with accuracy, convenience and confidence.

This volume is an important contribution to the field of hysteroscopy. It is both a comprehensive presentation of the available instruments as well as a detailed presentation of the diagnostic techniques and surgical procedures that are now accepted by our specialty for the treatment of intrauterine pathology. In addition to the standard material on hysteroscopy, this volume is unique in its emphasis on fibrohysteroscopy. The editors have had a particular interest in flexible hysteroscopy and, indeed, have been pioneers in the development and the introduction of fibrohysteroscopy into modern gynecologic practice. The readers of this volume, whether they be young physicians, practicing gynecologists or experts, will certainly benefit from the practical and useful information compiled by the editors of this volume in all areas of hysteroscopy but, especially, in the area of flexible hysteroscopy, that up until this time has been under-represented in gynecologic literature.
The technique of hysteroscopy is a skill-based technique, and requires careful attention to detail as well as patience and practice. In addition to the chapters contributed by Drs. Blanc and Marty, the solicited chapters are all written by recognized experts who are international authorities in the field of gynecologic endoscopy and minimally invasive surgery. Therefore, the authors are all writing from personal experience and are presenting the state of the art of diagnostic and surgical hysteroscopy. This collective experience of a large number of international experts is invaluable to individuals who wish to acquire the skills necessary to practice modern hysteroscopy.

This text is truly comprehensive. I indicated earlier that one unique feature of this volume is the material on flexible hysteroscopy. The editors, however, have not neglected the history of hysteroscopy nor the basic information necessary for the practice of hysteroscopy. They have also developed the volume to focus on the use of the hysteroscopy for the removal of dislocated intrauterine devices, for hysteroscopic metroplasty, for division of intrauterine adhesions, resection of submucous fibroids and removal of intrauterine polyps, as well as endometrial ablation for the treatment abnormal uterine bleeding. In addition, newer dimensions of hysteroscopy are also presented, such as falloposcopy for visualization of the fallopian tubes. This text, therefore, provides the reader not only with fundamentals but also with specialized and advanced information. It is my belief that this volume will become an important international classic textbook in the field of hysteroscopy. There is no question that hysteroscopy has already assumed an important place in the practice of gynecology and gynecologic surgery. As noted earlier, hysteroscopy affords a high level of accuracy in detecting intra-uterine pathology and is indicated whenever intrauterine disease is suspected. Today, this is often performed in an ambulatory setting and, therefore, the emphasis of this text on office procedures is, clearly, of great value. This is particularly true with the expansion of office hysteroscopy to include surgical procedures. This volume presents these new areas of hysteroscopy to the reader in a concise and informative fashion. Dr. B. Blanc and R. Marty are to be complimented. They are true pioneers in the field and have shared their experience and wisdom with us.

This important text, with its unique emphasis on flexible hysteroscopy, is a welcome addition to the field of hysteroscopy. It is, indeed, a valued resource for all of us in clinical practice and will improve the quality of hysteroscopic procedures that we provide to our patients presently and in the future.

John J. Sciarra, MD, PhD
Thomas J. Watkins Professor and Chairman
Department of Obstetrics and Gynecology
Northwestern University Medical School
Chicago, Illinois USA
Immediate Past-President
International Society for Gynecologic Endoscopy

# Preface

It is a honour and a pleasure to have been asked to write the introduction of such an interesting book. The expertise of Prof. B. Blanc in the field of hysteroscopy is widely known and he has been fortunate enough to be in the position of adding to his own experience and contribution information gained from various authors, particularly well selected themselves.

This book represents indeed a very valuable set of documents, sometimes quite original, concerning all aspects of hysteroscopy. The historical considerations are particularly informative ; however the main parts of the book are those concerning the technical and the clinical aspects of this procedure.

As far as the technical aspects are concerned, very precise descriptions of all the various instruments (rigid or flexible, including microhysteroscopy) are given, as well as an exhaustive description of the sources of light, of the video recording, the anaesthesia, the ancillary procedures. The use of hysteroscopy in office settings as an ambulatory diagnostic or minor operative procedure is clearly exposed, as well as the major operative aspects of hysteroscopy. Detailed information is given concerning the selected instrumentation and the reasons for choice, the distending media, the irrigation process, the use of high frequency energy, the electrodes, the biopsy forceps, the decontamination and the sterilisation of instrumentation.

Besides this technical information, the clinical field relevant to the use of hysteroscopy particularly holds the attention of the reader. All clinical situations where hysteroscopic procedures may be undertaken are scrupulously described and the indications are exposed and discussed with great details and objectivity: endometrial hormonal influences, polyps, adenomyosis, endometrial abnormalities, fibroids, intra uterine adhesions, as well as the types of interventions such as endometrial resection, endometrectomy and metroplasty.

A point of particular interest is the fact that for some important clinical situations, or therapeutic procedures, several chapters are written by different authors, thus giving a varied picture of the clinical and surgical approaches.

Another important fact is the full and precise description of the possible complications which may occur: traumatic, infectious, hemorragic, or those due to the fluid used for distension.

Less important but also interesting are the chapters dealing with IUD removal, preparation for IVF or falloposcopy.
This book of Bernard Blanc, well illustrated and which includes many useful references and statistics is undoubtedly a book of high theoretical and practical interest which needs to be carefully read by those involved in this very specific gynecologic procedure.

Claude Sureau
Honorary President of the French Academy of Medicine
Former President of the International Federation of Gynaecology and Obstetrics

# Table of Contents

# History of hysteroscopy

B. Blanc

Duplay and Clado [1] published the first book concerning hysteroscopy in 1898, but the true pioneer in the field of hysteroscopy was Charles David [2] who devised an endoscope made up of a system of lenses with a lamp protected by glass which enhanced visualization during the whole procedure.

In 1928, Gauss [3] published his findings on the use of fluids to rinse and distend the uterine cavity. In 1934, Schroder identified the level of intrauterine pressure necessary for best visualization without intratubal passage by positioning the drip at 65 cm distance above the patient creating a safe 30 mm mercury pressure.

From 1970 onwards, diagnostic hysteroscopy became a more efficient method for three reasons:
- "Hot" light was replaced by "cold" light. Light transmission no longer depended on an internal lamp of limited intensity but on a fiber glass system. Vulmière [5] eliminated the infrared rays which generated heat and used a cold light source filtered into fiberoptic cables;
- The endoscopic optical system was refined by Hopkins [6] who replaced the thin lenses in the tubes by thick lenses separated by air spaces. The resulting luminosity made for smaller endoscopical equipment;
- An elaborate insufflator was used to reduce the $CO_2$ flow and pressure rates, thus lessening chances of accidents due to intravascular dissemination of $CO_2$ and resulting in better uterine distension [7, 8]. Yet, the cervical suction cup used to prevent $CO_2$ from leaking out and the handling of the equipment were delicate. Cervical dilation were necessary to get the equipment through the cervical canal and thus implied anaesthesia. As the equipment had to be pushed through the cervical canal, bleeding was likely to occur and more $CO_2$ or fluid had to be pumped in.

Hamou [9, 10] used a lesser but continuous $CO_2$ flow rate which permitted easier and safer endo-cervical and then endouterine distension. With Hamou's micro-hysteroscope, the endocervical canal was slowly dilated with a smaller amount of gradually insufflated carbon dioxide ($CO_2$) and the micro-cavity filled with $CO_2$ in front of the optical system ensured visualization during the whole procedure.

Constant efforts are currently being made to reduce the size of the hysteroscopes which combine rigidity with fiber glass light transmission. Endoscopes combining flexibility and coherent glass fibers have also been introduced into gynaecological practice. Cornier [11] adapted and refined the equipment used by gastroenterologists for gynaecological usage. Several kinds of flexible diagnostic hysteroscopes are currently available. Their small calibre (outside diameters from 2 to 3 mm) is particularly adapt to the exploration of the uterine cavity for office setting and should contribute to the development of office gynaecology.

## History of surgical hysteroscopy

The first known hysteroscopic resection was performed by Commander Pantaleoni [12] as far back as July 14th 1869. He treated an endometrial polyp with a hysteroscope whose external calibre was approximately 30 fr (about 11 mm). The endometrial polyp was cauterized with silver nitrate and the outcome was satisfactory. The patient was apparently cured.

The use of a resectoscope has been a great asset for the development of hysteroscopical surgery. The resectoscope is equipped with a system of continuous irrigation of the uterine cavity and a quick fluid turnover. The resection loop can be moved back and forth in an anterior-posterior movement. The uterine cavity is thus constantly rinsed and drained and every endoscopical move is under eye control.

The equipment derived from Iglesias resectoscope [13] was used for the first time in the uterine cavity by Neuwirth in 1978 [14]. The resectoscope can be adapted to all kinds of intra-cavitary pathologies such as endometrial polyps, submucous fibroids or uterine septa. The dual-channel irrigating system provides high quality visualization and ensures high quality endoscopical surgery.

## Methods of uterine distension

Uterine distension may be obtained with $CO_2$ but this method has now been discontinued and fluids are preferred. Distilled water was ruled out because of osmotic reasons. Chlorate of sodium advocated by Mohri [15] is now only used with classical surgical equipment (scissors) when no electrical knife is possible because of risks of electrical arc. It can be used when resecting uterine septa or synechiae.

The recent introduction of glycine has greatly improved uterine distension by providing clear visualization of the uterine cavity. The solution prevents the electric current from being transmitted to the loop in case of surgical hysteroscopy by the resectoscope. The glycine solution is the most commonly used fluid in France. Other fluids (dextran, hyskon-sorbitol) are more often used in English-speaking countries.

## References

1. Duplay S and Clado S: Traité d'hystéroscopie, instrumentation, technique opératoire, études cliniques, Rennes, 1898, Simon.
2. David Ch: L'endoscopie utérine (hytséroscopie). Applications au diagnostic et au traitement des affections intra-utérines, master's thesis, University of Paris, Paris, 1908, G. Jacques.
3. Gauss GJ: Hysteroskopie, Arch Gynäkol 133:18, 1928
4. Shrœder C: Über den Aufbau und die Leistungen der Hysteroskopie, Arch Gynäkol 156:407, 1934
5. Vulmière J, Fourestier M, Gladu A. Hystéroscopie de contact. Perfectionnement à l'endoscopie médicale. Presse médicale. 60:1292, 1952.
6. Hopkins H. Optical principles of the endoscope. In Berci G (ed) Endoscopy New York: Appleton-Century-Crofts, p 3-26, 1976.
7. Porto R, Gaujoux J. Une nouvelle méthode d'hystéroscopie: Instrumentation et technique. J Gynecol Obstet Biol Reprod. 1:691, 1972.
8. Lindemann HJ, Mohr J. $CO_2$ hysteroscopy: Diagnosis and treatment. AM J Obstet Gynecol. 124:129, 1976.
9-10 Hamou JE. Microendoscopy and contact endoscopy. Brevet français 79, 04168 Paris 1979. International patent, PCT/FR80/0024 Paris, 1980. United States patent, 4,385,810. Washington, 1983.
12. Pantaleoni D. On endoscopic examination of the cavity of the womb. Med Press Circ. 8;26, 1869.
13. Iglesias JJ, Sporer A, Gellmann AC. New Iglesias resectoscope with continuous irrigation and simultaneous suction. J. Urol, 114:929, 1975.
14. Neuwirth RS. Amin HK. Excision of submucous fibrooids with hysteroscopic control. AM J Obstet Gynecol. 126:95-99, 1976.
15. Mohri T, Mohri C. Hysteroscopy. World Gynecol Obstet. 6:48,1954.

# Hierarchy of explorations

B. Blanc

For a long time the means of exploration of the uterine cavity were restricted to endometrium biopsies and the combined dilation and curettage for a biopsy, or DC for American authors. During the past ten years, exploratory procedures have multiplied with the advances of endovaginal probes and hysteroscopy. Specialists, however, disagree as to what is the best exploratory method amongst the ones routinely used. It is necessary to compare and assess results, failures, complications and costs of each method.

## Sonography

The abdominal approach of pelvic sonography is not invasive. It is reproducible and gives excellent results to visualize aspects of the genital tract such as walls, uterine lining, outlines, abnormalities and adnexal pathologies. The endovaginal probe provides a precise assessment of the endometrium and the endo-uterine cavity.

In 1991, Schaaps [1] reported the results of a series of 120 patients who suffered from severe bleeding. They were assessed by endovaginal sonography and hysteroscopy. There were 21 false-negative cases out of 110 cases for which sonography and hysteroscopy results were compared (20%). Seven false-positive cases included 5 submucous myomas and 2 cases of hypertrophied endometrium. In 70% of the cases, data from the sonography and endoscopical observations coincided.

| Normal | 43 |
|---|---|
| Atrophy | 13 |
| Hypertrophy | 12 |
| Myoma | 10 |
| Malformation | 1 |
| Total | 79 |
| Correlations sonography/ hysteroscopy | 70% |

These false-negatives and positives have to be compared with the 10 cases of hysteroscopical exams that could not be undertaken in an office setting.

Rudigoz [2, 3] compared the results of vaginal sonography and hysteroscopy in 80 patients who suffered from menometrorrhagia. Out of 44 patients with endocavitary lesions, three false-negative cases were found with vaginal sonography (2 polyps and one case of hyperplasy of the endometrium).

Fedele [4] performed a vaginal sonographic assessment associated with a hysteroscopical exam on 70 patients, previous to a hysterectomy. The results are as follows:

| | Sensibility | Specificity |
|---|---|---|
| Transvaginal sonography | 100% | 94% |
| Hysteroscopy | 100% | 96% |

The predictive value of a lesion discovered through sonography and hysteroscopy is 81% and 87%, respectively.

We carried out a prospective study concerning 230 patients with severe bleeding or sterility problems and the results were as follows:
- 230 patients (218 cases of metrorrhagia, 12 sterility cases);
- 3 cases for which hysteroscopy was impossible (1.3%);
- Correlations 214/230 (93%);
- 12 false negative cases (9 polyps, 1 fibroid, 2 cases of thick endometrium);
- 4 false positive cases (2 polyps, 2 fibroids).

Endovaginal sonography is an excellent diagnostic approach. The use of contrasting fluids in the case of hysterosonography seems to improve the efficiency of the transvaginal sonography. Rudigoz and Gaucher [5], working on a prospective series of 104 patients enrolled for severe bleeding problems, compared the results obtained by hysterosonography with those obtained by hysterography and transvaginal sonography. Unfortunately, three incidents occurred during instillation.

| | Sensibility | Specificity |
|---|---|---|
| Hysterosonography | 94% | 98% |
| Hysterography | 67% | 94% |
| Transvaginal sonography | 77% | 93% |

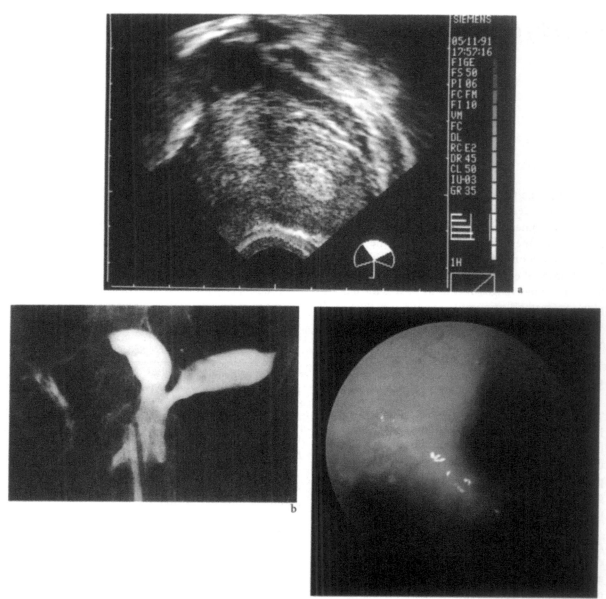

Fig. 1. Uterine septa of the same patient: a) endovaginal ultrasonography; b) hysterosalpingography; c) hysteroscopy

## Hysterosalpingography

Hysterosalpingography remains an efficient exploratory procedure. By using soluble solutions risk factors due to allergic complications have been cut down [6-8]. One indication for hysterography is severe bleeding as the endometrium and the uterine cavity can be easily assessed. As there are no precise histological correlations, and histological tests have to be carried out as well.

Hysterography generates a high rate of false positives as compared with hysteroscopy and transvaginal sonotomography. Pelvic masses do not qualify for exploratory hysterography. Contraindications include pregnancy and infection. Previous infection should be reported by the patient and antibiotic treatment should be associated to the hysterography procedure.

## Hysteroscopy

Diagnostic hysteroscopy is to be performed in an office setting. Hysteroscopic surgery should be developed now that miniature rigid hysteroscopes (ODs 5 mm, 4 mm and 2.5 mm) and hysterofibroscopes (OD 3,5 mm) are available. Its advantages are well known. It is a simple, quick, innocuous and low cost procedure [9-11]. Pregnancy and infection are contraindications. It is impossible to undertake hysteroscopy as an office procedure in about 1 to 5% of the cases. Many authors have tried to correlate the findings of hysteroscopy and hysterography (see Table 1) as divergences occur in about 30-40% of the cases. Discrepancies are rare in muscular or fibrous lesions (fibroids and synechia) and are very frequent in the assessment of endometrium pathologies.

|  | Parent [9] | Hamou [10] | Blanc [11] |
|---|---|---|---|
| Uterine Polyps | 46% | 62% | 60% |
| Submucous Fibroids | 91% | 74% | 88% |
| Hyperplasy | 38% | 45% | 38% |
| Synechies |  | 58% | 90% |

## Histological study

It can be carried out with Novak's metallic cannula, micro-cannulas, Cornier's small pipette or curette. The DC is a blind technique that should be given up. Mucous lesions such as polyps and localized hyperplasia cannot be completely excised by curettage and muscular lesions such as sub-mucous lesions cannot be reached and excised.

**Table 2.** Residual lesions after D&C in [11]

| Author | Ingelamn | Word | Burnett | Antoine | Hamou |
|---|---|---|---|---|---|
| Year | 1957 | 1958 | 1964 | 1980 | 1983 |
| Number | 124 | 512 | 30 | 188 | 42 |
| Res lesions | 81 | 49 | 6 | 68 | 23 |

**Table 1.** Hysterography/hysteroscopy correlations [10]

| Histological study | ? | Norment | Englund | Endstroem | Porto | Parent | Hamou Blanc |
|---|---|---|---|---|---|---|---|
| Year | 1956 | 1957 | 1970 | 1974 | 1978 | 1983 | 1992 |
| Number | 50 | 21 | 30 | 130 | 71 | 142 | 220 |
| Confirmation + 60% | ? | 52.4% | 53.3% | 70% | 75% | 61% | 65% |
| Confirmation − 40% | ? | 47.6% | 46.7% | 30% | 25% | 39% | 35% |

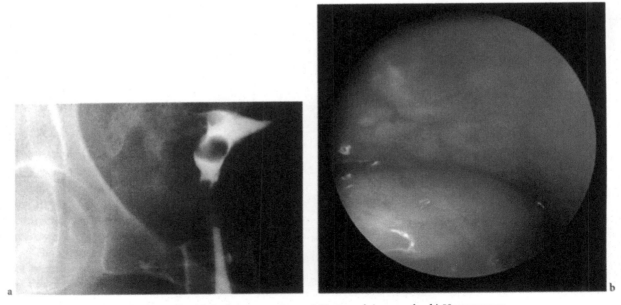

**Fig. 2.** Different aspects of uterine fibroids in the same patient: a) Hysterosalpingography; b) Hysteroscopy

## Conclusion

When confronted with menstrual disorders such as menorrhagia, menometrorrhagia and metrorrhagia or in post menopausal metrorrhagia, it is first necessary to assess the pelvic organs before any diagnostic is reached or any therapeutic procedure is attempted. A first attempt of pelvic and in particular transvaginal sonography has to be performed on an outpatient basis because they are reproducible and innocuous. Outpatient hysteroscopy can be performed to confirm the presence of an endo-uterine lesion. Hysterography remains the necessary procedure in case of suspected adenomyosis (diverticular images, rectitude of the walls and erecta tubes). Hysterosalpingography is the first intention procedure. Hysteroscopy is to be offered if there is a radiological endocavitary anomaly.

## References

1. Shaaps JP, Dubois M, Voise M (1991) Qu'attendre de l'échographie de la cavité utérine? Contraception Fertilité Sexualité 19: 929-934
2. Rudigoz RC, Frobert C, You SE et al (1991) Place de l'échographie vaginale dans l'exploration des méno-métrorragies de la période d'activité génitale. Entretiens de Bichat 1991, Chirurgie pp 91-92
3. Rudigoz RC, Frobert C, Chassagrand FR, Gaucherand P (1992) Place de l'échographie par voie vaginale dans l'exploration des ménorragies de la période d'activité génitale. J Gynecol Obstet Biol Reprod (Paris) 21: 644-650
4. Fedele L, Bianchi S, Dorta M et al (1991) Transvaginal ultrasonography versus hysteroscopy in the diagnosis of uterine subsarcoma myoma. Obstet Gynecol 775: 745-748
5. Gaucher P, Rudigoz RC, Sourour S et al (1993) L'hystérographie avec contraste liquidien. Une technique d'étude de l'endomètre et de la cavité utérine. 36èmes Assises Nationales de la Société Française de Gynécologie, Grenoble pp 20-22
6. Blanc B (1983) Atlas d'hystérosalpingographie comparée. Corrélations entre hystérosalpingographie, échographie, hystéroscopie et cœlioscopie. Sandoz, Rueil Malmaison
7. Tristan H, Benmussa M (1984) Atlas d'hystérosalpingographie. 2ème ed, Masson Paris
8. Musset R, Netter A, Potout P, Rioux JE (1977) Précis d'hystérosalpingographie. Presse de l'Université, Laval, Québec
9. Parent B, Guedj H, Barbet J, Nodarian P (1985) Hystéroscopie. Maloine, Paris
10. Hamou J (1991) Hysteroscopy and microcolpohysteroscopy. Appleton & Langee, Norwalk
11. Blanc B, Boubli L (1996) Endoscopie utérine. Pradel, Paris

# Anaesthesia in ambulatory hysteroscopy

D. Samson

Ambulatory surgery has developed exponentially over the last 20 years. While the surgical technique remains more or less the same whether the patient is hospitalized or not, the anaesthesia is altogether different. There are several reasons for this development:
- cost control;
- patients' choice;
- improvement of anaesthetic agents;
- better cost-saving/efficiency ratio.

In this chapter we are going to describe the principles and different possible methods of anaesthesia.

## Pre-anaesthesia examination and patient's selection

A pre-anaesthetic consultation is done remotely from the hysteroscopy. It usually concerns young women ASA 1 or 2 and the first interview enables:
- to evaluate the risk;
- to detect pre-existing pathologies;
- to obtain an enlightened consent of the patient for the suggested type of anaesthesia;
- the ratifying of constraints for ambulatory anaesthesia: attendants, telephone, accompaniment.
Complementary objectives include:
- a psychological preparation of the patient by an oral and written information;
- a pharmacological preparation by a premedication.

## The patient's preparation [1]

Preoperative fasting for 4 to 6 hours is compulsory for all patients. A medical check-up before operation comprises a blood analysis, with a cell count and chemistry, these patients often suffering from anaemia.

The premedication is based on the administration of an anti-histaminic (Hydroxyzine) besides a sedative as this allows to diminish the risk of vomiting [2, 3].

We limit the time for all ambulatory hysteroscopies to 1 hour and the post-operative disorders are few.

The main problem to be feared consists in metabolic complications in relation with the administration of Glycocolle (aqueous solution of Glycine 1,5%). This clear and non-conductive solution is, in fact, the medium we use for distending the uterus.

The re-absorption of Glycocolle in the blood circulation is the greatest complication of the procedure [4-6].

The first symptoms are neurological:
- visual problems followed by convulsions and coma. These are due either to hyponatraemia or to direct toxicity of Glycine wich turns into Amonia;
- hypervolaemia may lead to pulmonary oedema;
- on the biological ground this syndrome consists in hyponatraemia which may be of major importance associated with a fall in protidaemia and haematocrit.

Safety rules rely on:
- a careful control of Glycocolle input and output: immediate discontinuation in case of perforation of the uterus;
- no hyperpression while using this solution;
- careful clinical supervision and biological control if necessary.

Loco-regional anaesthesia allows an early detection of Glycine infiltration in the blood-vessels [7].

## General anaesthesia

General anaesthesia must fulfill different objectives [1]:
- rapid induction with no excitement phenomena;
- good recovery;
- management of post-operative pain, nausea and vomiting.

### Drugs used

Most of the time induction consists in an intravenous anaesthetic with a rapid action. Propofol has replaced barbiturics and benzodiazepines in ambulatory procedures due to its superior quality in recovery.

This drug will be used as induction agent or most often when performing a totally intra-venous technique, which is reported to have diminished post-operative nausea and vomiting facilitating an earlier return home [8].

## Volatile anaesthetics [9]

Volatile anaesthetics enable to maintain anaesthesia with spontaneous or controlled ventilation.

Their quick action and elimination allow an easy variation of the degree of anesthesia. The pharmacological characteristics of the two most recent volatile anaesthetics are very useful in ambulatory procedures:
- sevoflurane allows a rapid induction using an oxygen mask;
- desflurane allows an early recovery more rapidly than using other halogen drugs.

Nitrous oxyde, when chosen, enables to reduce the amount; this of the other anesthetic agents used is interesting considering its low cost, though its incidence in post-operative nausea is controversial [10].

## Central analgesics

Morphinomimetics allow to reduce pain and abnormal movements observed when injecting narcotics (Propofol, Etomidate). They diminish the hemodynamic response to anaesthetic or surgical stimulations, and at low dosage allow a recovery quicker than with an inhaling technique.

Alfentanyl and Remifentanil are two interesting molecules in this indication. Curare is not necessary to perform this act. When practising general anaesthesia, the airway is usually controlled by a laryngeal mask, unless otherwise indicated.

## Spinal anaesthesia

The aim is to obtain an anaesthesia extending as far as T1O since the sensibility of the uterine fundus projects to this level.

In all cases, the judicious choice of the local anaesthetic should avoid using a catheter.

Before leaving, the patients must have recovered sensibility, a normal motricity and be able to pass urine normally.

Persistance of a certain degree of sympathic block and orthostatic hypotension rarely gives rise to an ambulatory problem.

Two controls of the mean blood pressure at short intervals, in the standing position and having a result of no less than 10% of their basic value are necessary for the patient to leave the hospital.

In ambulatory surgery, the main problem is headaches following punction of the dura mater. They prevent patients from having a normal activity and delay their return to work [11, 12].

The frequency of this oncoming is low (< 0.5%) even in young women when pencil-shaped needles (Sprotte or Whitacre) of small gauge ($\leq$ 25 G) are used. We use plain bupivacaïne 0.5% in a range of 10 to 12.5 mg.

## Paracervical block [13, 14]

The aim of this technique is to block transmission to the paracervical ganglions which project to the medullary level of T10 L1.

This block is performed on the patient in gynaecological position. After disinfecting the vagina, a speculum is placed in situ in order to expose the vaginal fornices.

The needle is introduced in the right or left lateral vaginal fornices near the cervix at 3 and 9 o'clock position, then at 4 and 8 o'clock.

The correct positioning of the needle is obtained when the operator feels a loss of resistance to the injection. If after insertion the needle as far as the first stop, this feeling is not obtained, the operator passes on to the second stop. The injection will be done only after an aspiration test, and 15 ml to 20 ml of local anaesthetic will be used.

## Material

A needle with a security tip of Kobak type, wich due to its system allows a penetration of the vaginal wall not more than 3,5 or 7 mm, will be used.

## Choice of the local anaesthetic

We use 15 to 20 ml of either Lidocaine 1,5% or Mepivacaine 1%.

The anaesthesia obtained seems the same with any solution. The main problem of this technique is that it is not possible to anaesthetize of the vagina. Therefore, the operator must be very delicate when manipulating the hysteroscope. Anaesthesia lasts 30 to 45 minutes. The succes rate is about 80% to 90%.

## Complications [15, 16]

- Neuropathy caused by damage to the sciatic nerve if the needle is introduced too deeply;
- paracervical abcess;
- hematoma of the parametrium.
  The contra-indications of these techniques are:
- patient's refusal;
- coagulation anomalies;
- evolutive neurological disease;
- B.A.V.;
- sepsis.

The principal advantage of loco-regional anaesthesia techniques is the early detection of the passage of Glycocolle in the vascular system.

## References

1. Ostman PL, While PF (1996) Anesthésie Ambulatoire. In Miller Anesthésie. Flammarion, Paris, p 2218
2. Merily HW (1982) Criteria for selection of ambulatory surgical patients and guide lines for anesthetic management - A retrospective study. Anesth Analg 61:921-926
3. Boon JH, Hopkins D (1996) Hydroxyzine premedication: does it provide better anxiolysis than a placebo? S Afr Med J 86:661-666
4. Badetti C, Aknin P, N'Guyen C, Boubli L, Blanc B, Manelli JC (1993) Biological modifications during operative hysteroscopy under glycine irrigation. Ann Fr Anesth Reanim 12:365-371
5. D'Acosto J, Ali NM, Maier D (1990) Absorption of irrigating solution during hysteroscopic metroplasty. Anesthesiology 72:379-380
6. Arvieux C, Peyrin JC, Delchelette E, Davin JL, Naud G, Faure G (1984) Insuffisance rénale aiguë au décours de la chirurgie endo-urétrale sous irrigation de glycocolle. J Urologie 90:107-110
7. Dubois JC, Hamou J (1985) Intérêt de l'anesthésie loco-régionale dans la pratique de l'hystéroscopie. Contracep Fertil Sex 13:399-402
8. Mc Collum JSC, Milligan KR, Dundee JW (1998) The Antiemetic effect of propofol. Anesthesia 43:239-240
9. Alexander GD, Skupshi JN, Brown FM (1984) The role of nitrous oxide in post operative nausea and vomiting. Anesth Analg 83:175
10. Ghouri AF, Bodner M, While PF (1991) Recovery profile after desflurane nitrous oxide versus isoflurane nitrous oxide in outpatients. Anesthesiology 75:197
11. Smith EA, Thorburn J, Duckworth RA, Reid JA (1994) A comparison of 25G and 27G with acre needles for caesarean section. Anesthesia 49:859-862
12. Halpern S, Preston R (1994) Postdural puncture headache and spinal needle design. Metaanalysis, Anesthesiology 81:1376-1383
13. Lecron L (1980) Bloc Paracervical. In: Anesthesie loco-regionale. Ed Arnette, Paris, pp 887-892
14. Kobak AJ, Sadove MS (1961) Combined paracervical and pudendal nerve blocks, a simple form of transvaginal regional anesthesia. Ann J Obst Gyn 81:72
15. Gaylord TG, Pearson JW (1982) Neuropathy following paracervical block in the obstetric patient. Obstet Gynecol 60:524-5255
16. Mercado AO, Naz JF, Ataya KM (1989) Post abortal paracervical abcess as a complication of paracervical bloc anesthesia. J Reprod Med 34:247-2499

# Diagnostic hysteroscopy

B. BLANC, R. de MONTGOLFIER

## Description of the different models

There is a whole range of equipment available for diagnostic hysteroscopy. The first generation hysteroscopes with ODs of 5.2 mm are still in use and provide good quality hysteroscopy. Yet the procedure is painful in one case out of two.

The new minihysteroscopes, with ODs of less than 3 mm for the sheaths and of less than 2 mm for the lenses are more comfortable for exploration in office setting and failures are very rare, even though the observation of the uterine cavity is limited. Thus reliability of the diagnosis of small-sized lesions, hyperplasia and other proliferating abnormalities of the endometrium has to be assessed.

Hysterofibroscopy affords another valuable option with its flexible endoscope. Exploration of the uterine cavity under most circumstances is easy and satisfactory with that equipment.

The ODs range from 5.2 mm, 4 mm, to 3.5 mm. Light is transmitted through a system of lenses (Fig. 1) with ODs of 4 mm to 2.8 mm, according to the instrument. The minihysteroscopes are 25 cm long with a 90° wide field of view. They are 30° Foroblique and allow frontal and lateral visualization of the uterine cavity. The tapered distal tip is designed for smooth non-traumatic insertion into the endo-cervical canal but may lead to cases of false track with beginners. The endoscope locks into the sheath with a system of pins and holes. Gaskets around the holes may deteriorate and become brittle and porous and have to be frequently replaced. The equipment is easily autoclavable and immersible in disinfectant solutions; therefore it is convenient for routine use.

## Miniscopes

A miniscope is a minihysteroscope with an OD of 2.5 mm. Light is transmitted through fiberoptics with ODs of 1.2 mm (Fig. 2). An operating channel with an OD of 3.7 mm can be locked onto the minihysteroscope. It carries two coaxial channels of 3 Fr for ancillary equipment such as scissors, pliers and biopsy pliers to be inserted.

## Flexible hysterofibroscopes

The Olympus (HYF-P) diagnostic flexible hysterofibroscope is made up of four parts: a jacket, a sheath, a distal rotating tip and a light cord with a plug.

The *jacket* located on the proximal extremity contains:
- the proximal optical system with the eye-piece and focusing knob;
- the operating channel inlet;
- the proximal end of the fibroscope sheath.

The *main sheath* is flexible from handle to tip and contains the optical components for image transmission, the bundle of light fibers and the operating channel. The sheath is waterproof. It is made up of a steel blade whose degrees of flexibility, length and width vary according to the HiTech material it is made of.

The *distal bending tip* allows axial visualization and can be rotated up and down and to and fro depending on how operator maneuvers the insertion tube. It has an atraumatic edge. At the distal end, the objective lens can be seen under the operating channel outlet surrounded by the light fiberglass system.

All the optical connections are in the cable which is part of the jacket and is equipped with its specific *electric cord and plug*.

The Olympus HYF-P apparatus has an OD of 3.5 mm. With its bevelled bending tip, insertion is smooth and no manipulation of the cervix is required during the procedure. Insertion is obtained through gentle rotating and bending movements from the tip of the fibroscope. The optical system has an OD of 2.2 mm. A coaxial channel in the endoscope can be used for $CO_2$ insufflation or fluid irrigation, and in theory for insertion of micro biopsy pliers. The tip of the fibroscope can be bent in any direction with an up 100°, down 100° angulation

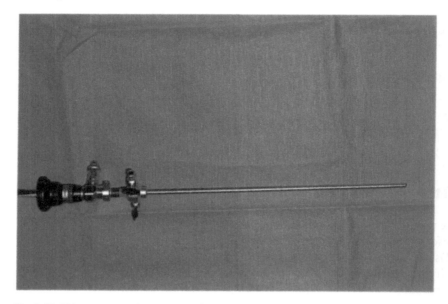

**Fig. 1.** Rigid hysteroscope (OD 4 mm, Olympus). Light is transmitted through a system of lenses

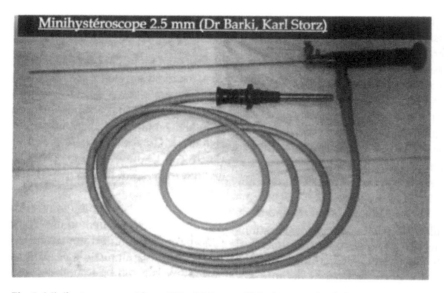

**Fig. 2.** Minihysteroscope with an OD of 1.2 mm. Light is transmitted through fiberoptics with ODs of 2.5 mm

range controlled by a lever attached to the handle of the equipment. This device allows a complete exploration of the uterine cavity even in the case of an intra-cavitary lesion. It is possible to introduce the tip of the fibroscope between the uterine edge and the lesion so as to observe the fundus of the uterine cavity.

The equipment is provided with a shock-proof case, is portable and self-contained. The endoscope incorporates the fiber optics and its own cold light source. Light transmission through coaxial fibers ensures the flexibility of the equipment. The ancillary equipment includes biopsy pliers (3 Fr) and a brush for cytological tests.

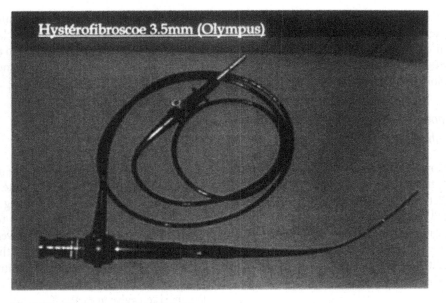

**Fig. 3.** Flexible hysteroscope OD 2.9-3.5 mm

The optical system features two kinds of bundles, a bundle of non-coherent glass fibers for light transmission and a bundle of coherent fibers for image transmission. Convergent lenses located at the proximal and distal ends of the bundles of fibers send images which are transmitted to the eye-piece at the proximal end of the bundle. Images are made up of as many dots as the fibers present. Fibers transmit images whatever flexion they are submitted to.

Several models of hysterofibroscopes are currently available (Fugi, Karlstorz, Leisegang, Machida, Wolf, etc). They differ each of here for the sizes and materials they are made of.

## Light sources

Light sources commonly used are in the 150 to 400 Watts range. It is better to use a self-regulated 250 Watts source which adapts to the prevailing conditions. Some light fountains use a xenon source for superior illumination, but they are not necessary in routine practice.

## Video camera and video monitor

A video camera and monitor have become a must. The patient is thus able to participate in the observation of the lesions. The surgeon is spared uncomfortable positions, and findings can be easily recorded for research and teaching purposes.

## Distension media

### $CO_2$ or carbon dioxide

It is necessary to have a $CO_2$ source with a double control of the flowrate and pressure. Mortal casualties with the use of $CO_2$ as reported in the literature can always be traced to the absence of control in the flowrate and pressure. The flowrate must not exceed 100 ml/min and intrauterine pressure must be under 100 mmHg for a safe $CO_2$ hysteroscopic procedure.

Three types of equipment are available and differ according to what comes first, control of $CO_2$ intrauterine flowrate or pressure, or both.

### *The constant pressure insufflator (distributed by Wisap)*

The pressure is preset to 100 mmHg and the flowrate rises from 0 to 80 ml/min. The small quantity of $CO_2$ delivered ranges between 30 to 40 ml and produces a slow but sufficient endo-cervical distension. $CO_2$ peritoneal transfer is small and shoulder pains are rare.

### *The constant flow insufflator (distributed by Storz, hysteroflator)*

The flowrate is preset to 40 ml/min and intrauterine pressure rises to a maximum of 180 mmHg. When the maximum is reached, a safety valve shuts off the inflow. The quantity of $CO_2$ delivered is more important and can reach 60 to 70 ml, thus producing a better distension of the endo-cervical canal, but shoulder pains are more important particularly if the procedure is long.

### The variable flow and pressure insufflator (distributed by Storz, microhysteroflator)

The instrument allows for continuous control of both the $CO_2$ flowrate and intrauterine pressure, ensuring complete safety. Both gas flow and pressure can be adapted to each particular case and any cervical or tubal leak is automatically compensated so as to maintain a constant equilibrium. The total quantity of insufflated $CO_2$ is usually about 50 ml. The risk of shoulder pains is small.

### Fluids

Diagnostic hysteroscopy can be performed with fluids such as normal saline (NS) or glycine. NS is to be preferred as it is cheaper and its optical qualities are excellent. The infection risk is negligible when the patient is infection-free. A thorough cervico-vaginal desinfection is sufficient. It is preferable to use a constant drip rather than a syringe on demand. We have recourse to the former technique when confronted with blood loss so as to rinse the uterine cavity. When there is a small quantity of blood, hysteroscopy can be performed using fluids as distension media. This procedure is less painful than gas insufflation as it distends the uterine walls more gradually. With fluids, the endo-cervical canal is progressively distended, and the internal os of the endocol opens under fluid pressure. The uterine cavity is gradually distended and visualization is excellent. The general aspect, however, is different as the endometrium floats on the surface of the fluid. The mucosa anomalies are easily on view.

## Diagnostic hysteroscopy: an office examination

### Preparation and technique

For diagnostic hysteroscopy to be widely adopted by gynecological surgeons, it should be a safe, innocuous and reproducible procedure. Diagnostic hysteroscopy is performed on an out-patient basis as a complement of the pelvic examination. It is offered during the consultation if exploration of the uterine cavity proves necessary. It is performed in the safest conditions possible, to be described later on and without premedication or anesthesia so as to ensure the ambulatory quality of the performance and to avoid the stress of the patient.

### The date

For menstruating women who are not using oral contraceptives, the appropriate date is during the preovulatory days. For menstruating women whose menstrual periods last between four to five days, the best date for a hysteroscopy is between the seventh and twelfth days of the cycle when the endocervical canal is slightly open and the isthmus hypotonic. Penetration and progression of the endoscope into the uterine cavity are easy. The endometrium in the early proliferative phase is thin and observation of the uterine cavity is excellent. There are no risks of unsuspected pregnancies.

For patients using oral contraceptives, the date is irrelevant except in the case of sequential contraceptives when the examination should be performed during the first oestrogenic phase.

In case of an emergency, the hysteroscopic procedure can be performed during the premenstruation phase. It is a more delicate procedure as the internal os of the cervix and the isthmus are hypertonic and resist penetration by the endoscope. The endometrium is thicker and observation of abnormal mucous tissues such as small polyps or hyperplasia of the endometrium is more difficult.

For postmenopausal women on hormonal replacement therapies, hysteroscopy is performed during the oestrogenic phase of the treatment. For postmenopausal women without hormonal replacement therapies, it is preferable and sometimes necessary to administer an eight-day local oestrogenic treatment or a four-day general oestrogenic treatment before the procedure.

### The place

The office setting is ideal. The gynecologist needs the help of an assistant for the practical realisation of the examination. A specific office in a private or public hospital is convenient. An operating theatre seems to be the worst setting possible; it nevertheless, is preferable for a diagnostic hysteroscopy under general anesthesia.

## Preparation for the examination

The psychological preparation is essential. The patient should be given a simple explanation of the procedure and should be reassured. During the examination, continuous conversation with the patient ("verbal anesthesia") is essential so as to ensure the smooth unfolding of the procedure. The patient assumes the lithotomy position. It is convenient but not necessary to have a tilt table in the case of uterine anteversion or retroversion. The sterile material necessary for the performance of a diagnostic hysteroscopy is laid out on a trolley next to the examination table. The instruments include a Collins speculum, vaginal pliers with smooth edges, Pozzi forceps, swabs, cotton and the hysteroscope. The material is hidden from the patient's view under a sterile cover so as to reduce her anxiety.

## Technique of diagnostic hysteroscopy with a hysterofibroscope

The patient assumes the lithotomy position. A pelvic examination before the hysteroscopy is necessary to assess the volume and position of the uterus. After the speculum is inserted, a cervico-vaginal disinfection is performed. It is preferable to use a non foaming antiseptic solution for better visualization. We use a Dakin solution, or a non foaming Betadine solution or a saline solution. The exploration of the uterine cavity can be realized with $CO_2$ insufflation or with liquid media. The gradual fluid flow allows a satisfactory dilation of the cervical canal. The vision of the uterine cavity is not altered by the fluid and there are few infection risks because of the small quantity of fluid pumped into the uterine cavity. The fluid used is a saline solution.

If examination is performed using $CO_2$, the gas line is connected to the instrument. Flowrate and pressure have to be strictly controlled. When the $CO_2$ insufflation or the saline perfusion starts, the extremity of the fibroscope is placed on the exterior os. Pozzi forceps on the cervix are not usually necessary because the procedure is painless with the thin, flexible fibroscope (3.5 mm).

The speculum is placed in a precisely symmetrical position level with the cervical lips for a better passive dilation of the cervix. The technique of the endoscopic examination is different from the technique used with rigid hysteroscopes. For the right-handed operator, the handle of the fibroscope is held in the right hand with the thumb on the lever controlling

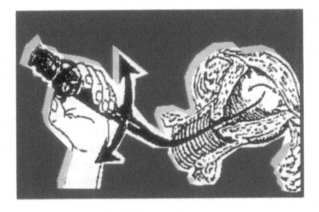

**Fig. 4.** Technique of flexible hysteroscopy. There is no need to use Pozzi forceps

the bending distal tip of the instrument, while the left hand holds the endoscope. The distal tip of the fibroscope can be moved with an angulation of 100° up and down and to and fro. The right-handed operator will gently push the tip of the endoscope into the cervical canal using the left hand. There is no need to use Pozzi forceps on the cervix (Fig. 4). By rotating the right wrist and moving it to and fro and up and down, the operator moves the endoscope in any direction. The progressing endoscope should always be kept in the axis of the endocervical canal. It is possible to do so thanks to the bending distal tip and the rotation of the wrist. The exploration of the endocervical canal is easy if the extremity of the endoscope is in line with the axis of the canal and of the uterine isthmus.

The operator directs the endoscope by moving the right wrist and bending the distal tip so that the endo cervical canal or the isthmus stays in the middle of the screen. The left hand keeps the proximal end of the endoscope in contact with the external os.

The isthmus is easily negotiated contrary to what happens with rigid hysteroscopes. The thin fibroscope (3.5 mm) is nearly always compatible with the size of the uterine isthmus.

The evaluation of the uterine cavity begins with a panoramic view, followed by identification of the two tubal ostia and assessment of the uterine walls, of the fundus and observation of the two tubal ostia on a few millimeters. The exploration of the uterus, particularly in case of an intra-cavitary lesion, is greatly facilitated by the flexible hysteroscope and its bending tip.

The endoscope tip can be steered around an intracavitary lesion to explore it from all angles and observe the endometrium behind the lesion. It is possible to assess the thickness of the endometrium by applying pressure with the distal tip of the endoscope into the mucosa of the uterus and evaluate the resulting imprint in comparison with the size of the endoscope.

The procedure is generally painless and does not last more than 3 minutes. No anesthesia either general or local is necessary except in some particular cases. Because the endoscope is so flexible, it is impossible to perforate the uterus. The only possible incident is the absence of good visualization which may be due to three reasons:

1. the tip of the endoscope is blurred by secretions and has to be cleaned;
2. the tip of the endoscope may be in contact with the fundus or with a uterus wall; thus, the endoscope has to be slightly withdrawn;
3. there may not be enough intrauterine pressure to create a space in the uterine cavity. The pressure has to be slightly increased while keeping it within safe limits.

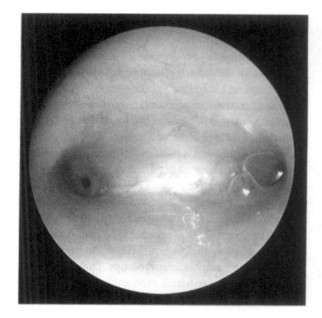

**Fig 5.** Diagnostic hysteroscopy with rigid hysteroscope and $CO_2$ insufflation, normal cavity. Note the tubal ostia.

## Technique of diagnostic hysteroscopy with rigid hysteroscopes (Fig. 5)

A pelvic examination always comes first to assess the volume and position of the uterus.

Then, a speculum is inserted. The cervix is cleaned and the cervico-vaginal cavity disinfected with a non foaming antiseptic solution. Pozzi prehension forceps are placed on the cervix between 12 and 6 o'clock. In case of a severely retroverted uterus, Pozzi forceps are placed at 6 o'clock and gentle traction is exerted so as to try and straighten out the uterus.

In some favorable cases, with a flaccid external orifice and an easily accessible endo-cervical canal, diagnostic hysteroscopy is possible without prehension of the cervix. On the contrary, it is sometimes necessary to use two Pozzi forceps with an incompetent cervix.

### The examination

Diagnostic hysteroscopy unfolds in three phases:
1-the anterograde cervico-isthmic phase;
2-the uterus phase;
3-the retrograde isthmo-cervical phase.

#### The anterograde cervico-isthmic phase

The light source and the $CO_2$ or saline sources are connected to the outside sheath of the hysteroscope.

The right-handed operator seizes the hysteroscope in the right hand and directs it towards the outside orifice of the cervix. With the left hand, he/she holds the cervix with the Pozzi pliers with gentle traction. The endoscope is progressively inserted under direct visual or monitor control. Gentle progression is guided by the distension of the two walls of the endo-cervical canal. The endoscope is inserted in the internal orifice of the cervix and can then penetrate into the uterine cavity.

In some cases the progression is impeded or even stopped. At the level of the inside orifice of the endocol, dilation is sometimes difficult. No force should be used through the orifice to avoid a false passage or cramps or bleeding. If the inside orifice is closed, the surgeon should wait for a $CO_2$ or NACL "bubble" to create a micro-cavity resulting in progressive dilation in front of the tip of the endoscope. The beginner needs to adjust to the 20 to 30° off-axis Foroblique view afforded by the endoscope to avoid false passages.

#### The uterine phase

After passage of the hysteroscope through the endocervical canal, the uterine cavity distended by $CO_2$ or NACL is reached. The examination of the uterine cavity begins with a panoramic view to check any anomalies. The tubal ostia should be located. If there are no important endo-uterine lesions, the operator should assess the state of the endometrium, its thickness, vascularisation and the aspect of the tubal ostia. The exploration of the uterine cavity is facilitated by the 90° wide field of vision and by the forobliquity which allows visualization of the whole uterine cavity with a single movement of the optical system. If there is an important endo-cavitary lesion, the operator assesses its location, volume, vascularisation and connections with the uterine muscle, and its situation with regard to the tubal ostia.

**The retrograde isthmo-cervical phase**

It is an essential moment for the exploration of the endocol, since its walls are poorly visualized when the hysteroscope is introduced in an anterograde position. After the exploration of the uterine cavity, the endoscopist observes the lateral walls of the endocol as they unfold at the retrograde passage of the endoscope, looking for marginal mucous synechiae or small-sized polyps which may have gone unnoticed up to that moment.

## Patient tolerance

A rigid diagnostic hysteroscope (OD of 5.2 mm) with $CO_2$ insufflation was used on an outpatient basis in a prospective study we carried out with a series of 1000 patients.
- 40% of the patients found the examination painless;
- 25% of the patients complained of uterine cramps;
- 20% of the patients complained of shoulder pains;
- 10% of the patients complained of important pelvic cramps or shoulder pains and would have preferred general anesthesia;
- 5% required a local or general anesthesia.

So, in our series, 40% patients found office diagnostic hysteroscopy a painless procedure. Most of them were multipara. Five to 7% of the patients required some kind of anesthesia. For 55% of the patients, the examination proved painful; they were mostly primipara or menopausal patients.

The study was repeated with the addition of fluids. In a series of 200 hysteroscopies performed with a rigid hysteroscope (OD 5 mm) with the perfusion of a saline solution, on the same outpatient basis, the results were as follows: 158 patients (79%) found the procedure painless or a little uncomfortable, and 34 found the procedure painful. We had 8 failures.

Patient tolerance is improved with liquid media. The distension of the cervical canal and endocol is progressive. With the drip of the perfusion placed 80 cm above the table, the effect of gravity results in regular distension. With a syringe, distension is brutal and painful and should be used only to improve visualization for hysteroscopies performed during bleeding.

## Incidents

Incidents mostly occur with rigid hysteroscopes. There may be several reasons.

### Stenosis

The inside orifice of the endo-cervical canal cannot be negotiated because of a difficult stenosal condition (nullipara or untreated menopausal women). It is possible to cautiously perform progressive dilatation with soft bougies of ODs from 2 to 5 mm with or without local anesthesia.

### False passage

A false passage occurs when the different phases of the procedure have not been properly respected. In that case, the endoscope is withdrawn and re-positioned in the axis of the endocol. Most often the false track is of no consequence and the procedure is continued. If the false track is important, if the patient bleeds or has cramps, it is better to stop the procedure and schedule another hysteroscopy after two cycles.

### Bleeding

There is blood inside the uterine cavity because of a lesion of the mucosa created by the endoscope. The extremity of the endoscope is cleaned and the patient reassured. The examination is continued with added caution. In some cases the use of fluids facilitates the examination.

### Incompetent cervix

An incompetent cervix prevents the distension of the uterine cavity. In most cases, the hysteroscopy can be performed by reducing the $CO_2$ flow or NACL to obtain a constant and progressive distension. In some exceptional cases, the two lips of the cervix have to be held by Pozzi pliers.

## Biopsies

### Rigid hysteroscopes

In theory there are two techniques with rigid hysteroscopes, but in practice only blind biopsies are possible.

*Biopsies under visual control* can be performed with a pair of rigid pliers (OD 1 mm) parallel to a hysteroscope (OD 4 to 5 mm). The advantage of this technique lies in the targeted biopsy which theoretically reduces false negative results. However, it requires the patient's active collaboration and favorable local conditions. The procedure takes place during the preovulatory period, between the 10th and the 12th day of the cycle and the hysteroscope (OD 5 mm) is pushed past the endocervical canal and the isthmus. If a pair of pliers (OD 1 mm) is added, the canal has to be further distended and the patient often requires a local anesthesia so that the procedure becomes more difficult and less easily reproducible. The specimens being often small, they do not provide enough tissues for a thorough histopathologic evaluation.

*Blind biopsies* are realized with a Novak cannula directed at abnormal areas previously observed by a diagnostic hysteroscopy.

### Hysteroscopes with double channels

There are several rigid hysteroscopes with optical systems (ODs of 1.2 to 3 mm) and a collateral channel (OD of 1.8 mm) inside a sheath (ODs of 4.5 to 5.5 mm). The instruments are equipped with a double stream of fluids which allows a perfect visualization of the uterine cavity. Biopsies can be taken under visual control by introducing a pair of pliers (OD 1.7) into the coaxial channel (OD 1.8, 5 fr). The specimens seem to be sizable enough for an adequate histopathologic evaluation. The instruments are currently being evaluated

### Flexible diagnostic hysteroscopes

It is theoretically possible to use the coaxial ($CO_2$ and NACL) insufflation channel through the means of a special stopcock and to introduce a pair of biopsy pliers (OD 1 mm). The biopsy sample is then taken under visual control. The hysteroscope is positioned facing the exact place for the biopsies to be taken. The biopsy can only be performed when the jaws of the pliers can be opened. The specimens, however,

(2.5 mm, 3 for the 3 fr biopsies) may not provide enough tissues for a reliable and reproducible evaluation.

It is always possible to perform a blind biopsy with a Cornier curette or a "vacurette" after the endo uterine exploration. It is then necessary to wait for two or three minutes after the end of the examination to perform the biopsy. The curette is best used when the uterine cavity is empty of $CO_2$ or the fluids. This type of biopsy is indicated when there are no localised lesions. An endocervical smear can be taken by introducing a cyto-brush into the operating channel (OD 1.2 mm) and gently pushing the brush to and fro.

## Indications of the diagnostic hysteroscopy

Since diagnostic hysteroscopy is little invasive and can be realized on an outpatient basis, its indications have multiplied.

- In all the cases in which visual control is necessary to complete the findings of an abnormal or insufficient hysterography, or pelvic and/or vaginal sonography or inadequate biopsy.
- To evaluate anomalies of the menstrual cycle (metrorrhagia, secondary menorrhagia) or post menopausal metrorrhagia (Fig. 6). We think this procedure should be performed in case of any abnormal bleeding during the menstrual cycle which has not been improved by a symptomatic or hormonal treatment. A diagnostic hysteroscopy is useful to confirm or infirm the presence of an endocavitary lesion. During the procedure, it is possible to collect adequate data about the state and aspect of the endometrium and detect abnormal areas suitable for biopsies. In the case of small lesions, it avoids useless progestative treatments. In case of neoplasic lesions, it avoids dangerous and falsely reassuring treatments.
- Infertility.

Diagnostic hysteroscopy is not as efficient as hysterography because it does not adequately assess tubal permeability. The development of microfibers will probably bring a solution by improving transcervical fallopian endoscopy on an outpatient basis.

## Abnormal uterine bleeding in menstruating women

Abnormal uterine bleeding is the most common indication for diagnostic hysteroscopy. Its frequency varies between 20 to 80% according to the authors.

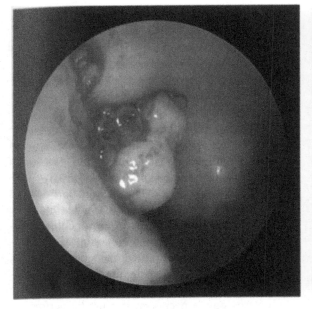

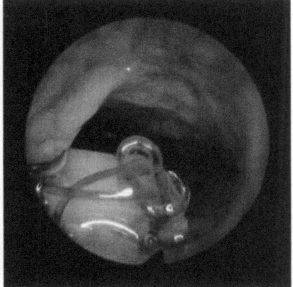

**Fig. 6.** Rigid hysteroscopy. Menometrorrhagia and intracavitary fibroid

**Fig. 7.** Bleeding due to IUD

Diagnostic hysteroscopy is one method of evaluation amongst several other exploratory means and should be compared to them:

- Diagnostic hysteroscopy is a more efficient method of evaluation of the uterine cavity than hysterography;
- Endovaginal ultrasonography and more recently sonohysterography should come first in any abnormal uterine bleeding. Endovaginal ultrasonography provides a documented analysis of the endometrium and the myometrium and confirms or infirms the presence of an intracavitary lesion and its connections with the myometrium. It is not an entirely reliable evaluation for small lesions (under 1 cm) or lesions near or around the cornua, or localised hyperplasia. With diagnostic hysteroscopy, it is always possible to confirm the diagnostic of endocavitary lesions and their accessibility to an endoscopic treatment (polyps, intracavitary or submucous fibroids);
- Adenomyosis is more easily detected by hysterography than by diagnostic hysteroscopy. This affection can be suspected through clinical signs such as abnormal menstrual cycles, dysmenorrhea, a globally increased uterus which is fibrous without being distorted. With ultrasonography, endocavitary anomalies are not detected; however, rounded intramyometrial anechogenous zones near the uterine cavity surrounded by mucosal hypertrophy

may be detected in certain cases. Hysterography should be preferred because its images of diverticuli, rigid edges and ectasia of tuba uterina have been well documented. There are no identifiable hysteroscopic signs of adenomyosis, except the glandular ostia, which are not easily visible except during the immediate post menstrual period and exceptional submucous adenomyosis blebs;

- Bleeding in women under contraceptive treatments represents 5% of the indications. Exploration procedure can be indicated when the usual medical treatment fails (change of pill) and menstrual bleeding persists. Vaginal ultrasonography is used to assess the endometrium. Hysteroscopy is used to evaluate the atrophy or subatrophy of the endometrium and a localised thickening of endometrium due to a polyp or a small submucous fibroid;
- Bleeding due to intrauterine devices (Fig. 7) represents 5% of the indications as illustrated in the literature. Diagnostic hysteroscopy is useful in the evaluation of the position of the IUD or to perceive endometrial or fibromatous pathologies.
- Post termination bleeding is not really a diagnostic hysteroscopy indication; however, it may be useful after an elective abortion in case of postoperative complications or after a molar pregnancy when the endometrium and uterine cavity have been evaluated by vaginal ultrasonography.

## Abnormal uterine bleeding in the post menopausal period

Hysterography has been replaced by hysteroscopic examination which is a far more comfortable procedure to confirm the data collected by endovaginal ultrasonography which is always performed first. In 50% of the cases endocavitary lesions are detected in patients under hormonal-replacement therapy and in 60% of the cases in the absence of hormonal-replacement therapy.

## Infertility

The findings of hysteroscopy should be completed by hysterosalpingography which provides reliable data about the state of the tubes and their permeability.

In the endo-cervical tract, hysteroscopy can detect endo cervical pathologies such as mucous or fibrous polyps, synechiae and bifid cervixes.

In the endouterine cavity, hysteroscopy can detect a septate uterus, synechiae, fibrous polyps, anomalies of the endometrium, endometritis, osseous metaplasia and vascular dystrophy. Diagnostic hysteroscopy should be part of the systematic investigation of infertility and *in vitro* fecundation process.

## *Other indications*

Hysteroscopy is prescribed before a myomectomy to assess the state of the uterine cavity and not pass by an endo cavitary fibroid needing a specific hysteroscopic treatment.

After an endouterine resection, hysteroscopy is an indication for a young woman who desires a pregnancy to assess the state of the uterine cavity and the aspect of the endometrium scar. The existence of iatrogenous mucous synechiae (8.5% in our experience), technical imperfections such as remains of fibroids or displacement of an interstitial fibroid towards the uterine cavity can be discovered.

## Contraindications

Contraindications are not specific and are the usual of any endouterine maneuver except in case of:
-    pregnancy. If there is any clinical doubt, a plasmatic pregnancy test should be performed;
-    an evolutive genital infection;
-    heavy uterine bleeding which is a major contraindication for carbon oxide hysteroscopy because of risks of pulmonary embolism. The presence of blood is also an important drawback when exploring the uterine cavity. The examination cannot be completed and the hysteroscopy should be continued with a fluid perfusion of saline solution to make sure there are no lesions. If the procedure is performed under general anesthesia, $CO_2$ should be avoided because of risks of pulmonary embolism. If a pre-surgery diagnostic hysteroscopy is necessary, it must be performed with a fluid perfusion.

## References

1.    Hamou JE (1991) Hysteroscopy and microlposcopy. Appleton, and lange edit. Norwalk San Matro
2.    Blanc B, Boubli L (1991) Manuel d'hystéroscopie opératoire. Vigot ed, Paris
3.    Mussoto P (1993) Les défits de la flexibilité en hystéroscopie, ses apports diagnostiques et thérapeutiques en gynécologie obstétrique, perspectives d'avenir. Thèse médecine, Faculté de médecine de Bobigny, Université Paris XIII 1-6
4.    Taylor S Hystéroscopie diagnostique ambulatoire, Technique d'examen. Diplôme européen d'hystéroscopie. Livre des communications p 1-11
5.    Marty R, Amouroux J, De Brux J (1992) The targeted endometrial biopsy during flexible endoscopy technic and result. International congres of gynecologic endoscopy. Seoul Korea, book of abstract L 25-61

# Office fibrohysteroscopy

R. MARTY, L. CARBILLON, M. UZAN

Conventional rigid hysteroscopy started in 1869 with Pantaleoni (Great Britain). The first fibroscope was presented 94 years later by Mohri and Mohri (Japan) in 1963. For the last 36 years, fibrohysteroscopes have developed tremendously because of the continuous improvement of the optic fibers. This progress has allowed to manufacture ultraslim hysteroscopes with superior resolution and brightness, that enable the physician to work on an outpatient basis.

The technique of a flexible hysteroscopic examination is specific and varies from the technique employed with a conventional hysteroscope. The difference is based on the specific design features of the flexible hysteroscopes. A tenaculum is rarely needed to hold the cervix. In more than 95% of the cases in which only diagnostic hysteroscopy is being performed with a 3 mm or 3.6 mm, the gynecologist does not need to dilate the cervix and use anesthesia. Unlike the procedure with rigid endoscope, the patient does not require prostaglandine nor premedication [1]. In our experience, when using the 4.9 mm, the dilatation of the cervix is required in about 10% of the cases, mainly for postmenopausal patients or women who had a previous cervical surgery [2].

The best period for an office hysteroscopic procedure is the first phase of the cycle, because during the proliferative phase the menstruation is completed. When the endometrial lining is thin, the endoscopist is able to detect more easily small modifications that could be hidden during the postovulatory phase [3]. An emergency kit containing medications to treat potential problems, such as vasovagal reactions and bleeding, must be available in the office.

## Guidelines for the procedure

It is important to place the triangle mark in the eyepiece of the hysteroscope at 0° before the onset of the procedure. This allows the operator to know where the tip is oriented. Then, normal saline is infused and the tip of the instrument is placed in front of the external cervical os. The procedure may be divided in three steps. The progression inside the cervical canal (step one), the exploration of the uterine cavity (step two) and the withdrawal of the fibroscope (step three).

## Step one (progression inside the cervical canal)

As soon as the tip is inside the cervix, the progression through the cervical canal begins following the opening of the virtual cervical cavity by the distending media. The normal saline creates and opens a space which that can be used for the progression of the hysteroscope. This must be done gently and the operator must be careful to remain in the middle of the cervical canal avoiding to touch the walls. This type of progression is painless and does not provoke bleeding of the endometrium. Because of the frontal view of the fibroscope and its softness, the operator can avoid any cervical laceration or possible damages to the endometrium resulting in bleedings. There is no risk of perforation unlike that present with the rigid hysteroscope which has a sharp tip. The progression goes up to the internal cervical os by snaking the hysteroscope through the cervical canal [4]. During this first step, a careful exploration of the canal is easy, looking for a pathological aspect of the endometrium.

The accomplishment of this first step is eased by the judicious use of the flexible tip to adjust the shape of the hysteroscope in each individual anatomy.

## Step two (exploration of the uterine cavity)

When the hysteroscope arrives at the junction of the lower uterine segment and upper cervical canal, it is possible from this point to visualize the entire uterine cavity. It is mandatory to have a global panoramic view of the endometrial cavity before initiating its careful exploration.

During a panoramic evaluation, it is generally easy to locate both tubal ostia, to look for the general shape of the cavity and to look for the presence of any abnormal growth or for a global or partial distorsion of the uterine walls [5]. The uterine cavity has an arcuate shape and the walls and lateral portion are concave on all the surface. The two horns are clearly visible and sometimes one or both tubal ostia are not identified when the uterine cavity is greatly enlarged or distorted by endometrial myoma, or if the horn is too deep. In such a circumstance, the endoscopist must insert the fibroscope further in the fundus to identify the ostia.

Then, if the evaluation is normal, one must explore closely each different area: fundus, anterior and posterior wall, lateral portion, cornual area and tubal ostia, and finally the lower uterine segment. This exploration is eased by the use of the possibilities of the flexible hysteroscope, allowing to observe any part of the uterine cavity and to face any suspected endometrial area in the totality of the uterine cavity. The distal eye piece needs to be moved in any direction, either up or down or towards the patient thight, with a single movement of the physician's thumb from side to side and a gentle rotation of the physician's wrist. The entire cavity can always be properly visualized, minimizing patient's discomfort (Table 1).

A directed cytology or a targeted endometrial biopsy must be performed at the selected area if a pathology is discovered or if an endometrial abnomaly is founded. With the fibroscope, it is very easy to pass over a pathological growth or a synechia. In any patient, the full endometrial cavity may be explored and faced. A difficult or hidden area located behind a myoma or a large polyp or an extended synechia is easily reached, utilizing the bending capacity of the tip. A minutious and close evaluation of the tubal ostia is always possible with sometimes the ability to explore the first centimeter of the interstitial part of the tube.

An excellent visualization is always obtained with the normal saline infused through an appropriate IV tubing. The stopcock may be closed when the appropriate uterine distension is obtained. Later, when necessary, it is easy to reopen the stopcock a little while to restaure a suitable pressure. Because of the slight leakage of the normal saline around the hysteroscope in the cervical canal, the pressure is always optimal, avoiding the risk of a dangerous overload. This system works as well as continuous flow rigid diagnostic hysteroscope works.

---

### Special screening by the low preassure test

We have observed that the appropriate intrauterine pressure of the distending medium plays a great role for the correct visualization of the uterine cavity. We would point out two important facts:
- the appearance of the uterine cavity varies with its dilatation. If the pressure is raised, the colour diminishes as well as ondulations and projections do. The patterns of subepithelial vessels are less visible;
- when the endoscopist has observed a modification or a rigidity of an area during the first panoramic evaluation, this may be the consequence of an intramural myoma. Such a rupture in the shape may be detected more clearly at very low pressure for some submucous myoma close to the endometrial surface. The detection of small endometrial polyps is also easier using this screening.

---

### Step three (withdrawal of the fibroscope)

This is an important step. The cervical canal may be better visualized as the fibroscope is withdrawn at the

---

Table 1. Hysteroscopic evaluation of the endometrium

| Macroscopic appearance | Endometrial lining | Thickness | Vascular pattern | Homogenicity | Intrauterine growths |
|---|---|---|---|---|---|
| Smooth Irregular Polypoid | Abnormal or suspicious endometrial area Adenomyosis appearance | Thin Thick Variable (area) | None Pattern regular or not Vascular caliber irregular or not Corkscrew vascular aspect Oozing | Homogeneous Heterogeneous Special area | Hypertrophia Mucous polyp Fibrous polyp Submucous myoma Adenocancer |

end of the procedure. This must be done slowly and progressively until the external cervical os is reached. In many occasions, we have discovered a pathology missed during the initial insertion. A small polyp or a focal endometrial lesion can be detected.

We have conducted a *retrospective study on N = 500 patients* who had ambulatory protocols performed at the University Hospital (Hôpital Avicenne) by three different operators.

A polyp or an endometrial cervical anomaly was missed in *N = 17* patients during steps one and two and discovered later during the step three. This rate of *3,4%* comes, most of the time, from an incorrect protocol. The reason is a bad technique, because the progression was done too fast or because the tip of the hysteroscope was too close to the cervical wall or the observation began only when the hysteroscope was arrived at the internal cervical os. Another reason is that, in most of the cases, the missed anomaly was a tiny polyp or a small focal endometrial lesion.

## Appearance of the endometrial lining

The visual appearance of the endometrium changes according to the phases of the menstrual cycle. In the follicular period, the epithelium is thin yellowish with a little vascularization. Later, during the secretory phase, the endometrium becomes thicker and takes a fluffy aspect with a red coloration [6]. The hystero-scopic appearance of the endometrium during the cycle may be divided into five periods. A good description of the cyclic changes of the endometrium has been done by Sugimoto [7].

The regenerative phase shows a yellowish endometrial surface without blood vessels and scattered or local spots may be present. The regenerative endometrium is less than 2 mm thickness.

The second phase is mid proliferative. The surface is livid and sometimes yellowish spots are observed (glandular ostia). Then, during the mid cycle the active growth of the endometrium is demonstrated by the presence of many glandular ostia scattered on the surface, strawberry like coloured, and presenting rough ondulations. During the secretory phase, the endometrium is reddish yellow colour red and subepithelial vessels are seen through the translucent stroma. A polypoid appearance is present. When the involutional phase comes, one can observe a wrinkled pattern with blood vessels easily visible and blood spots. Table 2 shows the various modifications of the endometrial lining [8-10].

## Postmenopausal endometrial appearance

If the patient does not receive the hormonal replacement therapy, the endometrial lining becomes very thin, flat and smooth. It looks yellowish white.

**Table 2.** Hysteroscopic and sonographic cyclic appearance of the endometrium

| Phase | Regenerative | Mid proliferative | Mid cycle | Secretory | Involutional | Menopausal |
|---|---|---|---|---|---|---|
| Day of the cycle | 6-8 | 10-12 | 17 | 20 | 25 | - |
| Hysteroscopy | | | | | | |
| Ondulation folds | gentle / none | slight uneveness irregular | rough / + | + polypoid projection | wrinckled pattern soft appearance | none none |
| Glandular ostia | shallow | visible all surface | many scattered on surface | hardly visible | no | none |
| Colour | yellowish red | livid | livid strawberry aspect | reddish yellow | whitered | light yellow |
| Blood vessels | none | none | rare | visible | visible with blood spots | clearly discernable |
| Sonography | | | | | | |
| Thickness (mm) | 4-6 | 8-10 | 12-13 | 14-15 | decreases | < or = 4 |
| Echogenicity | hypo | hypo | target appearance | becomes hyper starting from the basal layer | hyper (totality) | hyper (irregular) |

Sometimes cystic glands protrude. The course of small vessels is clearly discernable.

## Technical hitches (Table 3)

The gynecologist may face various problems during the hysteroscopic procedure: a difficulty to introduce the endoscope, or the impossibility to obtain a clear panoramic view of the uterine cavity; sometimes an insufficient uterine distention or a poor image. The Table 3 shows how to resolve these problems.

## Special cases

### Postmenopausal patients

In some postmenopausal women with an important cervical atrophia [11], it may be necessary to prepare the patients with a *preoperative treatment with oestro-*

*gen vaginal pellets* for three weeks, in order to soften the atrophic *cervix* or scarred cervix. Sometimes, even after this preparation, the insertion of the hysteroscope remains impossible. Then it is necessary to perform a cervical dilatation to reach 3 mm, which is enough to introduce the minifibrohysteroscope.

### Scarred cervix and cervical stenosis

Some women have undergone a previous cervical conization or cryotherapy, electro- or laser therapy. In such a condition, the gynecologist must perform, prior to the hysteroscopic procedure, a careful examination of the external cervical os with a small plastic or *rubber probe*. If the diameter is less than 3 mm, it may be necessary to dilate the *cervix* up to this size. Most of the time this can be done progressively. *The rate of cervical stenosis* in our practice is *about 5%*. If the patient feels uncomfortable, the best is to intro-

Table 3. Technical hitches

| | | |
|---|---|---|
| **Insertion** (step1) | | |
| • **Difficult** | *Pusillanimous patient*............................................ | *Perform a paracervical block* |
| • **Impossible** | *External cervical os < 3 mm* | *Stiffen the tip* |
| | | *Try the HYF-XP* |
| | | *Sound and dilate up to 3 mm* |
| **Cervical progression** (step1) | | *If failure = laminaria* |
| | *Stenotic cervical canal* .......................................... | *Stiffen the tip* |
| | .......................................... | *Wait after each small progression* |
| **Difficult or poor visibility** (step1) | *Possible synechia* | |
| | *Polyp or malformation* ......................................... | *Meticulous third step* |
| **Panoramic view** (step2) **Inadequate** | *Inadequate uterine distension* .............................. | *cf. below* |
| | *Presence of mucous, debris, clots or tissue* ........... | *wash to clear the cavity* |
| | *One or two tubal ostia not visualized*.................. | *pull back the fibroscope, look for the existence of septum synechia or large myoma* |
| **Uterine distension** | | |
| **Absent** | *No intrauterine pressure*........................................ | *check tubing and stopcock* |
| **Not sufficient** | *Pressure too low* ..................................................... | *elevate the plastic bag open the stopcock* |
| **Inconstant** | *Input flow < leakage*.............................................. | *increase the input flow* |
| **Image** | | |
| **Red or hazy** | *Tip on the fundus or uterine wall*......................... | *pull back the fibroscope* |
| | *Tip pressed on a pathologic growth* ...................... | *withdraw the endoscope* |
| | *Blood or debris on the lens* ................................. | *pull back the endoscope and clear the lens* |
| **White or dazzling** | *Tip too close to the endometrium*.......................... | *withdraw and change approach* |

duce a laminaria. This means that the patient requires a one-day hospitalization.

## Patients with spotting or moderate metrorrhagia

In such a condition, the choice of *normal saline 0,9%* as distending medium is mandatory. The irrigation will allow to evacuate the clots and debris and clear the view. This is not possible with a $CO_2$ distension. In such a patient, it is useful to get an endometrial sampling.

## Patients under Tamoxifen Therapy

Many patients who had a prior breast therapy for cancer receive postoperatively a treatment with Tamoxifen [12]. Most of these patients are postmenopausal and a careful evaluation of the cervix must be done prior a hysteroscopy. If necessary, a cervical dilatation must be done before endoscopy. A targeted endometrial biopsy must always be performed on any suspicious area. This treatment raises the problem of the screening of polyps and endometrial carcinoma or precursors. Many detailed articles have been published during the last years and the results are *controversial*. Some physicians recommend a vaginal ultrasound only on symptomatic patients during the treatment; some others perform a vaginal ultrasound on every patient, and others recommend a hysteroscopic uterine evaluation.

*In our University Hospital* (Hôpital Avicenne), we have decided that *every patient* who is going to receive Tamoxifen therapy must have a *fibrohysteroscopy, prior to initial of the treatment.*

In such a condition, if an endometrial pathology exists, it can be immediately treated. If not, the treatment is initiated. For the follow up of the treated patients, we perform a vaginal *ultrasound* each year and, if the endometrial thickness is more or equal to *4 mm* (double layer technique), we perform another fibrohysteroscopy.

## Symptomatic patients on hormonal replacement therapy

Hysteroscopy is a frequent indication in these patients suffering of spotting or metrorrhagia. If the treatment is sequential, one must choose the first part of the cycle to avoid the thicker endometrial second phase. A targeted endometrial *biopsy* must be performed to evaluate the hormonal response *in the fundus*. This is mandatory to adapt the hormonal treatment to each individual [13].

## Patients on IVF protocol

These patients have an hysteroscopic investigation scheduled as first or second intension depending on the teams. This exploration must be scheduled at day 11-14 and a targeted endometrial biopsy must be performed at the same time *on the fundus* to evaluate the hormonal status of the endometrium.

## IVF Protocol

Infertility is the second indication for hysteroscopy after abnormal uterine bleeding. The value of the hysteroscopic evaluation and reevaluation in patients with failed IVF is important. Because the failure rate of embryo transfer is the stage of the *in vitro* fertilization (IVF) procedure that has the highest failure rate, it is important to detect endometrial and structural abnormalities to decrease the rate of embryo transfer failure. Hysteroscopic evaluation and treatment for the IVF procedure are of extreme importance, because the *reduction of intrauterine abnormalities will reduce the IVF-IT failure rate [14].*

## Embryo transfer

In connexion with the Assisted Medical Reproduction Department of our University Hospital (Jean Verdier), we have discussed the opportunity to perform a hysteroscopy to facilitate the transfer. Sometimes, in selected cases, this transfer is not possible because the cannula cannot clear the cervical canal when too much angled, tortuous or partially obstructed by a synechia. The *cannula* containing the embryo could be introduced *into the operating channel* of the HYF-1T (4.9) to clear the cervical canal before leaving the embryo in the uterine cavity. *The tip* of the fibroscope should be *stopped* as soon as the *internal cervical os* is reached. Then the catheter could be easily introduced alone in the uterine cavity.

The reliability of this protocol requires a confirmation by some selected cases.

## Report on a printed form

When the procedure is over, it is very useful to fulfill a detailed sheet reporting the hysteroscopic procedure.

If a pathology is discovered, a brief description must be done and the lesion must be localized on the sketch. When a targeted endometrial biopsy is perfor-med, the chosen area must be indicated on the sketch. A *copy* of this report sheet must be *sent to the patholo-gist* with the tissue samples (Table 4).

Table 4.

---

## HOPITAL JEAN VERDIER
Service de gynécologie obstétrique – Pr. Michèle UZAN

## FIBROHYSTEROSCOPY REPORT

Surgeon :

Date :

Name :

Age :

Type of Fibro :

Indication :

Last Period :

Distending media :     $CO_2$     Normal Saline     Glycocol     Other

Cervical Canal :

Isthmus :

Fundus :

❖ Right tubal ostium and cornua
❖ Left tubal ostium and cornua

Uterine cavity :

Endometrial Lining :

**Biopsy** :

---

**Table 5.** Office fibrohysteroscopy

| Instrumentation | |
|---|---|
| ■ Minifibrohysteroscope : HYF-P | • Caliber: 3.5 mm<br>• Operating channel: 1.2 mm<br>• Steerable tip 100° up and down<br>• Axial view with a field angle 90° |
| ■ Minifibrohysteroscope : HYF-XP | • Calibrer: 3 mm |
| ■ Xenon light source | |
| ■ Ancillary instrumentation<br>(outer diameter 3-French) | • Cytobrush<br>• Selection of several biopsy forceps with various jaws<br>  - rat tooth<br>  - mouse tooth<br>  - alligator, etc<br>• Lasso forceps<br>• Basket forceps<br>• Monopolar electrode ($CO_2$ insufflation required) |
| ■ Isotonic saline | • Bag (with appropriate tubing)<br>distention by gravity (≤ 1.50 m above patient)<br>• Syringe (with appropriate tubing) |
| ■ Optional | • Camera<br>• $CO_2$ hysteroflator<br>• Tenaculum |

## Necessary instrumentation

For office diagnostic evaluation, the necessary instrumentation is listed on Table 5.

## Patient tolerance

An American study conducted by Bradley and Widricht under conditions similar to the French study, determined patient tolerance to flexible hysteroscopy on the following scale:  1 = easily acceptable discomfort or minimal discomfort;  2 = acceptable discomfort, uncomfortable but easily bearable; 3 = tolerable discomfort, equivalent to menstrual crampe and spasme; 4 = barely touchable, tolerable for a short time only, and  5 = intolerable pain, bad enough to stop the procedure. Acceptance of the procedure, corresponding to the first three groups, was found in *84% of patients, while 12.4% accepted the conditions of the procedure for a short period (group 4) and 3.6% stopped the procedure because of intolerable pain. The results of this American study were comparable to the French experience [15].

Our results are also very close to this American study. We have observed that it is very important to focus the attention of the patient during the procedure on the video screen. After some necessary explanations on the progress of the procedure, the endo-scopist must comment the image on the screen and explain its different steps, while performing it. We have never been forced to stop a targeted endometrial biopsy, even with three sampling. We have observed that the sampling of endometrial tissue by aspiration (pipelle or suction curretage) causes more discomfort than targeted endometrial biopsy during hysteroscopy.

## Office hysteroscopy, analgesia or local anesthesia

In a great majority of the cases, no systematic sedative nor medication is required as the procedure is practically painless. In some specific patients when the cervix must be dilated prior to the hysteroscopic procedure, we sometimes perform a paracervical block. About 4 ml of a local anesthesia is injected at the base of each uterosacral ligament. The results of a French National Survey (N = 35.289) in 1998, gave 80% of procedures without anesthesia. In our experience over twelve years, the *rate of local anesthesia ranges around 5%* [16].

## Importance of the low intrauterine pressure test

This test takes place at the end of step two before pulling back the fibroscope inside the cervical canal. This test is very useful if a myoma is suspected or when a suspicious endometrial area has been detected during the procedure. The endoscopist decreases the intrauterine pressure and wait and observe until the two uterine walls are almost together. During this manoeuvre, a careful observation of the endometrial lining is recommended to look for a local convex area; this appearance is very revealing of an *interstitial myoma* close to the endometrial lining and *becoming shortly submucous*. This signal may not exist during the normal intrauterine pressure.

Another interest of this manoeuvre is the better observation of a suspicious endometrial area discovered during the procedure. The test allows to have a better observation of its *vascular pattern* than that not visible because of too much intrauterine pressure. It is recommended to perform a vaginal ultrasound if this was not done prior to the hysteroscopic examination. We have started to experience this test when a patient was referred to us with a previous vaginal ultrasound showing an interstitial myoma located close to the endometrium but yet not submucous.

This test gives also useful information when a distorsion of the uterine cavity has been observed during the procedure or when an abnomaly is detected in the general concavity of the uterine shape.

## Retrospective study: our experience

For the last twelve years, we have used three types of fibrohysteroscopes from Olympus with a great success: the HYF-P and the HYF-1T. For the last 18 months, we have evaluated and used the mini HYF-XP (3 mm). The uterine distension is always performed with normal saline 0.9% perfused by gravity. The procedure is carried out with a cold light source Xenon and always with a light sensitive video camera.

Among a serie of 1.113 patients who had a diagnostic procedure on an outpatient basis with a cytobrushing or a targeted endometrial biopsy (Table 6), 917 had a targeted endometrial biopsy and 196 only a cytobrushing. The average duration was eight minutes, including biopsies, and no complication occurred (Table 7).

Two decisional charts (Tables 8 and 9) may be consulted when the hysteroscopist during the procedure finds a suspicious area or a pathological growth.

Table 6.

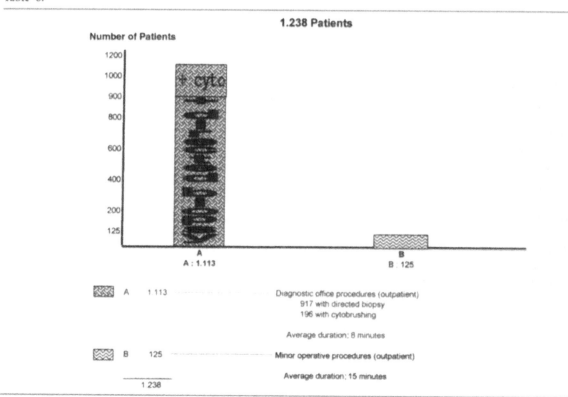

Table 7.

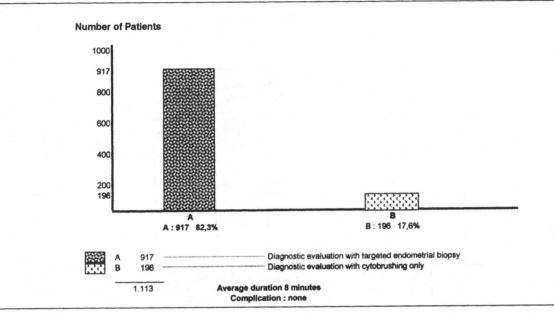

**Number of Patients**

A : 917  82,3%          B : 196  17,6%

A    917 ............................................................. Diagnostic evaluation with targeted endometrial biopsy
B    196 ............................................................. Diagnostic evaluation with cytobrushing only

1.113          **Average duration 8 minutes**
               **Complication : none**

Table 8.

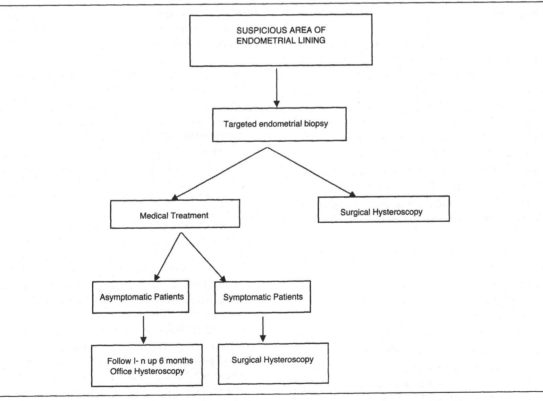

Table 9.

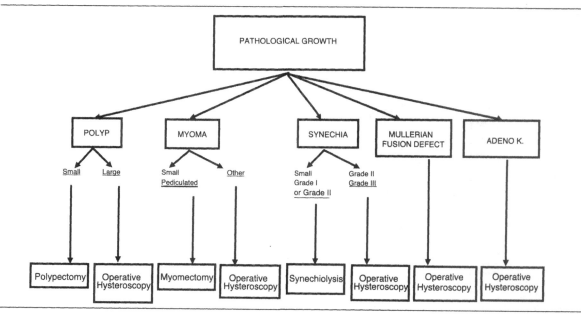

## References

1. Loffer FD (1996) Techniques for Diagnostic Rigid Hysteroscopy. In: Isaacson KB (ed) Office Hysteroscopy. Mosby-Year Book, St Louis, USA, 55, 56

2. Mussuto P (1993) Les defis de la flexibilité en hysteroscopie. Ses apports diagnostiques et thérapeutiques en gynécologie obstétrique: des perspectives d'avenir. Thèse pour le Doctorat en Médecine. Faculté de Médecine Broussais Hôtel-Dieu, pp 127, 128

3. Valle RF (1997) A Manual of Clinical Hysteroscopy. Parthenon Publishing, New York, p 50

4. Marty R (1995) Fibrohystéroscopie au Cabinet médical (8 ans de pratique). Gynécologie Obstétrique Pratique 7: 13-14

5. Blanc B, Boubli L (1996) Endoscopie Utérine. Ed Pradel, Paris, p 21

6. Marty R (1996) Nine Years of Experience with flexible hysteroscopy. Office Hysteroscopy. Mosby-Year Book, St Louis, USA, pp 61, 62

7. Sugimoto O (1978) Diagnostic and Therapeutic Hysteroscopy. Igaku-Shoin, Tokyo, pp 39-49

8. Ardaens Y (1996) Endomètre au cours du cycle menstruel. Apport de l'écho doppler couleur vaginal. Gynécologie Obstétrique Pratique 87: 10

9. Rudigoz RC, Salle B (1995) Echographie et endomètre. Reproduction Humaine et Hormones. 8(1-2): 65-67

10. Haag T, Manhes H (1995) Instant de l'echo doppler couleur dans la surveillance de l'endomètre postménopausique. Références en Gynécologie 43(4): 369-376

11. Marty R, Valle RF (1995) Eight years' experience performing procedures with flexible hysteroscopes. J Am Assoc Gynecol Laparosc 3(1): 116

12. Marty R (1997) Technique de l'Hystéroscopie souple de consultation. Série de 1000 cas. La Revue du Praticien. Gynécologie et Obstétrique 2: 23-26

13. Marty R (1998) Diagnostic fibrohysteroscopic evaluation of perimenopausal and postmenopausal uterine bleeding: a comparative study with Belgian and Japanese data. J Am Assoc Gynecol Laparosc 5(1): 69-73

14. Dicker D, Ashkenazi J, Feldberg D, Fahri J, Shalev J, Ben-Rafael Z (1992) The value of repeat hysteroscopic evaluation in patients with failed in vitro fertilization transfer cycles. Fertility and Sterility. 58(4): 833-835

15. Marty R (1996) Nine Years of Experience with flexible hysteroscopy. In Office Hysteroscopy. Mosby-Year Book, St Louis, USA, 70-71

16. Marty R, de Mouzon J (2001) The use of the fibrohysteroscope in ambulatory patients for diagnostic and minor operative procedures. French National Survey conducted by Le Club Gynécologique d'Endoscopie Flexible. Global Congress of Gynecologic Endoscopy 30th Annual Meeting of the AAGL, San Francisco/California, November 2001, Book of Abstracts August 2001, vol. 8 n° S 41, n° 136

## Phisiological aspects

These photos were made with the 3.5 mm fibrohysteroscope (HYF type P)
The « weft » aspect (« moiré » effect) does not exist anymore with the new 3 mm fibrohysteroscope (HYF type XP), because the number of optic fibers is increased by 1.6 and they have a smaller diameter.

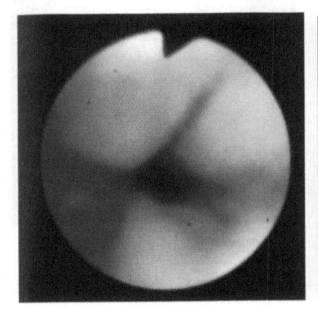

Fig. 1.  External cervical ostium

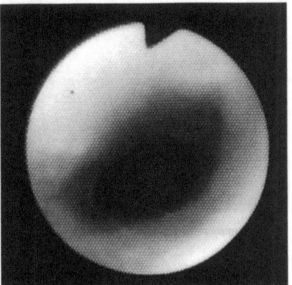

Fig. 2.  Cervical canal

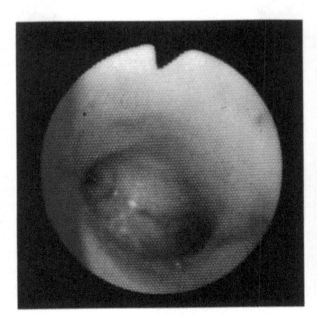

Fig. 3.  Uterine cavity from internal cervical ostium

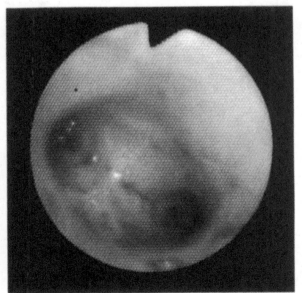

Fig. 4.  Uterine cavity from the middle of the cavity

## Physiological aspects II

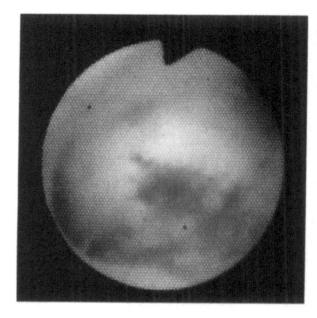

Fig. 5. Postmenopausal fundus and tubal ostia

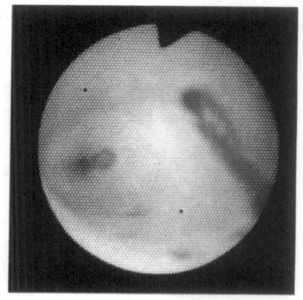

Fig. 6. Right cornua

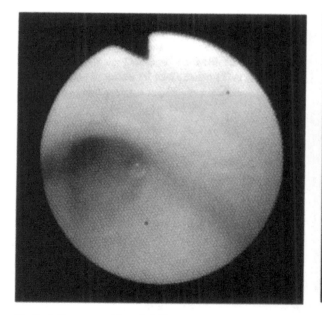

Fig. 7. Left cornua with arch fold

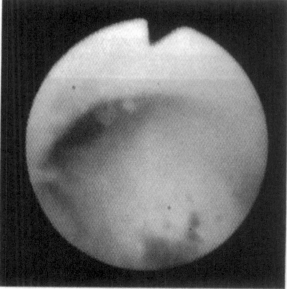

Fig. 8. Right tubal ostium and deep cornua

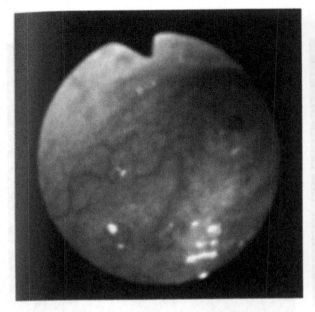

Fig. 9. Left tubal ostium and hypervascularization of the cornua

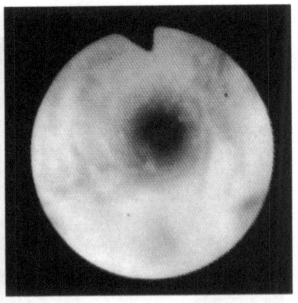

Fig. 10. Close view of the right tubal ostium – Before the envertion of a Katayama catheter

## Pathology

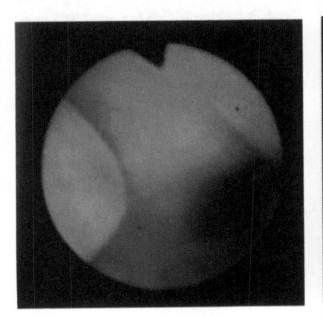

Fig. 1. Endometrial polyp near left tubal ostium

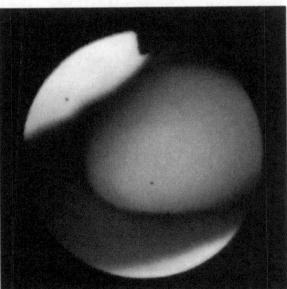

Fig. 2. Pediculated polyp on the fundus

## Pathology II

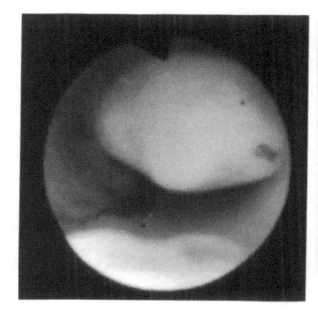

**Fig. 3.** Polyp near internal cervical ostium

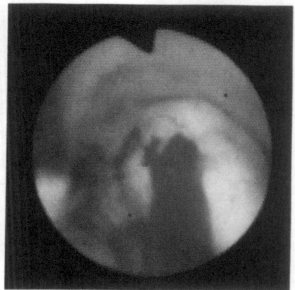

**Fig. 4.** Polyp with bleeding on the surface

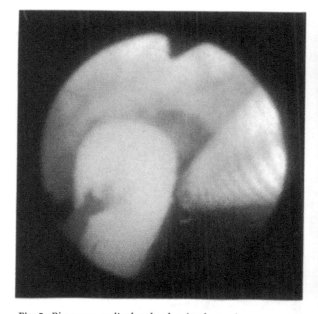

**Fig. 5.** Biopsy on pediculated polyp (at the tase)

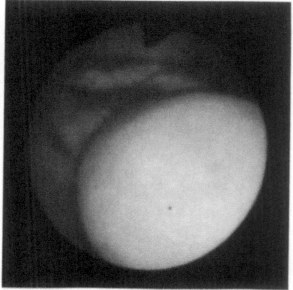

**Fig. 6.** Submucous myoma

## Pathology III

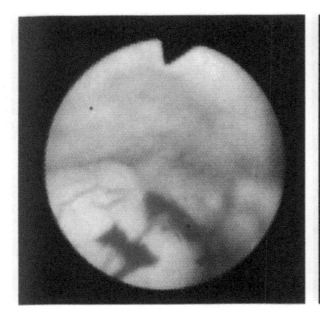

**Fig. 7.** Myoma. Slight vascularization of the surface

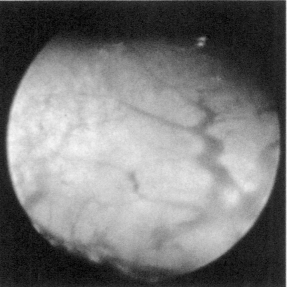

**Fig. 8.** Vascular network of myoma

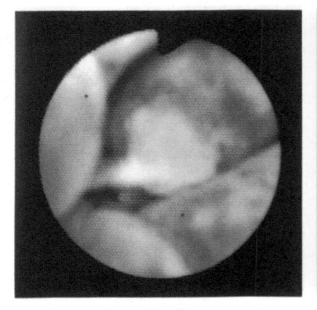

**Fig. 9.** Myomas on the posterior wall

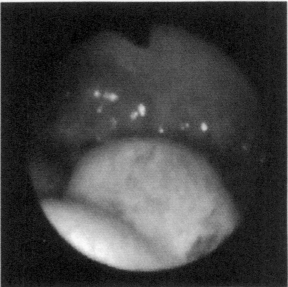

**Fig. 10.** Myoma near the fundus

## Pathology IV

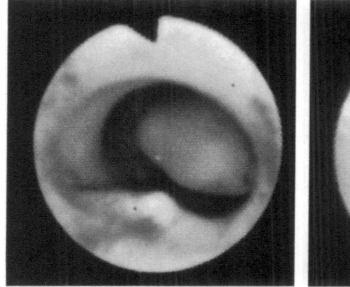

**Fig. 11.** Myoma of the fundus and sessile polyp at the isthmus

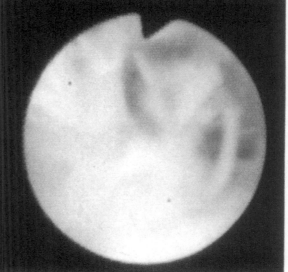

**Fig. 12.** Endometrial ossification (post abortum)

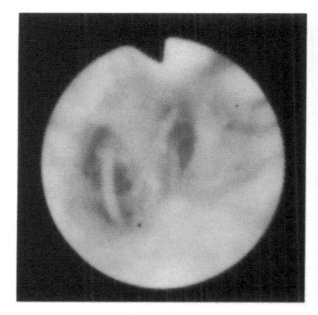

**Fig. 13.** Details of endometrial ossification

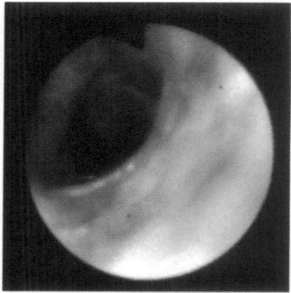

**Fig. 14.** Hemi-uterus *(right)* + septum + right tubal ostium

# Pathology V

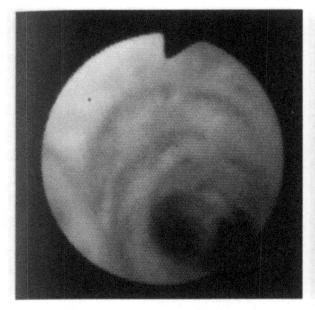

Fig. 15. Left hemi-uterus + septum + left tubal ostium

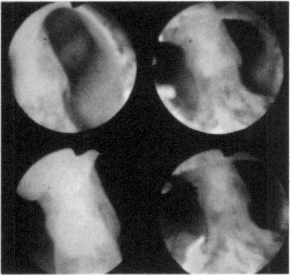

Fig. 16. Septum and hemi-uterus

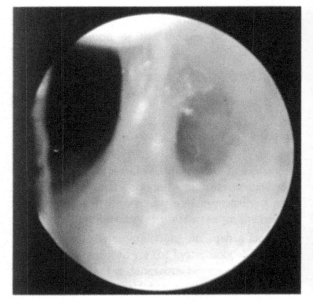

Fig. 17. Synechia grade I/II

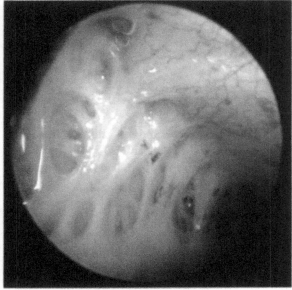

Fig. 18. Synechia early grade II - Lateral

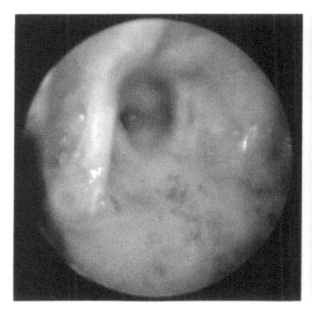

**Fig. 19.** Synechia grade III - uterine cavity

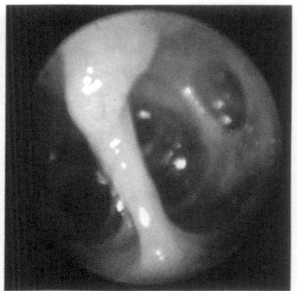

**Fig. 20.** Multiple synechia - grade II and III

# Decontamination, disinfection and sterilization of the hysteroscopes

R. MARTY

The risk of serious infections during the performance of a hysteroscopy in out-patients' departments can be avoided by strictly following the rules of decontamination, disinfection and sterilization.

In Europe, with the emergence of the prion (Creutzfeldt-Jakob) and the tremendous increase of office hysteroscopy, the risk of nosocomial infections is increased. An official French epidemiologic study (1996) reports an incidence of 1,03/106 for prion, of 110.000 persons alive for HIV and of 1,3% (women) for hepatitis C. In a French report on 13.360 surgical procedures (1996) the evaluation of the infection after incision shows 1,9% in gynecology obstetrics, including 32% staphylococci, 18% Escherichia coli and 13% Enterobacteria [1].

In France, according to the legislation, the surgeon must "take care of the correct sterilization and decontamination of the instrumentation he/she is using and of the elimination of the medical waste" (French Legislation, 1996).

## Etiopathogeny

There are two ways of transmission of an infection through a hysteroscope:

a) Endogenous (autoinfection). The hysteroscope carries a vaginal germ into the uterine cavity. A good vaginal disinfection and eventually a prophylactic antibiotherapy greatly reduce the risk.

b) Exogenous (heteroinfection). In such a case, the germ is introduced via the hysteroscope. This way of transmission is dangerous because the gynecologist could ignore a potential pathology of the patient, such as hepatitis B, C or HIV.

During the procedure of hysteroscopy, various factors are increasing the risk of infection:

- the opening of the cervical canal;
- the introduction of the scope inside the uterine cavity;
- the insufflation of $CO_2$ or a liquid distention media;
- a possible scratch of the endometrium during the progression of the tip of the hysteroscope inside the uterine canal leading to a possible introduction of micro-organisms to the blood stream, initiating a iatrogenic infection (sexually transmitted disease).

These different factors have been already detailed a few years ago by Gadonnaix et al. in the volume "Hystéroscopie et infections nosocomiales".

Since fibrohysteroscopes scarcely require a cervical dilatation (very small diameter, 3 mm) and are supple, they offer less possibilities to scratch the endometrium and cause a iatrogenic infection.

## Bacteria

They may be Neisseria gonorrhoeae, Mycobacterium tuberculosis or Treponema pallidum. They may come from the cervico-vaginal population and when they arrive in the uterus, they react as opportunistic bacteria.

- Bacteria aerobia: Streptococcus, Staphylococcus, Escherichia coli, Gardnerella vaginalis etc.
- Bacteria anaerobia: difficult to diagnose.
- Mycoplasma hominis or Ureaplasma urealyticum trachomatis, which are responsible for salpingitis and sterility. They require a treatment only if they are above a fixed level.
- Chlamydia. This intracellular bacteria, difficult to detect, is responsible of a great number of sterility. It may be diagnosed after a long time of insidious infection damaging the tubes.
- Virus. They are numerous: Herpes I and II, Hepatitis B, and C, HIV 1 and 2, Papillomavirus (0,2 to 7% of the female population).
- Parasites and mushrooms. They may coexist with Trichomonas vaginalis, Candida etc.

## Principles of disinfection and sterilization

The hysteroscope is classified as a "semi-critical" medical device, because it comes into contact with mucous membranes [2].

According to the European Safety Standard to be used, the sterilization has three major steps which must be followed: decontamination, disinfection, and sterilization.

### Decontamination

This operation allows to momentarily eliminate, kill or inhibit the micro-organisms. This is a phase of bacteriostasis or fungistasis.

### Disinfection

Allows to kill or eliminate momentarily micro-organisms and also to inactivate viruses. The results of the disinfection are limited to the micro-organism existing at the moment of the disinfection. This phase is a step of destruction of the germs.

### Sterilization

This final step must eliminate all microbes and viruses. After this final step, the hysteroscope must be protected by a suitable packaging to remain sterile.

The three steps of sterilization are listed and explained in Table 1 (European Instructions, 1996).

If these procedures are possible for both rigid and fibrohysteroscopes for the steps one and two, the sterilization may be different for the third step. If the steam sterilization is the best for rigid hysteroscopes, the cold disinfection must be used for fibrohysteroscopes. One must keep in mind that the destruction of the prion requires autoclaving at 134° C for eighteen minutes.

## Protocol of disinfection and sterilization

### Step 1 – Precleaning procedure

This first step concerns both rigid and flexible hysteroscopes; it is a precleaning procedure. One must use clear water and a cleaning solution. This solution must be a detergent able to digest organic material and protein on contact. One must alternate irrigating and rinsing the hysteroscope with the detergent and with clear water. This phase lasts about five minutes.

### Step 2 – Cleaning procedure and liquid high level disinfection procedure

It concerns both rigid and flexible hysteroscopes. This procedure must use an enzymatic solution without aldehyde. The detergent (Alkazyme or Phago lase in France) is diluted in water in a bin at a correct temperature (dilution recommended by the manufacturer). Alkazyme is the detergent and disinfectant most frequently used in France; the alkaline pH with a proteolytic enzyme removes the biofilm, splites up the proteines and optimizes the disinfection. It must be used at 0,5% of concentration for a least fifteen minutes.

Details of this high level disinfection are as follows: (3)

- immerse the hysteroscope in the disinfectant immersion bin and pump disinfectant through the channel with a syringe;
- allow the scope to remain in the solution for the recommended immersion time;
- following disinfection, remove the scope and irrigate the channel with water until thoroughly rinsed;
- rinse the scope externally and place it in an immersion bin filled with water. Allow it to soak to remove all disinfectant;
- if tap water is used, the rinse must be followed by 70% alcohol washing, since tap water may inoculate the inside lumen of the channel with waterborne micro-organism that could incubate;
- remove the scope and place it on a clean, dry surface;
- run air through the channel until all moisture has been expelled and the channel is dry;
- wipe the outside surface of the scope until dry;
- store so as to prevent recontamination or damage. Never store in foam material because fungus is known to grow in these areas.

This immersion phase should last fifteen minutes.

Alkazyme may be also introduced in an ultrasound bin. It is important to remember that the excellent quality of the sterilization depends totally on the quality of the cleaning. The duration for step 1 + step 2 procedure is about twenty minutes.

### Step 3 – Sterilization or cold disinfection grade 3

### Rigid hysteroscopes

The European Safety Rules (1995) recommend eighteen minutes at 134° C for autoclaving. In such a condition, the prion is destroyed. The steam sterilization is the most suitable for rigid endoscopes. One must use demineralized water to avoid corrosion of the instruments. The cold sterilization procedure may also be used for rigid hysteroscopes. The whole duration of autoclaving for the full cycle depends on the type of instrumentation. For the three phases including rise of temperature and pressure, sterilization and drying, time required is about sixty minutes (Table 2).

### Fibrohysteroscopes

Flexible hysteroscopes do not stand autoclaving and must be disinfected by cold procedure, in order to obtain a "level 3" disinfection, which includes effects on bacteria, viruses and spores. The soaking time requires sixty minutes in diluted glutaraldehyde.

Table 1.

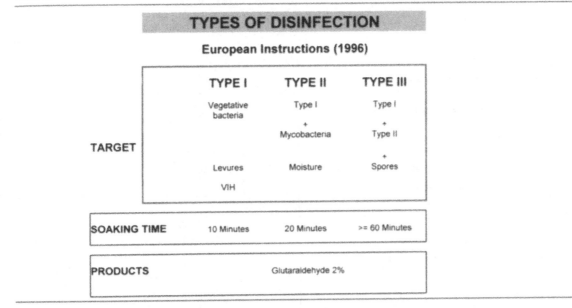

Table 2. European protocol instructions for decontamination, disinfection and sterilization

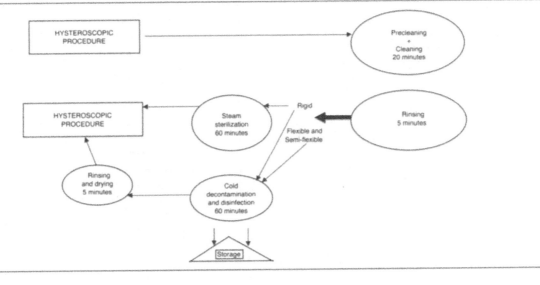

Glutaraldehyde at 2% is a chemical germicide indicated for high level and cold disinfection. The most commonly used in France and Europe is Cidex.

After the disinfection, the hysteroscopes must be rinsed carefully to remove the disinfectant. A chemical colitis from absorption of glutaraldehyde could occur if the endoscope is not adequately rinsed [4] and [5].

The scheme of the full procedure is on Table 2 [6].

## Ancillary instrumentation

All the ancillary instrumentation has to be sterilized as well (Table 3). Biopsy forceps must follow the same steps as the hysteroscopes and be steam sterilized.

Since they are rigid, they can perfectly stand this type of procedure if they are carefully cleaned and disinfected before the sterilization. For the other instruments, such as cytobrush, etc., they must be purchased as disposable items [7].

## Alternative methods for sterilization

Glutaraldehyde 2% (Cidex) is the most used in Europe as a chemical germicide to achieve high level disinfection by immersion (Figs. 1-3). But there are other possibilities to achieve disinfection and sterilization. These procedures are uncommon in Europe and need expensive machines.

**Table 3.** Sterilization of the ancillary instrumentation processes

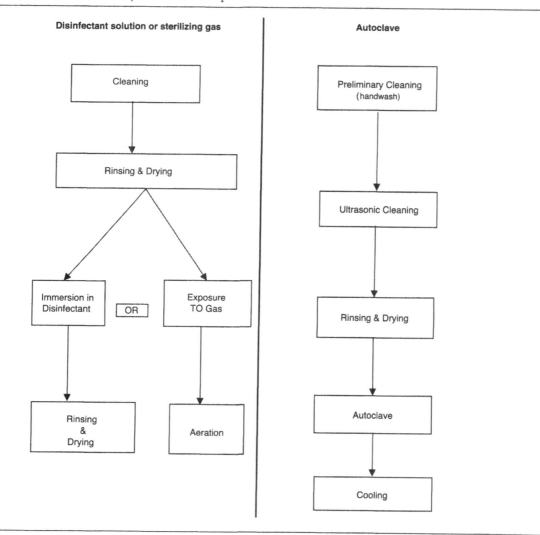

## Ethyline oxide gas sterilization (ETO-CFC)

If correctly cleaned and dryed, the fibrohysteroscope can withstand this type of sterilization.

## Paracetic acid

This procedure is a low temperature sterilization technique. A precleaning is required. The length of the cycle is 30 minutes for the endoscopic reprocessing. It requires an endoscopic reprocessing system.

## Hydrogen peroxide gas plasma

This is a low temperature sterilization technique, too. This procedure is only for rigid endoscopes and the cycle lasts 60 minutes.

Other techniques have been proposed, but they need verification and more studies.

## How to organize an hysteroscopic consultation: practical considerations

There are several possibilities to organize a hysteroscopic procedure depending on the type of hysteroscope available and on the place where the examination must be performed.

## Office setting

If only one hysteroscope is available, either rigid or flexible, the reprocessing time lasts about ninety minutes. An alternating method is suggested in Table 4 for such a situation. This means that the gynecologist

**Table 4.** Hysteroscopic consultation alternating method

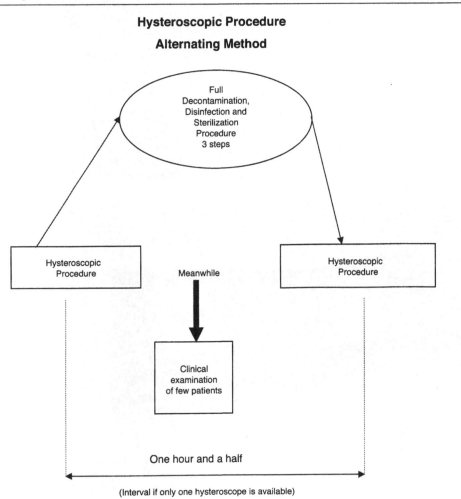

can perform a procedure <u>every hour and a half</u>. In a case like this, the presence of a least two consultants in the interval between one hysteroscopy and the next, should be planned (Table 4).

If two hysteroscopes are available, this allows more adaptability. We must point out the fact that the cold sterilization process allows to start the sixty minutes soaking at any time, even if one hysteroscope is already on process; this is impossible when steam sterilization is used.

## Private Hospital or University Hospital

In such a situation, the instrumentation available is generally more important with two or more endoscopes, both rigid and flexible. Consequently, the organization is much easier and more nurses are available for the sterilization procedure.

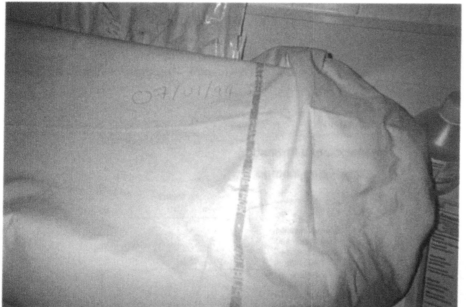

**Fig. 1.** The date of glutaraldehyde preparation must be indicated (for ex., January 07, 1999)

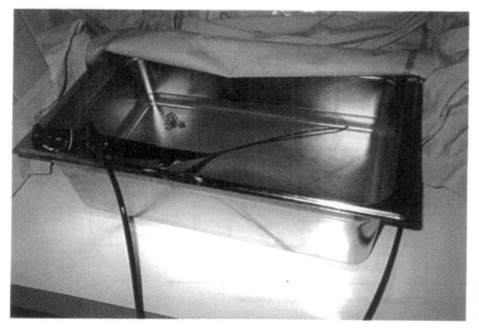

**Fig. 2.** Bin with Cidex. Fibrohysteroscope and stopcock

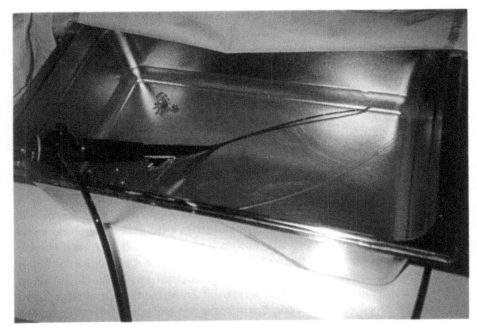

**Fig. 3.** Fibrohysteroscope soaking in glutaraldehyde with a 3-French flexible biopsy forceps

## Conclusion

Because hysteroscopic procedures can be dangerous, the nurses who handle the equipment must have a proper care and maintenance of the endoscopes to ensure a maximum security. The staff should be well trained and able to strictly follow the recommended procedure for each step of the sterilization process. The timing of each step must be respected, the correct concentration of detergent or sterilizing product must be obtained for the soaking bins and the storage has to be appropriate. A safe hysteroscopic procedure, apart from the skill of the operator, requires a perfect sterilization process.

## References

1. Aynaud, Durand (1998) Les bonnes habitudes de stérilisation. 21ème Congrès National SFCPCV. Luneau Gynécologie, Paris

2. Spaulding EH (1968) Chemical disinfection of medical and surgical materials. In: Lawrence CA, Block SS (eds) Disinfection, sterilization and preservation. 3rd ed, Lea & Febiger, Philadelphia

3. Tempesta SO, Spencer MP (1996) Nursing implications for hysteroscopy in an outpatient setting. In: Isaacson Office Hysteroscopy. Mosby-Year Book, St-Louis (MO), pp 38-44

4. Jonas G, Mahoney A, Murray J, Gerther S (1988) Chemical colitis due to endoscope cleaning solutions: a mimic of pseudomembranous colitis. Gastroenterology 95:1403-1408

5. Mussuto P (1993) Les défis de la flexibilité en hystéroscopie. Ses apports diagnostiques et thérapeutiques en gynécologie obstétrique: des perspectives d'avenir. Thèse pour le Doctorat de Médecine, Faculté de Médecine Broussais Hôtel-Dieu, PA 060032:143-144

6. Le Cavorzin N (1992) Cleaning and disinfection protocol for endoscopes. Rev Infirm 42(16):40-42

7. Blanc B, Boubli L (1996) Hystéroscopie opératoire. Matériel et Technique. In: Blanc B, Boubli L (eds) Endoscopie Utérine. Pradel, Paris, pp 59-61

# Distending media for diagnostic and operative hysteroscopy

R. MARTY

The virtual space of the uterine cavity starts at the external cervical os and finishes at the fundus. This first portion is made of the cervical canal ended at the internal cervical os. Such a space is narrow and cannot be easily distended, being dilatation possible only in a small proportion. After the cervix, the uterine cavity is delimited by the fundus and the anterior and posterior walls. At the upper part, but laterally on both sides of the fundus, the tubal ostia are present opened to the right and left horn.

To perform a diagnostic or operative hysteroscopy, the gynecologist needs to have a panoramic view. In order to obtain a distention, we can choose among various distending media. This choice must take into consideration:

a) the type of instrumentation to be used (rigid, semi-rigid or flexible);
b) the size of the outer diameter of the endoscope;
c) the diameter of the operating channel.

Some hysteroscopes with a continuous flow are designed for the low viscosity fluids only. They have an inner sheath to provide a channel for introducing the distending media into the uterine cavity and they also have an outer sheath with holes at the distal end to remove the soiled distending media from the cavity.

On the contrary, fibrohysteroscopes have a single operating channel through which the distending media is introduced and the soiled media evacuated by leakage around the cervix with possibly a slight over-dilatation.

The distending media must be delivered under a pressure great enough to overcome the resistance of the myometrium. Another target is to keep the uterus distended enough for a good visualization with an appropriate infusion pressure of the media to compensate the outflow.

In France, normal saline media has become commonly used, replacing progressively the $CO_2$ [1]. Our last national survey reports $CO_2$ 26%, normal saline 70%, others 4%.

There are three types of distending media for the uterine cavity: carbon dioxyde, Hyskon and low viscosity fluids. Since the target is to obtain a panoramic view which requires uterine distention, potential complications relative to distention exist for all uterine procedures.

To avoid such complications, the gynecologist must follow the correct procedure and select the best media for each type of procedure. For example, $CO_2$ was commonly used for diagnostic, while low viscosity fluids are used more for operative procedures. With the introduction of the last generation minihysteroscopes, the diameters of operating channels are reduced to 1 mm and sheaths have a smaller diameter. This means the choice of the appropriate distending media.

Another choice must be made for the method to be used to insufflate these media. It may be a single plastic bag with appropriate tubing delivered by gravity, a syringe or a mechanical pump providing continuous pressure with variable flow. The hysteroscopist is able to set the exact amount of pressure desired and avoid the inconvenience of elevating the bag height enough to provide adequate gravity pressure.

Since the gynecologist can set an excessive pressure, this is potentially dangerous as compared with gravity which is much safer.

## Carbon dioxyde

Carbon dioxyde gas in gynecology was first used for tubal insufflation by Robin in 1920; later on, Lindemann (1971) introduced the use of controlled carbon dioxyde gas insufflation in hysteroscopy [2, 3]. Non conductible and non inflammable, $CO_2$ has the lowest viscosity of all media. This means that the size or length of the inflow channel is not a limiting factor. One important advantage is refraction index which is the same as air. The viscosity of $CO_2$ allows a good passage through the minihysteroscopes with a very small diameter sheath.

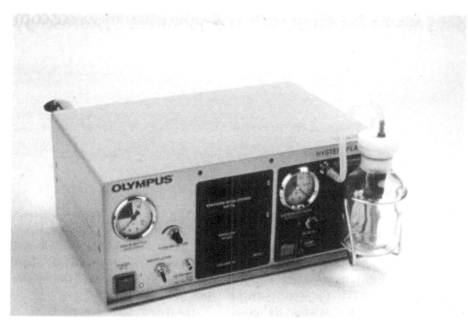

**Fig. 1.** CO$_2$ insufflator from Olympus

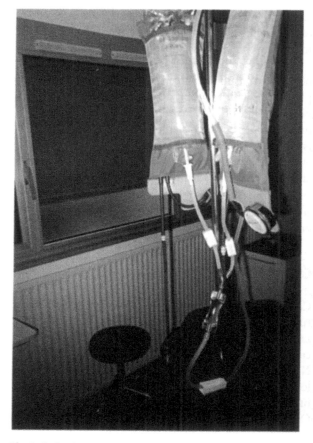

**Fig. 2.** Irrigation system

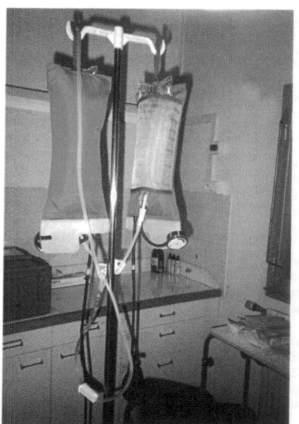

**Fig. 3.** Serum stand with 2 pockets of normal saline and pressure cuff

One must use insufflators specially designed for this purpose, delivering a <u>low flow and a low pressure</u> [4]. Many models are available, specifically designed for hysteroscopy; they can be used either for office or surgical procedures. Laparoscopic insufflators are unsuitable because they provide too much volume (liter/minute) and too much pressure.

The complications observed with $CO_2$ are largely attributable to the improper selection of the insufflation apparatus [5]. The maximum flow rate of $CO_2$ is 100 cc/minute and the maximum intrauterine pressure is 200 mmHg. Commonly, a flow rate of 50 cc is convenient and a pressure of 75/80 mmmHg is adequate for a good uterine distention.

Several models specifically designed are on the market from Storz, Olympus, (Fig. 1), Circon and others. They deliver low flow and low pressure. The gynecologist has a great choice among the manufacturers and may feel to choose the same manufacturer for the hysteroscope and the insufflator. Carbon dioxyde is a good medium for outpatient diagnostic hysteroscopy (Table 1). It does not damage the uterine cavity and is well tolerated by the patient under local anesthesia [6, 7].

The AAGL 1995 Membership Survey [8] reported $CO_2$ embolism rate 0.07°/°°, but details have not been given, and almost all the cases were observed during intrauterine surgery. The results are corroborated by a national French survey on fibrohysteroscopic diagnostic evaluation conducted by Le Club Gynécologique d'Endoscopie Flexible. Out of 35,269 patients examined [9], only one case of embolism is reported.

The disadvantages of $CO_2$ are:
- leakage from the cervix;
- creation of bubbles obscuring the view;
- film on the optic;
- flattening of the endometrium.

## Liquid distention media

Quinones [10] was a pioneer in the study of liquid media for the uterine distention. He developed the metallic bridge with two surgical channels, one to aspirate the blood or mucus, and the other one for biopsy forceps scissors or electrodes. He also developed an air compressor with a regular system to modify the amount of air introduced into the receptacle of glucose solution, and a manometer measuring the pressure of the air chamber in the fluid container.

### Hyskon

Hyskon (32% Dextran), is a clear crystal highly viscous with a molecular weight of 70,000. It can be administered through an intravenous tubing, using a large syringe or by mean of commercially available pumps. The pressure must be less than 150 mmHg. The distention of the uterine cavity requires about 10 ml.

Complications such as fluid overload or idiosyncratic reaction are not frequent, but if present, difficult to manage. During outpatient procedures for diagnostic, the complications are highly improbable.

Table 1. $CO_2$ normal saline use in out patient diagnostic hysteroscopy

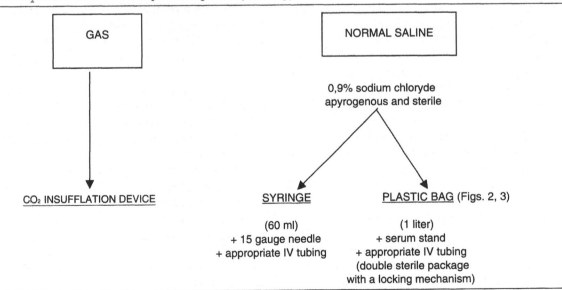

Hyskon is provided in bottles, as a solution of 32% Dextran 70 in 10% dextrose in water. It is electrolyte free, non conductible and biodegradable; furthermore, it is non miscible with blood [11]. These properties are very <u>interesting for patients presenting bleeding during diagnostic or operative procedures.</u>

Because of its viscosity, Hyskon <u>cannot be used</u> with <u>hysteroscopes designed for a continuous flow</u> or with <u>fibrohysteroscopes</u>. It must be used only with rigid hysteroscopes. A major disadvantage of the Hyskon is the fact that the solution is sticky and, when dry, it crystallizes inside the hysteroscope. So, it must be cleaned immediately. Hyskon cannot be used with the resectoscopes.

Dangerous complications are connected with Hyskon if the maximum volume exceeds 500 ml per case: overload, non cardiogenic pulmonary oedema [12], coagulopathy [13], or idiosyncratic anaphylactoid reaction [14]. For outpatient diagnostic evaluation, the volume of Hyskon does not exceed 30 or 40 ml, so complications are highly improbable.

## Low viscosity fluids

Continuous flow hysteroscopes are designed to make use of low viscosity fluids. These solutions are ideal for operative procedures. Various solutions are: glycine, sorbitol manitol, glucose at 5% and normal saline.

### Glycine

It is non hemolytic, non immunogenic and electrolyte free. It is provided in plastic bags (3 liters 5% solution with water). An adequate uterine distention is obtained with the bag elevated from 100 to 150 cm above the patient. This direct flow allows a good visualization though, at the moment, pump infusion systems are the most employed method [15].

Glycine is well-known by urologists and has been used for transurethral prostatic resection [16]. Water intoxication and pulmonary oedema have been reported at a rate of 1,4 for 1,000 hysteroscopic procedures [17]. Hyponatraemia is also a dangerous complication to be avoided by strictly monitoring the inflow and output.

It is important to obtain the right intrauterine pressure, in order to <u>avoid intravasation</u> of the fluid. Since the length of a diagnostic procedure ranges between five and ten minutes, the volume of the fluid is not important and cannot create complications.

### Sorbitol mannitol

They are both sugar. The solution is 2.7% sorbitol and 0.54% mannitol and it is non conductible. It is provided in 3 liter plastic bags. The interest is the short plasma half-life (15 minutes) of the mannitol and its effects as an osmotic diuretic [18]. This medium <u>allows "roller ball" endometrial ablation procedures to</u> be performed [19].

### Glucose 5%

It has the same optic characteristics as sorbitol mannitol.

### Distilled water

It could be used for diagnostic procedures, but it has tobe used for operative procedures, because intravasation can create hemolysis of the red blood cells. It is <u>not appropriate</u> for uterine distention.

### Normal saline

This medium contains electrolyte and must not be used for hysteroscopic electrical resection, since the electrical current creates undesired effects on the resectoscopic electrode [16].

This is an <u>excellent medium for diagnostic hysteroscopy</u> and is commonly used for <u>laser procedures</u> with rigid, semi-rigid or fibrohysteroscopes. It allows to perform minor operative procedures, such as polypectomy, targeted endometrial biopsies or ablation of submucous pediculated myoma. This isotonic, non viscous solution is delivered in plastic bags (Table 2).

One can also use a 60 ml syringe connected to the hysteroscope by appropriate tubing. The nursing assistant slowly pushes the syringe. If an assistant is not available, the bag can be hung within an insufflated blood pressure cuff to provide distention. It can also be administered by a mechanical pump.

It is an excellent medium to be used for diagnostic hysteroscopy and minor office operative procedures (Table 3) and commonly used during intrauterine laser procedures with rigid, semi-rigid or fibrohysteroscopes, for minor operative procedures such as polypectomy, targeted biopsies or myomectomy. The vision is excellent.

**Table 2.** Equipment for surgical procedures (uner general anesthesia)

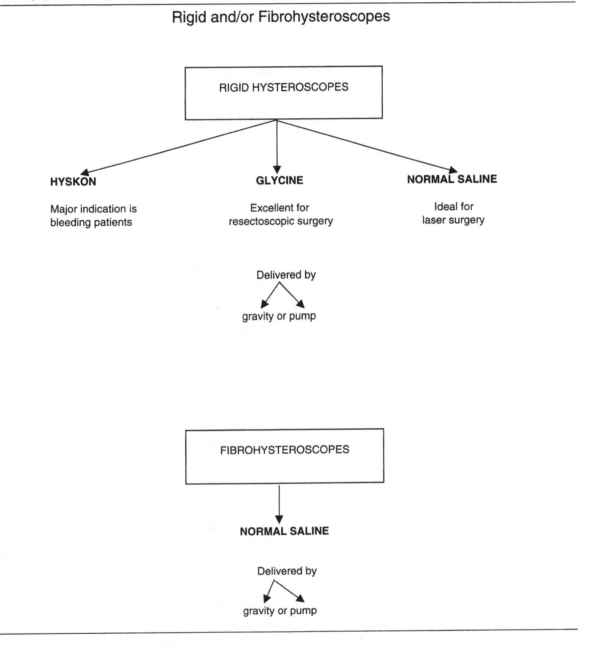

## Rigid and/or Fibrohysteroscopes

RIGID HYSTEROSCOPES

**HYSKON**

Major indication is
bleeding patients

**GLYCINE**

Excellent for
resectoscopic surgery

**NORMAL SALINE**

Ideal for
laser surgery

Delivered by

gravity or pump

FIBROHYSTEROSCOPES

**NORMAL SALINE**

Delivered by

gravity or pump

**Table 3.** Normal saline as the best choice for minor office operative procedures

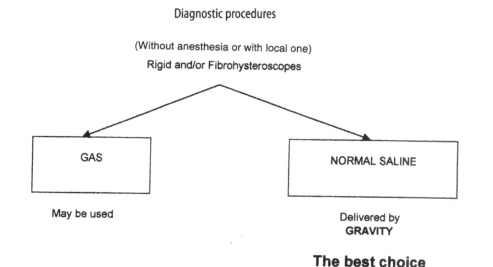

Diagnostic procedures

(Without anesthesia or with local one)
Rigid and/or Fibrohysteroscopes

| GAS | NORMAL SALINE |
|---|---|
| May be used | Delivered by **GRAVITY** |

**The best choice**

### Visualization

To achieve a clear visualization, the gynecologist has three possibilities:

### Continuous flow hysteroscopes

This concerns the rigid endoscopes. Adapters are available for current continuous flow hysteroscopes.

### Outflow catheter

It may be used via the operating channel of rigid hysteroscopes to create a kind of continuous flow.

### Overdilatation of the cervical canal

This is easy to realize and works well with the low viscosity fluid, such as normal saline. This process is excellent for the fibrohysteroscopes, but the endoscopist must perform a slight overdilatation to avoid too much leakage.

### Safety rules

Hysteroscopic diagnostic evaluation does not last a long time, less than five minutes in 71% of the cases and less than fifteen minutes for minor operative procedures [9]; it does not lead to open the vascular tree; consequently, complications due to fluid overload are very improbable.

The major complication may happen during surgical procedures, particularly myomectomy or endometrial resection. The gynecologist must keep in mind that the best way to avoid fluid overload is the use of an appropriate infusion pressure. The volume of the balance intake/output is essential in all operative cases, but with a pressure of 110 mmHg or less, problem are rare. An incidence of fluid overload of 0,4% has been reported on one large series [20], but it was during a laser surgery.

*Important remark:* the endoscopist must pay a special attention to clear bubbles from the IV tubing before its connection to the hysteroscope.

### Normal saline: The best choice

At first, it depends on the type of hysteroscope to be used and also on the type of procedure planned for the patient: diagnostic or surgical. After twelve years of experience with the fibrohysteroscopy, our choice is normal saline for both diagnostic and/or surgical procedures.

For surgery, the choice is obvious: one must use laser because the size of the operating channel of the fibrohysteroscope is 2.2 mm, and we can only introduce a bare Nd-Yag laser fiber (0.6 mm). This leaves 1.6 mm for the normal saline, which is perfect to obtain a good visibility.

For diagnostic procedures (Table IV), we believe that, even for rigid or semi-rigid hysteroscopes, the use of $CO_2$ for the uterine distention is not the best choice. Normal saline seems the most appropriate for the following reasons:

- Better tolerance of the patients for normal saline uterine distention than with $CO_2$ [21] has been demonstrated by several publications. A study on 157 cases has been published as a prospective randomized clinical trial to evaluate the acceptability and clinical efficacy of $CO_2$ and normal saline. The hysteroscopic view was similar regardless of the medium, but eight cases had to be converted to saline. The occurrence of bubbles was significantly greater with $CO_2$ ($p = 0.001$). Longer abdominal pain and shoulder tip pain were both significantly worse with $CO_2$ ($p = 0.001$ and $p = 0.007$, respectively). Durations were significantly longer for $CO_2$ ($p = 0.003$).
- Easily available all over the world.

### Better observation

Normal saline accentuates the uterine pathology if the procedure is performed in the proliferative phase.

Furthermore, it does not flatten the endometrium; when a submucous myoma is present, it is easier to localize and it is possible to have a precise measurement of the intracavitory invasion [21]. Finally, the endometrium is floating free in the liquid distention media, it facilitates the discovery and detection of small pathological areas.

### Avoiding possible problems and/or complications

By using normal saline, gas embolism is impossible. Furthermore:
- the procedure may be performed even if the patient is bleeding (apart from heavy bleeding);
- saline it provides a clear vision without film on the lens;
- it allows to wash the uterine cavity to get rid of mucus, clots or debris;
- it does not create bubbles obscuring the view [22];

- it does not create vascular modifications of the endometrium, such as red spots that may be observed with $CO_2$ when the procedure lasts too long.

### Saving money

Normal saline is very cheap and it saves the cost of a $CO_2$ insufflator.

### During surgical procedures

Normal saline is a perfect distention media when using the Nd-Yag laser (Table 2).

It is an appropriate for cooling ND-Yag sapphire tips, avoiding the danger of excessive absorption of gas.

The numerous advantages of the use of normal saline vs $CO_2$ for the uterine distention should convince the physician to always choose it to perform a hysteroscopic procedure, specially for office procedures or laser surgery.

## Mechanical pumps

Various pumps are available to supply fluids and thus to avoid complications. In France, the most commonly used are manufactured by Karl Storz and by Olympus. The first ones are able to deliver the glycine with a variable pressure and a variable flow. They are electronically controlled to obtain a permanent regulation of the intrauterine pressure.

The pump we are generally using is the Uteromat Fluid Control from Olympus. This pump provides a constant monitoring and display of inflow fluid volume and fluid loss.

Another good pump is proposed by Circon; it has a "Circon Dolphin system" providing a real time fluid deficit and intrauterine pressure information with alarms and warnings. The flow is non pulsatile and controlled by the surgeon.

As a matter of fact, there is a choice of various fluid pumps manufactured by various factories. The difficulty is that the true intrauterine pressure is not measured by a majority of the available insufflating systems. Even if it were possible, the operator should use the least infusion pressure necessary to distend the uterus and prevent bleeding into the medium [23, 24].

Apart from the cost, pumps are not necessarily safer than gravity, because some can be set to use excessive pressure. So, continuous flow pumps may create excessive pressure. The use of commercially available

## Golden and safety rules for diagnostic and minor operative procedures

Do not ignore contraindications. Furthermore:
- strictly follow the decontamination, disinfection and sterilization procedure;
- choose the smallest hysteroscope available;
- omit the tenaculum;
- avoid a cervical dilatation;
- choose normal saline for uterine distention;
- clear off the bubbles in the tubing connected to the operating channel;
- avoid to damage or scratch the endometrium;
- avoid excessive pressure for the distending media;
- proceed gently and slowly.

fluid pumps <u>does not guarantee protection of fluid overload</u>. They are very useful, but the endoscopist must always keep in mind that the continuation of excessive pressure with the open vascular tree leads to excessive absorption.

## References

1. Marty R (1999) Evaluation de la Fibrohystéroscopie diagnostique. La Revue du Praticien. Gynécologie et Obstétrique. Ed JB Baillière, in press
2. Gallinat A (1984) Carbon Dioxyde Hysteroscopy: Principles and Physiology. In: Hysteroscopy principles and Practice. JB Lippincott, Philadelphia: Siegler AM, Lindemann HJ (eds), pp 45-47
3. Robin IC (1947) Uterotubal insufflation. Mosby St-Louis (CV)
4. Loffer FD (1993) Complications of distending media. World Congress of Gynecologic Endoscopy. Syllabus Postgraduate Course VI. AAGL, California, pp 41-70
5. Rioux JE (1984) Methods of Uterine Distention. In: Hysteroscopy Principles and Practice. JB Lippincott, Philadelphia: Siegler AM, Lindemann HJ (eds), pp 37-40
6. Porter MB, Brumsted JR (1996) Uterine Distention. In: Isaacson KB (ed) Office Hysteroscopy. Mosby-Year Book, St-Louis, pp 45-53
7. De Jong P, Doel F, Falconer A (1990) Outpatient Diagnostic Hysteroscopy. Br J Obstet Gynecol 97: 299-303
8. AAGL Survey (1995) J Am Assoc Gynecol Laparosc 2(2): 131-133
9. Marty R, Demouzon J (1999) The use of the fibrohysteroscope in ambulatory patients for diagnostic and minor operative procedures. French National Survey conducted by Le Club Gynécologique d'Endoscopie Flexible. Global Congress of Gynecologic. Endoscopy 30th Annual Meeting of the AAGL, San Francisco/California, November 2001, Book of Abstracts August 2001 vol. 8 n° 3, S41, n° 136
10. Quinones RG (1984) Hysteroscopy with a New Fluid Technique. In: Hysteroscopy Principles and Practice. JB Lippincott, Philadelphia, pp 41-43
11. Porter MB, Brunmsted JR (1996) Uterine Distention. In: Office Hysteroscopy Edited by KB Isaacson. St-Louis, Mosby-Year Book, pp 45-53
12. Leake JF, Morphy AA, Zacur HR (1987) Non cardiogenic pulmonary oedema or complication of operative hysteroscopy. Fertil Steril 48(3):497-499
13. Vercellini P et al (1992) Hypervolemia pulmonary oedema and severe coagulopathy after intrauterine instillation. Obstet Gynecol 79(5):838-839
14. Ahmed et al (1991) Anaphylactic reaction of intrauterine 32% Dextran 70 instillation. Fertil Steril 55(5): 1014-1016
15. Blanc B, Boubli L (1996) Les dispositifs d'insufflation des fluides. In: Endoscopie Utérine. Blanc B, Boubli L (eds), Ed Pradel, Paris, p 55
16. Witz CA et al (1993) Complications associated with the absorption of hysteroscopic fluid media. Fertil Steril 60 (5): 745-756
17. AAGL Survey (1995) J Am Assoc Gynecol Laparosc. (2): l31-133
18. Van Boven MT, et al (1989) Dilutional Hyponatremia associated with intrauterine laser surgery. Anesthesiology 1:40-45
l9. Townend DE et al (1990) Roller ball coagulation of the endometrium. Obstet Gynecol 76(2):310-313
20. Garry R, Erian J, Grochnal S (1991) A Multicentric collaborative study into the treatment of menorrhagia by Nd-Yag laser ablation of the endometrium. Brit J Obstet Gynecol 98:357-362
21. Goldfarb HA (1996) Comparison of Carbon dioxyde with continuous flow technique for office hysteroscopy. J Am Assoc Gynecol Laparosc 3(4)
22. O'Connor H, Nagele F, Bournas N, Richardson R, Magos A (1996) The effects of $CO_2$ and normal saline on pain and visualization during outpatient hysteroscopy. Selected Scientific Abstracts of the World Congress of Hysteroscopy. AAGL Journal California 20-21
23. Loffer FD (1995) Complications of Hysteroscopy. J Am Assoc Gynecol Laparosc 3(1):12
24. Loffer FD (1994) The need to monitor intrauterine pressure. Myth or necessity? J Am Assoc Gynecol Laparosc 2:1-2

# Endometrial cytology and biopsy during fibrohysteroscopy

R. MARTY

The endometrial biopsy is essential before initiating medical or surgical procedure in the uterine environment. For years, biopsies were performed blindly, either with a full curettage or with a Novak cannula, to obtain a small sample of endometrium. Subsequently, an aspiration method was developed. The use of hysterography allowed gynecologists to more specifically locate pathologic lesions, but the high number (32%) of false positive and false negative results made this approach less than ideal [1]. Even the addition of ultrasound guidance did not eliminate false positive and false negative results (Table 1).

The greatest advance in providing an accurate diagnosis of endometrial pathology has been the hysteroscope and specially the fibrohysteroscope which allows the gynecologist to perform targeted endometrial biopsies (TEB) under direct vision. The panoramic view of the uterine cavity greatly increases accuracy in a manner offered by no other method [2].

Although any rigid hysteroscope can be used, if the diameter is large enough to perform the biopsy through the operating channel of the sheath, only a flexible hysteroscope (because its direction of view is forward, with a 100 degrees field of view and flexible tip bending up and down 100 degrees), allows the operator to move past obstacles in the uterine cavity [3]. Under these circumstances, the target may be approached from many more positions than would be possible with a rigid instrument, permitting exploration of hidden or obscure areas. This flexibility also results in less trauma to the endometrium. During the same procedure, a directed endometrial cytology may be obtained for the detection of cancer cells.

The directed biopsy is performed with a small biopsy forceps and the volume of the tissue sample is small. Because we deal with microbiopsies, we have been obliged to develop the suitable protocol to obtain a good reliability and a small rate of rejected

**Table 1.** Evolution of the endometrial biopsy

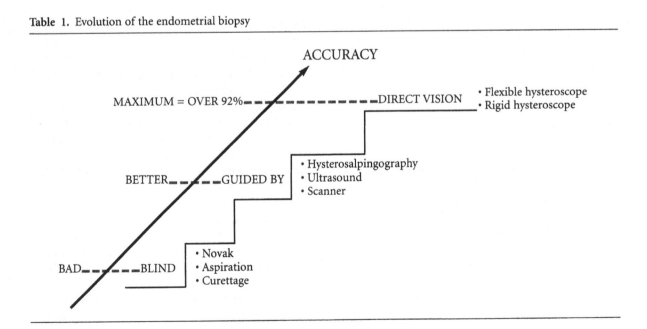

biopsies. We had the privilege to work during many years with Prof J. de Brux, ex-director of the Institute for Applied Pathology and Cytology, a pathologist greatly involved in gynecology. With his precious help and after three successive series of data collected over five years, we have developed a special protocol which, if correctly followed, allows a high reliability.

## Directed endometrial cytology

A good endometrial sampling has to avoid contamination from endocervix and vagina. Contamination provides sources of diagnostic error. Because the brush is pushed inside the operating channel, it does not exist any possibility of contamination. The sampling is easy and allows to obtain a representative sample of the entire endometrium or may be focalized in a small area. The major application is the early detection of endometrial carcinoma and its precursors. The cytologic sampling does not interferer with the concomitant histologic studies of the lesion [4]. We do not believe in the utility of endometrial cytology for the determination of the hormonal status. The only target is the detection of cancer cells.

### Protocol

We use a cytobrush (3-French) available from Cook, Olympus or many others [5]. The cytobrushing may be done on a special area associated with a TEB or the cells may be collected from the endometrial lining fundus, anterior or posterior uterine wall. It is easy to use the operating channel (1.2 mm) of the diagnostic hysteroscope. It may be useful to collect separately each uterine wall and the fundus and spread the cells on three separate slides. This fixation is the same as pap smear.

### Our French results

We routinely obtain around 70% of cytobrushing that can be interpreted by biological test and 30% of negative smears due to insufficient material, acellular smears or fibrocruoric material. The results are also dependent on the distension medium in which the cytologic brushings are performed. Furthermore, some material can be taken away by the flow of the liquid before it can be set. From a hormonal point of view, the endometrial cytology is much less interesting than the vaginal cytology.

In our experience, over more than 750 directed cytological brushing (not published), we have observed 19 positive results for malignancy, all confirmed by a combined biopsy (2,5%).

## Conclusion

To detect endometrial hyperplasia or cancer, the blind endometrial cytology does not give enough security, even with the Gravler jet washer (reliability 54,9% to 74,4%). Endometrial cytology does not allow differentiation of hyperplasia from endometrial carcinoma and is not helpful if the endometrial carcinoma is necrotic, infected or bloody. Therefore, since the cytological sampling is very easy to perform and it takes only some minutes, we suggest to do it in conjunction with a targeted endometrial biopsy, if a suspicious area is detected. This may be of a great help in the screening of patients at risk for endometrial carcinoma, particularly when the microbiopsy is of difficult interpretation. One must remind that a negative result has no predictive value.

## Reliability of targeted endometrial biopsy

### Our French experience (three successive series of data)

Between 1988 and 1992 we have evaluated the reliability of TEB using fibrohysteroscopy in 3 successive assays:
- The first evaluation (N = 89 biopsies) was reported in 1989 [6]. This series utilized a flexible biopsy forceps 1.7 mm in diameter (5-French diameter) and resulted in an accuracy of 80,2% with 19,9% rejected biopsies.
- A second report (N = 69 biopsies) was presented in 1990 to the AAGL International Meeting and utilized a flexible Olympus hysteroscope 3.5 mm in diameter and a flexible biopsy forceps 1 mm in diameter (Cook Company, 3-French diameter), and resulted in an accuracy of 82,8% with 12,4% rejected biopsies.
- A third report, completed in January 1992 evaluated N = 210 biopsies performed either with a 3-French or a 5-French flexible biopsy forceps, with an accuracy of 92,4% and 2,79% rejected biopsies [7].

The 368 biopsies collectively in these groups resulted in an average reliability greater than 85% with

11,3% rejected biopsies. Concerning the directed cytobrushing, an assay was also published (N = 113 patients) with a good concordance [8].

## Materials and methods

The 368 biopsies were taken from women who were either hospital or private patients. For hospital patients (CHU, Paris XIII) the samples were sent to Prof. Amouroux, Head and Chief of the Hospital, and for private patients the biopsies were interpreted by Prof. J. de Brux.

The two pathologists worked in two different departments and used individually selected criteria. In all women, a full curettage was performed immediately after the biopsy or during the following week. The age of the patients ranged from 19 to 83 years, with an average age of 44.03 years.

### The hysteroscopes

Two types of flexible hysteroscopes and forceps were used:
- the 3.5 mm HYF-P, the smallest hysteroscope, which was very convenient for an office hysteroscopy practice, having a 3.5 mm diameter, a working channel of 1.2 mm allowing the use of a 3-French flexible biopsy forceps. The average volume of the specimen was 0,85 mm$^3$;
- the 5 mm HYF-1T, a 4,9 mm diameter hysteroscope with a 2.2mm operating channel. The biopsy was performed with a 5-French flexible forceps, with various jaws. The standard cup shape was used, either fenestrated or not. The average volume of a specimen was 4 mm$^3$.

### Distending medium

The uterine cavity was dilated with normal saline, 0,9% by gravity.

## Results

The targeted endometrial biopsies were easily done as an office procedure. The volume of the biopsy considered as sufficient for interpretation of endometrial hyperplasia, polyp, endometritis and hormonal status of the patient, as well as malignancy, ranged from 0.85 mm$^3$ to 4 mm$^3$. The accuracy of diagnosis improved with the gradual experience of our two pathologists. Tables 2 & 3 demonstrate the fact that the accuracy increases regularly with the number of biopsies performed. At the same time, there was a significant decline in number of rejected biopsies with the use of multiple biopsies (Tables 2 and 3). We can notice that the reliability of targeted endometrial biopsy has increased regularly with a greater number of biopsies (1 to 3) and at the same time the rate of rejected biopsies has decreased.

### Rejection of biopsies

There were several reasons for rejection of biopsies and the rate of acceptance varied for the two pathologists. One recurring difficulty was an insufficient tissue sample; thus, a multiple biopsy technique was preferable. When only one sample per patient was collected, rejection of biopsies was 11,6%. When at least two biopsies were performed in each patient, only 2,3% of the biopsies were rejected.

Biopsy site was not a determining factor in rejection of the biopsy; however, the age of the patient and the previous treatment she had received (GnRH analogues) did play a role. On occasion, the use of a liquid distending medium made cell collection less effective during cytobrushing.

Biopsies were rejected when: 1) the specimen was taken only of the necrobiosis and/or coagulum; 2) the biopsies came from postmenopausal patients, in whom the endometrium had become thin and atrophic, and the stroma was fibrotic, and 3) the biopsies were performed in front of a submucous myoma that had an overlying atrophic endometrium.

### Choice of biopsy forceps

A cup biopsy forceps, either fenestrated or not fenestrated, provided a sufficient specimen in most cases. A mouse type biopsy forceps was preferable in menopausal or postmenopausal women, as well as in women with submucous myomas, because it bites more easily over atrophic endometrium. In patients with polyps, however, the alligator type forceps was preferable (Table 4).

There are different ways to perform a directed biopsy. The good choice of the forceps is mandatory to improve the quality of the biopsy (Table 5). Selecting the correct forceps involves taking into consideration tissue resistance and lesional topography [9].

**Table 2.** Importance of the number of biopsies (3 sucessive series of data)

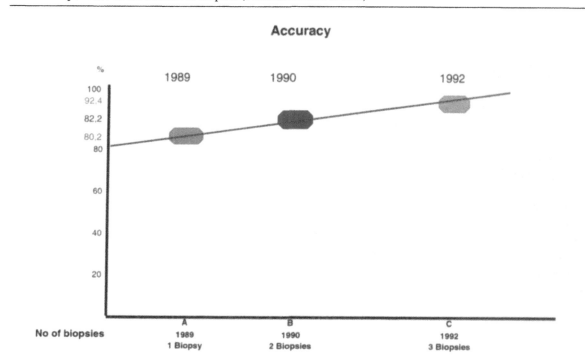

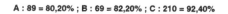

A : 89 = 80,20% ; B : 69 = 82,20% ; C : 210 = 92,40%

**Table 3.** Rejected biopsies

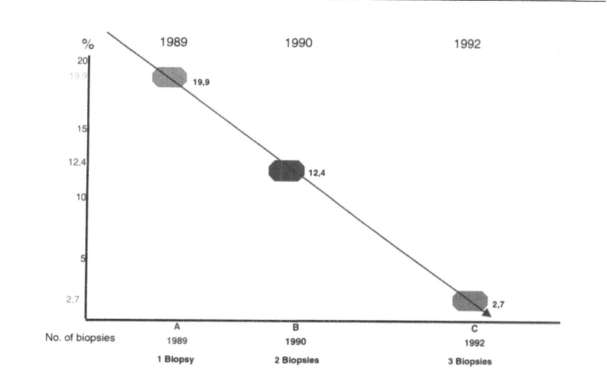

**Table 4.** Flexible hysteroscopy: the choice of the biopsy forceps (Olympus, Fuji, Cook). Outer diameter varies from 3-French (± 1m/m̀) to 5,2-French (1,7 m/m)

| Type of nozzle | Description |
|---|---|
| Standard cup | Classical |
| Elongated cup* | Greater volume of biopsy than standard |
| Rat tooth | Full hollow cup or oblong |
| Rat tooth with needle | Thin needle betwween the 2 jaws |
| Mouse tooth | Cup completed by two opposite hooks |
| Alligator | One or two mobile jaws |

\* Fenestrated or not

**Table 5.** Flexible hysteroscopy and microbiopsy

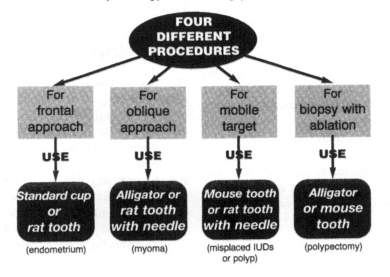

### Fixative medium

Because of its small size, the sample was stabilized with a liquid medium (Bouin). Although this caused some shrinkage, it allowed the best interpretation of the glycogenic change inside the epithelial cells.

### Discussion

The pathologist's skill choosing the appropriate biopsy size played a role in the correct interpretation of the procedure. The first pathologist founded that the 0.2 mm² to 3 mm² sample of tissue is sometimes too small to interpret; the second pathologist required only two or three glands to give an interpretation, while the other required more. Multiple biopsies are therefore desirable. Working with a pathologist who has specific experience in gynecology is important because, when evaluating the degree of malignancy of a tumor or looking for possible infection, skills required are more than those necessary for a simple evaluation of the hormonal status in an infertile patient.

The accuracy of targeted endometrial biopsy during hysteroscopy is better than D&C. Gimpelson, in 1988, founded in 60 out of 342 patients an accurate diagnostic missed by D&C Loffer, in 1989, in a serie of 187 patients with abnormal uterine bleeding, found the sensitivity of hysteroscopy and directed endometrial biopsy to be 90% as compared with 65% of D&C.

A serie of 273 biopsies has been performed in 142 patients during a study coordinated by Colafranceschi and Perino in 1991. These biopsies were performed with rigid hysteroscopes. An absolute concordance has been demonstrated in 88% of the cases (with a reference biopsy either of Novak or curettage). A percentage of 1,3% of the biopsies appeared to be too small to allow an accurate diagnosis in multiple biopsies, but in 9,9% of the cases the biopsy was not readable when only one was performed. Authors conclude that multible biopsies in the same patient allow an accurate diagnosis. In 1993, Altaras diagnosed 3 cases of endometrial carcinoma with hysteroscopy and directed biopsy on 40 cases with failed D&C.

A targeted endometrial biopsy eye-directed to the lesion is the main advantage of the diagnostic hysteroscopy. However, the sample volume is small, sometimes less than 1 mm$^3$ with a 3-French biopsy forceps, and this microbiopsy is not always well accepted by some pathologists who are not experienced in gynecology and microbiopsies.

The pathologist's observations will be enhanced if the gynecologist provides a detailed patient's history, including the indications for hysteroscopy, an accurate description of the visual findings at hysteroscopy and the exact location from which the sample was taken (Scheme 1).

## Practical advices and special recommendations for specific cases

### Hormonal status

The histological aspect of the endometrium is of most interest during days 20-23 of the cycle [10]. Best results were obtained when the biopsy was performed in the uterine fundus or in the area close to the tubal ostium and the hysteroscopist avoided the isthmic area or uterine anterior wall, which does not respond well to hormonal impregnation.

### Number of glands

Although the ideal number of glands taken during biopsy is controversial, we found that at least two or three glands were necessary to be sure that the stromal area could be seen.

### Menopause

Biopsy samples taken from the atrophic endometrium of a perimenopausal or postmenopausal woman are often fragmented or small, and the endometrium makes interpretation more difficult.

### Polyps

There are two types of polyps, one responding to hormonal stimulation and the second, in menopausal women, not responding. When the top of the polyp is inflamed and necrotic, the biopsy must be taken from the base.

### Endometrial hyperplasia

Curettage may not sample the entire endometrial lining, so histological or cytological severity may not be properly determined [11]. In our retrospective studies, we use De Brux classification [12] which has three grades: 1) polypoid endometrial hyperplasia; 2) endometrial dystrophia, glandulo-cystic hyperplasia and endometrial polyp, and 3) endometrial dysplasia (typical hyperplasia and *in situ* adenocarcinoma).

We use two further criteria for evaluation:
1) we observed whether the endometrial hypertrophia covers the entire surface of the uterine cavity or only a very small area;
2) diagnosis is made by histopathology and not by pathologic aspect. One must point out that the hysteroscopic evaluation allows to observe only hypertrophic endometrium (pathological aspect), but the diagnosis of endometrial hyperplasia must be made by the pathologist. Since we found a 77% rate of false positive and false negative with the hysterogram and ultrasound, we felt that a targeted endometrial biopsy during hysteroscopy was the best approach.

We noted the relative frequency of coexistent pathology. During hysteroscopy, endometrial hypertrophia may have been suggested by the thickness of the endometrium, but hidden in a small area of the cor-

Scheme 1.

Assistance Publique – Hôpitaux de Paris
## HOPITAL JEAN VERDIER
Service de gynécologie obstétrique – Pr. Michèle UZAN

## FIBROHYSTEROSCOPY REPORT

<u>Surgeon</u> :

<u>Date</u> :

<u>Name</u> :                                         <u>Indication</u> :

<u>Age</u> :                                          <u>Last Period</u> :

<u>Type of Fibro</u> :

<u>Distending media</u> :        $Co^2$      Normal Saline      Glycocol      Other

<u>Cervical Canal</u> :

<u>Isthmus</u> :

<u>Fundus</u> :

- ❖ Right tubal ostium and cornua
- ❖ Left tubal ostium and cornua

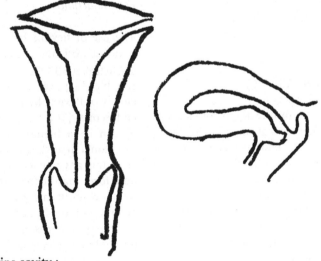

<u>Uterine cavity</u> :

<u>Endometrial Lining</u> :

**<u>Biopsy</u>** :

<u>Remarks</u> :

nua or behind a submucous myoma. For this reason, the hysteroscopist explored the full uterine cavity, observing any abnormal visual aspect of the endometrium or any local thickness.

## Myomas

Submucous myomas cause intrauterine filling defects and an enlarged uterine shadow on the hysterogram. Hysteroscopy permits a more precise analysis of size, location and attachment of the submucous tumor [13]. Targeted endometrial biopsy is most valuable before surgery in identifying changes in the sublining of the epithelium and coexistent pathology within the uterine cavity.

## Non specific endometritis

Non specific endometritis may be responsible for postmenopausal bleeding and frequently develops in an atrophic endometrium. In such cases, good tissue samples during curettage are difficult to obtain without the aid of targeted endometrial biopsy. Hysteroscopic visualization and biopsy are essential to differentiate a non specific endometritis from endometrial carcinoma. The biopsy may be performed in the selected area of epithelial shedding, where a fine network of subepithelial blood vessels can be seen through the thin surface epithelium.

## Intrauterine device (IUD) pathology

The endometrium close to or directly in contact with the IUD often shows a network of subepithelial blood vessels with blood clots - the endometrial response to a chronic inflammation; therefore, the biopsy must be performed in the area adjacent to the IUD and another sample should be taken after the IUD has been removed from the area of endometrium where it lies on. Such a biopsy shows microscopic hemorrhage and thrombosis, round cells and edematous stroma surrounded by normal tissue.

## Adenomyosis

The hysteroscopic diagnostic is not possible but some endoscopic findings may evoke the disease, such as the presence of small bluish or brownish spots giving a punctuate appearance to the endometrial lining.

When adenomyosis is suspected, the gynecologist must perform an MRI: 90% of uterus with adenomyosis can be detected by MRI [14].

The authentication must always be made by the pathologist. The detection of this disease is very important before endometrial resection; since this is an important cause (30%) of failure, the endoscopist must always perform, on each patient, a diagnostic evaluation with eye directed biopsies before the procedure and pay special attention to the cornual areas often missed by the operator.

## Adenocarcinoma

The microscopic diagnosis of adenocarcinoma may be difficult, and the pathologist should be familiar with the normal histology of the endometrium at the various phases of the cycle because a premenstrual endometrium may be mistaken for a carcinoma [15]. For the diffuse carcinoma involving a large area of the endometrial surface, visual diagnosis is easy because of the polypoid area with its roughness, occasional ulceration and protrusion of the surface and, later, necrosis. Detecting a circumscribed adenocarcinoma may be difficult if only a small surface of the endometrium is affected.

## *Personnal data*

The use of flexible hysteroscope increases the likelihood of noticing a small lesion. In an international comparative study (N = 981) on postmenopausal uterine bleeding, we have demonstrated the greatest accuracy of flexible hysteroscopes vs. rigid or semi-rigid endoscopes [16]. Furthermore, the carcinoma may be hidden by a benign pathology close to it. Adenocarcinoma may begin as a very localized polypoid growth in any portion of the uterine cavity. This polypoid form may be the only manifestation of the carcinoma, without any gross disease similar to what can be found on the hysterectomy specimen.

It may have less than 1 cm diameter with a negative endometrial cytology and a negative fractionated curettage [17]. The experience and skill of the hysteroscopist are of major importance in such a condition, and the accuracy of the pathologist's finding depends greatly on the quality of the biopsy. Another important consideration is that invasive carcinoma and/or endometrial intraepithelial neoplasia may coexist with hyperplasia in the same endometrium; thus, the pathologist must pay great attention to the cytological atypia [18].

## Before surgery

A targeted endometrial biopsy should always be performed prior to endoscopic surgery with electro- or laser therapy. These later procedures cause damage to the specimen, and coexistent pathology may be overlooked. Pathological diagnosis is impossible in more than 60% of the cases [19] after electro or laser surgery.

## After surgery

Partial endometrial resection was performed with a resector in 43 patients suffering from menometrorrhagia (32-67 years). Thermal effects were evaluated histologically in each patient, in order to assess the diagnostic reliability of the resected specimen. No case was spared from thermal injury, but with variable effects. Reliable diagnosis concordant with endometrial biopsy was still possible in 23 resected specimen (53%).

## The use of histopathology in hysteroscopy

The endometrial pathology is made of polyps, hyperplasia without cytologic atypia, endometrial cancers and hyperplasia with cytologic atypia. For Bergeron [20], hysteroscopy is the best way to detect a focal lesion and to obtain a really good targeted endometrial biopsy. Polyps are easily diagnosed and a polypectomy may be done during the procedure. Since the diagnostic of endometrial hyperplasia must be made only by histology, the importance of a reliable endometrial sampling is great. Since endometrial hyperplasia with cytologic atypia is often very localized, a biopsy under direct vision is the best reliable way to detect it.

In some specific cases, it is useful to perform a suction curettage after the directed biopsy has been done.

If an endometrial cancer is discovered, hysteroscopy is able to give a precise staging (cervical extension) and the tissue sample is of a major importance for the classification between differenciated or not. These information are necessary to decide the type of surgery to be made on the patient.

## Practical guidelines to perform targeted endometrial biopsy

When a targeted area is defined, the tip of the fibrohysteroscope is placed in front of it and the brake is activated to keep the good position. Then the selected biopsy forceps is pushed through the operating channel until the two jaws are visible outside the hystero-scope and opened. To obtain a good bite, the distance between the tip and the target must be just enough to perform the biopsy. It is useful to slightly push forward the biopsy forceps while the jaws are closed to get the sample.

To collect the biopsy sample from the jaws, the best way is to open the forceps jaws inside a small cup filled with sterile water and shake. Sometimes, it is useful to collect by aspiration the microbiopsy with a needle.

The specimen must be placed immediately in a fixation medium. Because of its small size, the best liquid for stabilization is Bouin which, although causes a minimal shrinkage, allows the best interpretation of the glycogenic charge inside the epithelial cells.

The highest reliability of microbiopsies depends on the scrupulous filling of specific guidelines (Table 6) already described by us in 1996 [21]. The hysteroscopist must keep in mind that any breach of the rules may led to decrease the reliability.

---

**Table 6.** Guidelines for microbiopsies (from [21])

Protocol

The hysteroscopist should:

- be experienced and skilled
- possess good mastery of the macroscopic appearance of intrauterine pathology
- choose the most appropriate forceps for each case
- obtain tissue for biopsy from a selected area in each pathologic lesion
- perform at least three biopsies
- select a pathologist well trained in gynecology and microbiopsy
- complete a sheet with a good description of the hysteroscopic findings, include the gross appearance, location of the pathology, and sites of the biopsies

---

The certainty of targeted endometrial biopsy during fibrohysteroscopy (92%) is comparable with the reliability obtained with the association of transvaginal sonohysterography and endometrial biopsy (95%). However, the great advantage of hysteroscopy is the study of the vascular endometrial pattern which gives sometimes valuable indication [22].

## Main indications for targeted endometrial biopsy during office hysteroscopy

We believe that the gynecologist must perform a biopsy if he/she is involved in the situations listed below.

## Preoperative and operative indications

During the direct visual confirmation and localization of a pathologic lesion before surgery:
- prior to an endometrial resection, it is mandatory to perform eye directed biopsies to look after a focal adenocarcinoma or adenomyosis. That could led to choose another surgical procedure;
- after the IUD ablation, eliminate an inflammatory endometrial process;
- grading of endometrial carcinoma and extension of a cervical cancer.

## During a medical treatment

Hormonal replacement therapy in symptomatic patients:
- tamoxifen for symptomatic patients or after an abnormal vaginal sonogram;
- progestin (during and after) if persistant bleeding without intrauterine growth is present;
- reevaluation after a medical treatment for endometrial hyperplasia.

## Unexpected hysteroscopic findings

Abnormal area in a normal uterine lining:
- suspicious neoformation with a doubtful visual correlation;
- endometrial hypertrophiae large or focal, to confirm endometrial hyperplasia and eventually a cytological atypia.

## In correlation with another investigation

Equivocal vaginal sonography without hysteroscopic visual correlation:
- abnormal hysterosalpingography without obvious hysteroscopic correlation;
- abnormal blind cytobrushing or endometrial biopsy.

## Infertility, sterility and IVF

- To establish the hormonal sensivity of the endometrium
- To evaluate the endometrial ability for nidation;
- To monitor the induction of ovulation.

## Miscellaneous

Postmenopausal bleeding without an obvious pathological hysteroscopic finding:

- Difficult or poor visualization of a specific endometrial area during hysteroscopic evaluation.

## Conclusion

For years, gynecologists performed blind endometrial biopsies using curettage or a Novak cannula, with poor accuracy. Later, the hysterosalpingogram, and then vaginal ultrasound and more recently, the Magnetic Resonance Imaging increased accuracy. For example, in the detection of an endometrial polyp, a study [23] founded 72% reliability. However, benign polyps cannot be reliably distinguished from polypoid endometrial cancer.

As compared with rigid or semirigid hysteroscopes, the flexible hysteroscope gives a more precise diagnosis and produces less trauma, owing to its softness and very small caliber. This avoids dilatation and use of anesthesia for most women. All area of the uterine cavity can be seen under direct frontal vision and obscure and hidden areas which could not be reached by a rigid scope can be viewed from various angles. Two or three biopsies are desirable for each patient. Directed cytobrushing is a useful adjunct procedure and close collaboration between the gynecologist and the pathologist is desirable.

The main problem remains the smallness of the volume of the biopsy (microbiopsy), and in the fact pathologists have not yet reached a consensus on minimal histologic criteria necessary to interpret a tissue sample. As it has been demonstrated by our successive assays and by various authors, it is mandatory to perform multiple biopsies (Table 7).

Targeted endometrial biopsy performed with fibrohysteroscopes is a reliable procedure (over 90%) if the endoscopist follows the suitable protocol.

The greatest accuracy is achieved when the hysteroscopist and the pathologist are skilled and have had a considerable experience with this technique.

Table 7. N° of biopsies per patient

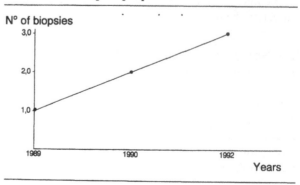

# References

1. Parent E, Guedj H, Barbot J, Nodarian P (1985) Hysteroscopic panoramic. Maloine, p 118
2. Valle R, Sciarra JJ (1979) Hysteroscopy. In: Harper, Row (eds) Chap 90
3. Marty R (1988) Experience with a new flexible hysteroscope. Int J Gynecol Obstet 27:97-99
4. Liang-Chetao (1993) Cytology of the normal endometrium and cytopathology of benign disorders, hyperplasia and neoplasia of the endometrium. A direct intrauterine sampling. ASCP Press, Cook Group Conference Indiana
5. Marty R, Mussuto P, Amouroux J et al (1990) Endometrial biopsy during office hysteroscopy with a 3-French flexible biopsy forceps: Evaluation of over 69 cases. AAGL International Congress, Book of Abstracts, p 157
6. Marty R, Amouroux J, Haouet S (1990) The reliability of endometrial biopsy performed during hysteroscopic evaluation of 89 cases. Int J Gynecol Obstet 34:151-155
7. Marty R, Amouroux J, De Brux J (1992) The targeted endometrial biopsy during flexible hysteroscopy. Technic and Results. International Congress of Gynecologic Endoscopy, Séoul, Korea, Book of Abstracts, p 61
8. Mussuto P (1993) Les défis de la flexibilité en hystéroscopie. Ses apports diagnostiques et thérapeutiques en gynécologie obstétrique: des perspectives d'avenir. Thèse pour le Doctorat en Médecine, Faculté de Médecine Broussais Hotel-Dieu, PA 060032
9. Marty R (1996) Nine Years of Experience with Flexible Hysteroscopy. In: Isaacson KB (ed) Mosby-Year Book, St. Louis, p 67
10. De Brux J (1971) L'endomètre. In Histopathologie Gynécologique. Masson & Co, Paris/Fance, p 143
11. Ferenczy A and Bergeron C (1989) Biology of the uterus. 2nd ed. Edited by M Wynn & WP Jollie. Plenum Medical Book, New-York and London, Library of Congress, pp 333-351
12. De Brux J (1971) Endometrial Hyperplasia. In Histopathologie Gynécologique. Masson & Company, Paris/France, pp 165-175
13. Siegler AM, Valle RF (1988) Therapeutic Hysteroscopic Procedures. In: Fertility and Sterility. American Fertility Society, USA, Alabama, vol 50, pp 685-701
14. Hoff FL (1998) Computed sonography and magnetic resonance imaging in Gynecology. In: Valle RF, A Manual of Clinical Hysteroscopy. Parthenon Publ Group, NY, chap 15, pp 135, 136
15. Novak and Woodruff (year) Novak's Gynecologic and Obstetric Pathology. 6th edit. NB Saunders, Philadelphia and London, pp 163-167
16. Marty R (1998) Diagnostic Fibrohysteroscopic Evaluation of Perimenopausal and Postmenopausal Uterine Bleeding: A Comparative Study with Belgian and Japanese Data. J Am Assoc Gynecol Laparosc 5 (1): pp 69-73
17. Sugimoto O (1978) Hysteroscopy Principle and practice. In: Diagnostic and Therapeutic Hysteroscopy. Igaku-Shoin, Tokyo, pp 157-161
18. Ferenczy A, Wynn RM, Jollie WP et al (1989) Biology of the uterus. In: Plenum Medical Book, New-York and London, p 334
19. Colafranceschi M, van Herandael B, Mencaglia L, Betochi S, Bolis JB, Hansch (1992) Endometrial Resection Histological Study. The Hysteroscope Newsletter of the European Society of Hysteroscopy, 3:5
20. Bergeron C (1995) Histopathologie appliquée à l'hystéroscopie. Gynécologie Internationale Hors Serie, p 9. Cours Européen d'Imagerie Gynécologique de Consultation
21. Marty R (1996) Nine Years of Experience with Flexible Hysteroscopy. In: Office Hysteroscopy Isaacson KB (ed) Mosby-Year Book, p 66
22. O'Connel LP et coll (1998) Triage of abnormal postmenopausal bleeding: a comparison of endometrial biopsy and transvaginal sonohysterography versus fractionnal curettage with hysteroscopy. Am J Obstet Gynecol, 178: 956-961
23. Hoff FL (1998) Computed tomography and magnetic resonance imaging in gynecology. In: A Manual of Clinical Hysteroscopy. Edited by RF Valle, Parthenon publishing Group, New-York, p 136

## PHYSIOLOGICAL ASPECTS
## CYTOLOGY AND PATHOLOGY COLLECTED DURING AMBULATORY PROCEDURES

These documents come from:

Professeur AMOUROUX, Chief of the Laboratoire d'Anatomopathologie, Hopital Avicenne, Centre Hospitalier Universitaire - Paris XIII
Docteur C. BERGERON, Director of the Institut de Pathologie et Cytologie Appliquée
Professeur J. de BRUX, Ex-Director of the Institut de Pathologie et Cytologie Appliquée
Docteur CERESA-MANOUX Anatomopathologiste, Hopital Jean Verdier, Centre Hospitalier Universitaire - Paris XII

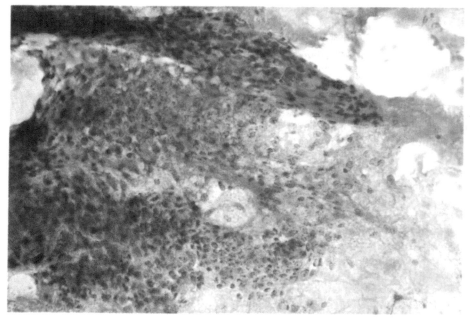

**Fig. 1.** Cytobrushing - Cycle + 19

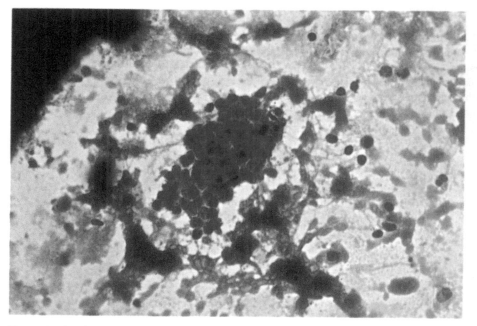

**Fig. 2.** Cytobrushing - Stimulated endometrium + mitose

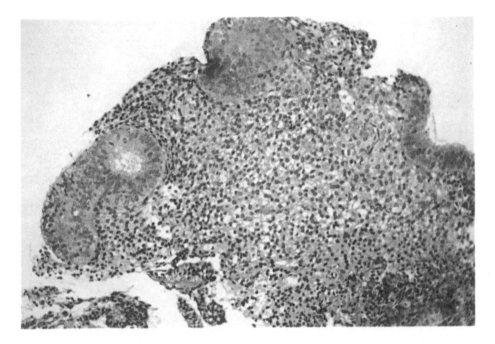

**Fig. 3.** Proliferative phase

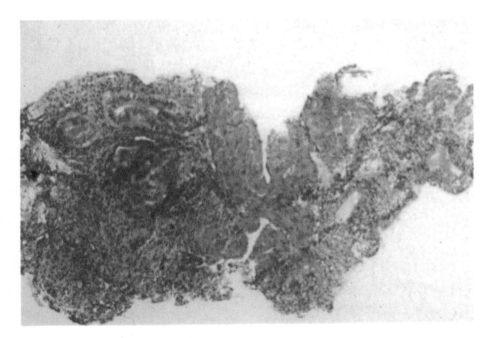

**Fig. 4.** Endometrial biopsy - Cycle + 14

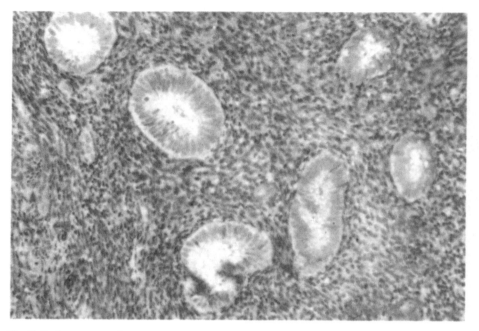

**Fig. 5.** Early secretory phase

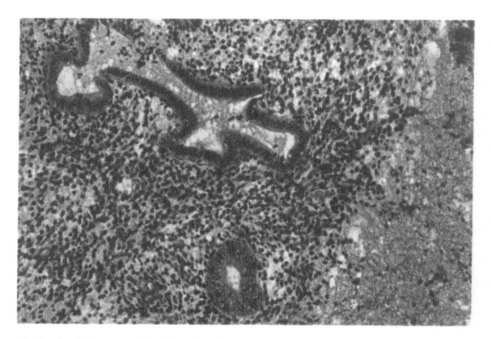

**Fig. 6.** Glandular tubes with proliferative cells

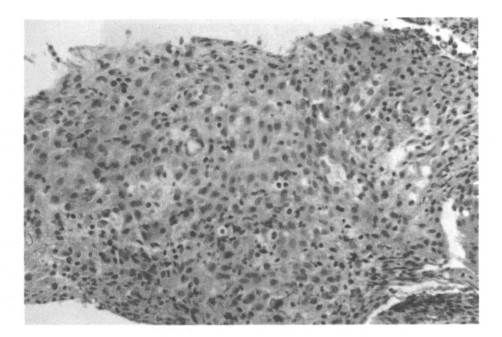

**Fig. 7.** Premenstrual phase

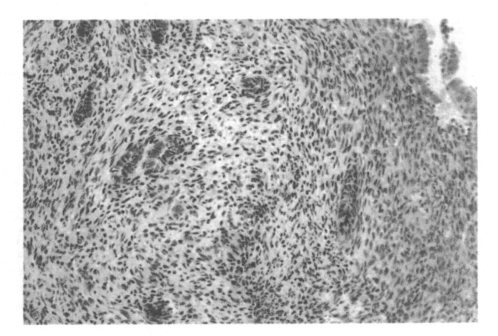

**Fig. 8.** Postmenopausal atrophia

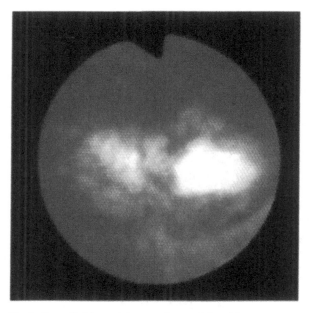

**Fig. 9.** Scar of a biopsy (olympus forceps 5 french)

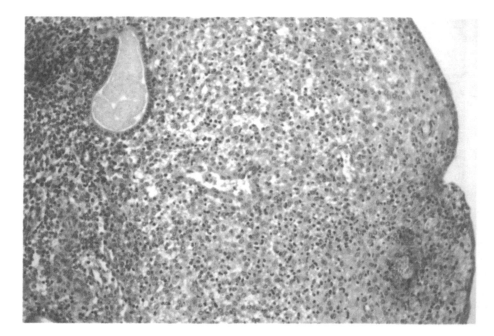

**Fig. 10.** Decidualisation

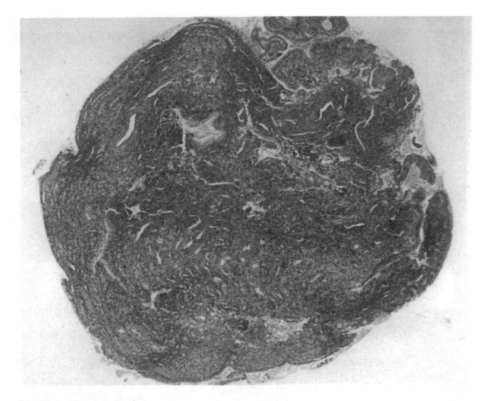

**Fig. 11.** Endocervical polyp

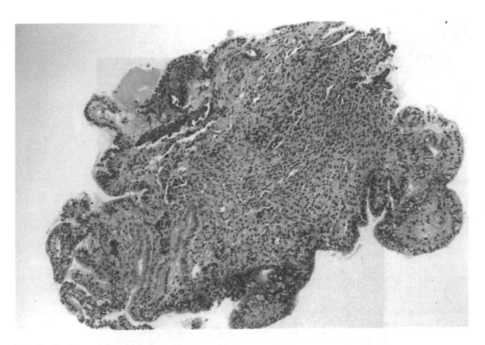

**Fig. 12.** Endometrial polyp

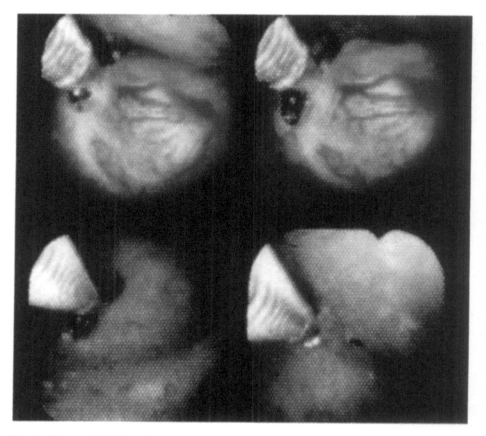

**Fig. 13.** Biopsy with Fujinon forceps

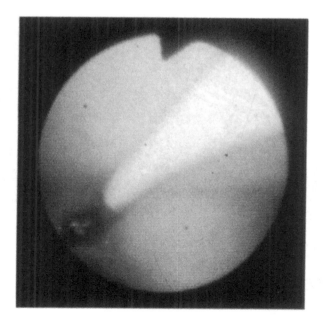

**Fig. 14.** Biopsy with the Olympus forceps

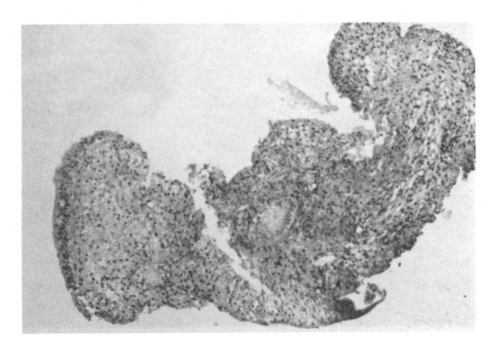

**Fig. 15.** Biopsy and polypectomy

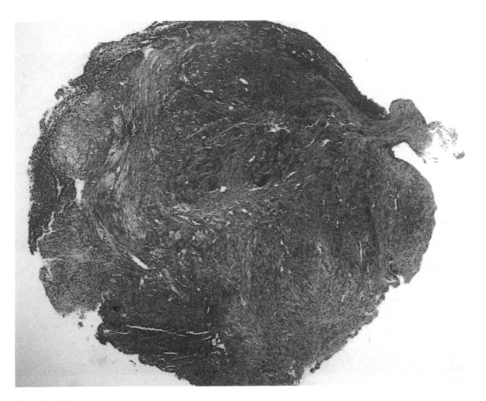

**Fig. 16.** Leiomyoma

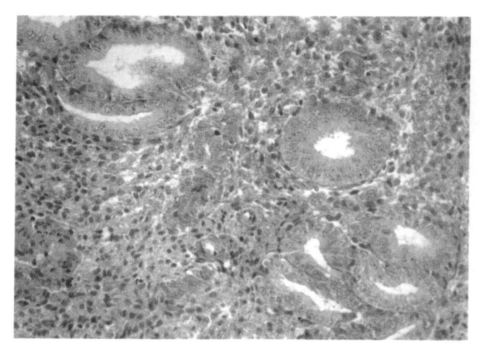

Fig. 17. Endometrial hyperplasia without cellular atypia

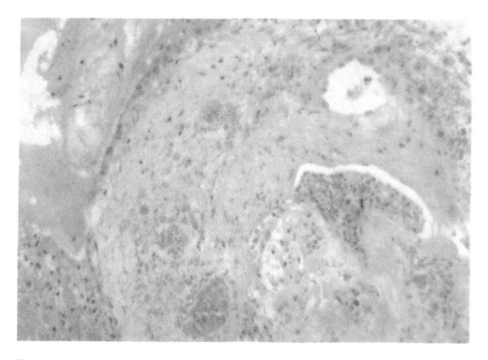

Fig. 18. Necrotic chorial villosity

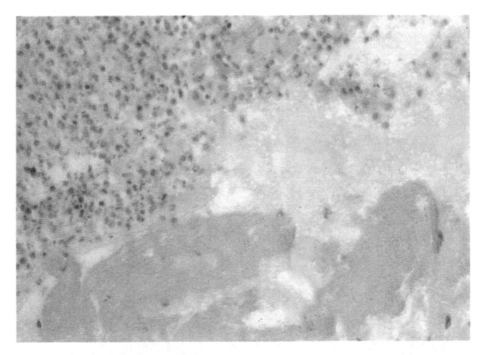

**Fig. 19.** Endometrial placenta retention

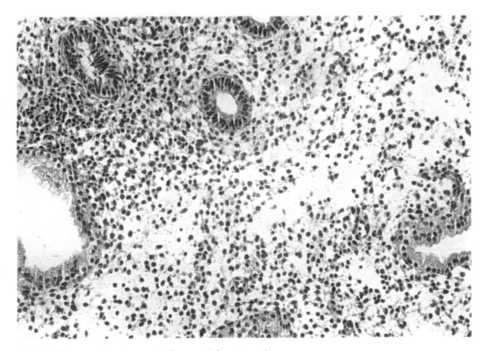

**Fig. 20.** Hormonal replacement therapy: inhomogeneity

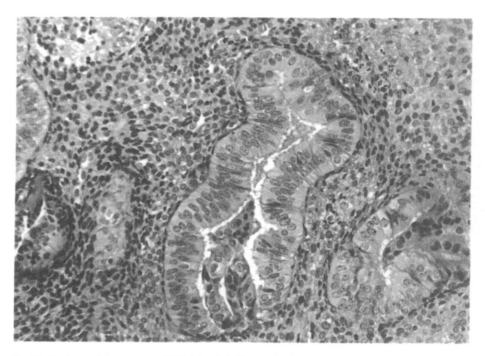

**Fig. 21.** Endometrial response to IUD (chonic inflammation)

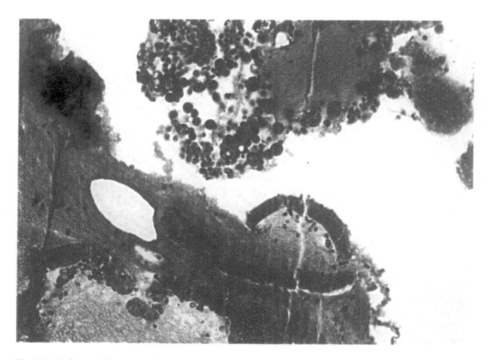

**Fig. 22.** Endometrial metastasis

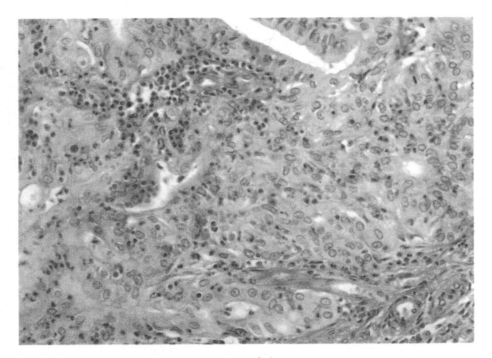

**Fig. 23.** Endometrial cancer ( Patient under Tamoxifen)

# Uterine evaluation by hysteroscopy in patients undergoing in vitro fertilization

J.N. Hugues, I. Cedrin-Durnerin, R. Marty, L. Carbillon, M. Uzan

The success rate of In Vitro Fertilization (IVF) procedure is partly dependent on the ability to transfer embryos within a uterine cavity appropriate for implantation. Indeed, it is has been shown that cervical canal, uterine cavity and endometrial abnomalities may interfer with embryo replacement and implantation [1]. However, the significance of mild intrauterine or cervical pathology is still unknown and the actual incidence of severe abnomalities has been differently appreciated [2, 3]. Consequently, the rationale for a systematic evaluation of the uterine cavity is still questionable. To address this issue, we will consider different clinical situations which are usually encountered in our clinical practice and we will discuss the exact place of hysteroscopy which is an useful tool to evaluate uterine cavity [4].

In women undergoing an IVF cycle for tubal, endometriosis-related or unexplained infertility, hysteroscopy usually takes place in the standard pre-IVF work-up including laparoscopy and allows a valuable evaluation of the uterine cavity. In these situations, hysteroscopic abnormalities seem to be frequent although the actual incidence differs largely from one study to another : 30% [5, 6], or 60% [1, 2], with a higher rate in elderly women over than 40 years [6]. Furthermore, a previous first trimester abortion was found to be the main risk for intra-uterine adhesions [7]. Thus, it seems reasonable to state that most of these abnormal findings detected by hysteroscopy (adhesions, polypes, myomas, hyperplasia, adenomyosis) should be treated before entering IVF program. Indeed, even if they are certainly not the primary cause of infertility, they may act as contributive factors which must be considered especially in elderly women who have an additive critical time limit. However, although Shamma et al. [8] showed that the pregnancy rate after IVF is lower in women with abnormal hysteroscopy, a prospective randomized study is needed to justify the therapeutic merit of hysteroscopy in IVF.

Furthermore, as it does appear in patients with tubal infertility that presence of hydrosalpinges has a negative impact on implantation rate through inflammatory disorders at the level of uterine cavity, hysteroscopic evaluation may be performed to visualize the endometrium and allow an oriented biopsy accordingly. In this particular case, hysteroscopy seems helpful to the final decision to remove the altered fallopian tubes before IVF procedure.

In women included in an IVF program mostly associated with micro-injection of spermatozoa (ICSI) for male infertility, the rationale for a systematic evaluation of uterine cavity is still a matter of debate. Indeed, when there is no reason to expect uterine abnormalities on grounds of gynaecology history (including previous miscarriages or exposure to Diethylstilbestrol), abnormal bleeding or clinically enlarged uterus, the main critical issue is to decide whether a systematic evaluation of uterine cavity should be performed and which one is the most appropriate. In our clinical practice, hysterography is recommended as a first line examination in these situations. According to the results, we decide if an hysteroscopy must be performed or not. This policy was designed to take into account the need for defining the most cost-effective pre-IVF work-up in women without any previous history of uterine pathology. It is likely that some uterine anormalities still remain unknown following hysterosalpingography but the precise false negative rate has not yet been clearly evaluated in this subgroup of women.

Hysteroscopic evaluation after failed IVF or ICSI cycles deserves another consideration. As reported by Dicker et al (1992), a significant number (18.2%) of uterine abnormalities can be detected in women who had failed to conceive during 3 or more IVF cycles while an initial hysteroscopy has been considered as normal. It is interesting to speculate whether the abnormal findings during repeat hysteroscopy evaluation were initially undiagnosed, misinterpreted or newly added disorders. In view of the nature of the abnormalities detected, mainly endometrial lesions (hyperplasia, polyps, endometritis), submucuous myomas and adhesions, it is likely that the process of ovulation induction as well as traumatic factors during the replacement procedure are partly involved in these uterine disorders and that progestogen or antibiotic therapies may be useful for optimizing the IVF procedure as suggested by Dicker et al. [9]. Thus, it may be stated that hysteroscopic evaluation of uterine cavity is required in patients with repeat implantation failure and this guideline is probably relevant to all patients with previous intrauterine manipulations including inseminations. Similarly, in patients with preclinical in-vitro fertilization abortions, hysteroscopy is an efficient mean for both identifying intrauterine pathology (partial uterine septum) and excluding adhesions [10]. In all situations, endometrial biopsy seems to be less effective than hysteroscopy for detecting uterine pathology [11].

In conclusion, it seems that hysteroscopy should be performed routinely in most of IVF candidates. However, while this examination may be easily performed on an outpatient basis under local anesthesia and is an innocuous procedure, it is still unknown whether it must be systematically proposed to women whose infertility is primarily related to male factor. Moreover, the interest of hysteroscopy as a therapeutic agent remains to be determined in prospective randomized studies. Finally, it has been recently suggested that saline contrast hysterosonography which is a simple, accurate and well-tolerated procedure could be an alternative method for detecting uterine abnomalities, avoiding invasive and expensive diagnostic hysteroscopy [12]. Further prospective comparative studies are required to evaluate their respective value for uterine cavity assessement.

# References

1.  Frydman R, Eibschitz I, Fernandez H, Hamou J. Uterine evaluation by microhysteroscopy in IVF candidates. Hum. Reprod. 1987, 2 : 481-485.

2.  Valle RF. (1980) Hysteroscopy in the evaluation of female infertility. Am. J. Obstet. Gynecol.  137 : 425-431.

3.  March CM. (1983) Hysteroscopy as an aid to diagnosis in female infertility. Clin. Obstet. Gynecol 26 : 302-309.

4.  Hamou J, Salat-Baroux J (1985) Advanced hysteroscopy and microhysteroscopy in 1000 patients. In: Siegler AM, Linderman HJ (eds) Hysteroscopy: principles and practice Lippincott, pp 63-77

5.  Mohr J, Lindermann HJ. (1977) Hysteroscopy in the infertile patient. J. Reprod. Med. 1977, 18 : 143-148.

6.  Dicker D, Goldmann JA, Ashkenazi J, Feldberg D, Dekel A (1990) The value of hysteroscopy in elderly women prior to in vitro fertilization-embryo transfer (IVF-ET): a comparative study. In vitro Fertilization and Embryo Transfer 7:267-270

7.  Golan A, Ron-El R, Herman A, Soffer Y, Bukowsky I, Caspi E. (1992) Diagnostic hysteroscopy : its value in an in-vitro fertilization/embryo transfer unit. Hum. Reprod. 7 : 1434-1444.

8.  Shamma FN, Lee G, Gutmann JN, Lavy G. (1992) The role of office hysteroscopy in in vitro fertilization. Fertil. Steril. 58 : 1237-1239.

9.  Dicker D, Ashkenazi J, Feldberg D, Farhi J, Shalev J, Ben-Rafael Z (1992) The value of repeat hysteroscopic evaluation in patients with failed in vitro fertilization transfer cycles. Fertil. Steril. 58 : 833-835.

10. Dicker D, Ashkenazi J, Dekel A, Orvieto R,    Feldberg D, Yeshaya A, Ben-Rafael Z (1996) The value of hysteroscopic evaluation in patients with preclinical fertilization abortions. Hum. Reprod. 11, 730-731.

11. La Sala GB, Montanari R, Dessanti L, Cigarini C, Sartori F (1998) The role of diagnostic hysteroscopy and endometrial biopsy in assisted reproductive technologies. Fertil. Steril 70 : 378-380.

12. Ayida G, Chamberlain P, Barlow, Kennedy S  ( 1 9 9 7 ) Uterine cavity assessment prior to in vitro fertilization : comparison of transvaginal scanning, salie contrast hysterosonography and hysteroscopy. Ultrasound Obstet. Gynecol. 10 : 59-62.

# Flexible or rigid hysteroscopes?

B. Blanc

Why choose a flexible hysteroscope?

## An ergonomic equipment

The distal tip allows an axial vision and can be aimed at the four directions, high, low, right and left according to the transverse or longitudinal position of the fiber. It is equipped with an atraumatic edge.

The HYP-P (Olympus) has an OD of 3.1 mm. Thanks to its flexible tip, no prehension of the cervix is necessary. Entry into the cervical channel is obtained thanks to combined rotating and flexing motions of the tip of the fibroscope. The optical system has an OD of 2 mm. The endoscope is equipped with a coaxial channel to insufflate $CO_2$ or fluids, and theoretically to accommodate biopsy micropliers.

Because of its bevelled tip, the fibroscope can be directed towards all the quadrants according to whether the fiber is positioned transversally or longitudinally. Thus, this device allows exploration of the whole uterine cavity even in case of intracavitary lesions.

Diagnostic hysteroscopy can be performed with saline or glycine solutions. Saline is preferable as it is less expensive; further more, its optical qualities are excellent and the infectious risks seem negligible when a thorough cervico-vaginal disinfection has been carried out and when there are no infectious contraindications. It is preferable to use a continuous perfusion rather than injection with and syringe as the sudden distension of the uterine walls is painful. The endocervical canal is progressively distended, the inside orifice of the endocol is slowly opened under the fluid pressure. The uterine cavity is progressively distended; vision is excellent and unchanged by the fluid. The procedure is painless and the quantity of insufflated liquid is small (15 cc). Vision is excellent and risks linked to the insufflation of $CO_2$ are eliminated. Loss of liquid through the cervix is small and does not perturb the examination: it is significant problem either for the patient or the gynecologist.

We carried out a randomised prospective study to compare advantages and drawbacks of the HYP-P fibroscopes and the rigid hysteroscope (OD of 4 mm) by randomly using $CO_2$ or NACL as distending media. The objectives of the study were to compare the feasibility of the ambulatory procedure without anesthesia, patients' pains and the diagnostic reliability for each endoscope.

For a similar diagnostic efficacy, the results showed that:

- the use of saline rather than $CO_2$ as a distending medium, whatever the kind of endoscope, increases patient's comfort (Table 1);
- the use of the fibroscope rather than a rigid hysteroscope is less painful for the patient whatever the distending medium, $CO_2$ or saline (Table 2).

So, practically the advantages of the fibroscope include:

- easy procedure and good patient tolerance as prehension of the cervix is not necessary;
- great security since risks of mechanical complications linked to a cervical wound caused by the cervical prehension pliers or uterine perforation are eliminated thanks to the flexible tip of the endoscope. The absence of forobliquity eliminates risks of false passages during the penetration of the cervix;
- excellent vision so the whole of the uterine cavity can be explored. The bevelled tip can be turned around to go from one side to the other. When there is an endocavitary lesion obstructing part of the cavity, it is easy to go around, behind or under it and explore the invisible part of the cavity;
- the small OD of the fibroscope (3 to 3.5 mm) allows the endoscopic procedure whatever the circumstances, either in a nullipara, a menopaused woman or in a severe cervical stenosis. In case of stenosis, a dilating bougie (OD of 1 or 2 mm) is usually enough to reduce the stenosis (cf Tables 1 & 2).

The tip of the endoscope allows minor therapeutic gestures such as adhesiolysis, in case of a central mucous synechia, and extraction of an IUD whose

Table 1.

| Fibroscope<br>Hysteroscope | OD | Distending<br>medium | Painless | Little painful | Very painful | Procedure<br>stopped |
|---|---|---|---|---|---|---|
| HYF-P | 3.5 mm | $CO_2$/gas | 102/167 | 42/167 | 20/167 | 3/167 |
| HYF-P | 3.5 mm | Saline | 753/993 | 187/993 | 44/993 | 9/993 |
| Rigid HSS | 4 mm | $CO_2$ R4 gas | 55/144 | 52/144 | 36/144 | 1/144 |
| Rigid HSS | 4 mm | $CO_2$ R4 liquid | 103/194 | 53/194 | 34/194 | 4/194 |

Table 2.

| Fibroscope<br>Hysteroscope | Distending<br>medium | Painless | Little painful | Very painful | Procedure<br>stopped |
|---|---|---|---|---|---|
| HYF-P | Gas | 61% | 25% | 12% | 2% |
| HYF-P | Fluid | 76% | 19% | 4% | 1% |
| Rigid HSS 4 mm | Gas | 38% | 36% | 25% | 1% |
| Rigid HSS 4 mm | Fluid | 53% | 27% | 18% | 2% |

thread has disappeared into the uterine cavity and is no longer visible.

Through the collateral channel (OD 12 mm), biopsy pliers of 3 French can be introduced for sample taking under visual control. With the use of saline, there are no risks of gaseous embolism though this is a rare occurrence and exclusively with $CO_2$.

## Conclusion

The fibroscope appears as the best compromise. Visibility is satisfactory so that no endocavitary lesions go unnoticed. The procedure is well accepted and tolerated. There are no risks and the use of saline is particularly well adapted to the endoscope.

# Hysteroscopy and hormonal treatment

B. Blanc, R. de Montgolfier

Hysteroscopy can be used either as a diagnostic or a therapeutic procedure in some cases of oral hormonal treatment, such as oral contraception, menstrual troubles, substitutive treatment of the menopause or anti-estrogen therapy. This examination, however is rarely used and, in any case, after a therapeutic cure has failed, most often to check the data collected by vaginal ultrasonography.

## Hysteroscopy and oral contraception

Indications include repeated metrorrhagia, different from spotting and persisting after change of pill. Thus, associated pathologies such as polyps or fibroids may be revealed. The mucosa is most often subatrophic with normodose contraceptives. In macroprogestative contraception, hysteroscopy often reveals a clearly marked atrophy with hypervascularisation (Fig. 1).

### Hysteroscopy and progestative treatment

Driguez et al. [1] reported these data. They particularly studied thickness of the muco sa and vascularisation.

### Hysteroscopy and hormonosubstitution

With a substitutive treatment of the menopause, the endometrium should be carefully monitored. Though endometrial prognosis is linked to the presence or ab-

sence of atypias, estrogenotherapy can induce prolonged hyperplasia so it has to be biologically assessed in case of metrorrhagia (Fig. 2). The substitutive treatment should have little impact on the mucosa. A subatrophic state is judged the best.

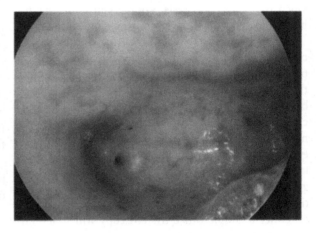

Fig 1. Bleeding due to macroprogestative contraception: atrophy with hypervascularisation

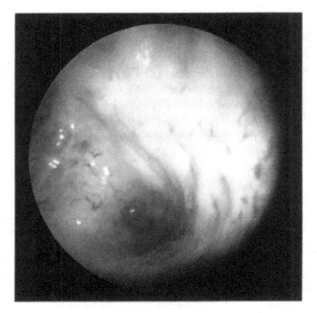

Fig 2. Metrorrhagia due to cyproterone acetate. Atrophy with fasciculated aspect

Table 1.

|  | Atrophy | Vessels |
|---|---|---|
| Norsteroids | +++ | no dilatation |
| Cyproterone ac | +++ (fasciculated aspect) | fragility |
| Nomegestrol ac | +++ | vasodilatation |
| Chlormadinone ac | + | network, no distension |
| Promegestone | + | normal |
| Progesterone | ++ | no dilatation |

Regulation is provided by the progestative component of the substitutive treatment. Diagnostic hysteroscopy is one of the different techniques of endometrial exploration. The best orientation test is vaginal ultrasonography, and histological tests afford reliable results when sample-collection is guided by endoscopical results.

Hysteroscopy should take place at the beginning of the cycle, when the patient is on a sequential pill. In this case, endoscopical evaluation is not performed when a treatment is first installed. Regulation is provided by the progestative component of the substitutive treatment. Diagnostic hysteroscopy is one of the many endometrial exploratory techniques. The key exam is vaginal ultrasonography and certainty is provided by histological tests, sample collection having been guided by endoscopical observations.

It can take place at any time for women under continuous treatment. In the latter case, the endoscopical evaluation is not prescribed at the beginning of the treatment, particularly if the menopause is recent because some sort of bleeding is frequent in those cases. Nevertheless, if bleeding persists after six months of treatment, there should be an endouterine evaluation even if the ultrasonography has not revealed any disorder. Ultrasonography, however, provides guide-lines for the conditions of endoscopic evaluation:

- either a simple office hysteroscopy which should reveal endometrial atrophy, or
- on the contrary, a hysteroscopic exam associated with biopsies in case of an expansive intracavitary process.

In this perspective, a pararegional block may be interesting, either from the beginning or during the procedure, particularly when the samples are collected with a small diameter (21 CH) hysteroscope.

Thus, it is no longer an office hysteroscopy but a surgical procedure to be performed in an operating theater, even if the risks are very low.

The hysteroscopic examination may reveal several abnormalities:

- intrauterine polyps or fibroids whose endoscopic cure is compatible with a continuing substitutive hormonal treatment;
- mucous pathologies either atrophic or, on the contrary, an abnormally thickened mucosa.

The endoscopical examination will provide information on the abnormalities, whether the lesions are homogeneous or not, and information on endometrial vascularisation. However, the most important information is given by directed histological biopsies. Heterogeneity of the endouterine surface, the so-called "leopard aspect" with thick zones and areas of different vascularisation is amongst the most common aspects observed during monitoring of a continuous combined substitutive treatment. The heterogeneous zones seem to correspond to heterogeneous hormonal receptivity accounting for intermittent bleeding, which is characteristic of the early phases of the treatment.

Different therapeutic protocols endeavour to meet the objectives of a long, safe and efficient substitutive hormonotherapy providing sufficient estrogenotherapy with no bleeding and no risks for the endometrium.

By combining hysteroscopic procedures and histological biopsies, David [2] was able to study the evolution of the endometrium through four cycles, with a substitutive protocol associating three cycles of estrogenotherapy alone (17ß estradiol 2 mg/j per day during 21 days) and then a fourth cycle associating 17B estradiol and 1 mg of norethisterone acetate.

Results appear in Table (cf. Table 2).

This study shows some important points:

- the first results of an isolated estrogenic impregnation appear as glandulo-cystic hyperplasia;
- the proportion of localised or diffuse abnormalities is the same, and thus the interest of hysteroscopy as a method of endometrial assessment is demonstrated;
- anomalies disappear with the four month treatment.

Table 2.

|  | Atrophy | Proliferative | Secretory phase | Diffuse glandulo-cystic hyperplasia | Localised glandulo-cystic hyperplasia |
|---|---|---|---|---|---|
| TO | 43.5% | 4.3% | 0 | 0 | 0 |
| 1st and 2nd cycle | 10.8-17.3% | 80.4-86.9% | 0 | 0 | 0 |
| 3rd cycle | 2.1-6.5% | 78.2-82.6% | 0 | 2,1-8.7% | 4,112-13% |
| 4th cycle | 2.1-4.3% | 2.1-4.3% | 73.9-80.4% | 0 | 0 |

## Tamoxifene treatment

The increase of breast cancers has led to an important development of the indications of antiestrogenes and particularly tamoxifene.

Tamoxifene with its antiestrogenic action on the breast has a more varied action on the endometrium with risks of several mucous pathologies.

Demuylder [3] reported that out of a series of 46 patients, 23 presented with endometrial pathologies with 13 polyps, 8 hyperplasia and 2 adenocarcinomas.

Lahti [4] compared two populations of patients with and without tamoxifene treatment.

The patients who received tamoxifene had a more voluminous uterus and a thicker endometrium.

Hysteroscopy showed endometrial thinness in 28% of the patients as against 87% in the group without tamoxifene. Endometrial polyps were more frequent in the group with treatment (36%) than in the group without treatment (10%). And finally, only one case of adenocarcinoma was found in the first group and two were observed in the group without treatment.

When a patient is treated with tamoxifene, there are two reliable and complementary investigations to be performed.

One is vaginal ultrasonography which may reveal a heterogenous mucosa due to the presence of small liquidzones.

The second is hysteroscopy. It is possible to detect a simple atrophy, polyps or neoplasic aspects but the most characteristic aspect is glandulocystic atrophy. Atrophy is suspected if the tip of the hysteroscope does not depress the mucosa. Cystic formations are like small vesicles; under chorion edema they are frequent and there may be some liquid in the uterine cavity. Vascularisation is not overdeveloped. These investigations are not systematic but they are necessary if there is bleeding (Fig. 3). Samples for histological tests should also be taken to round up the work-up.

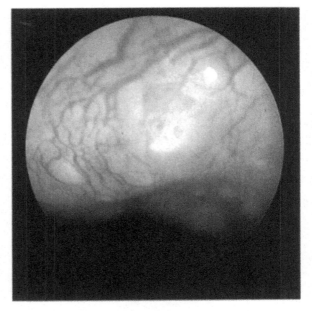

**Fig 3.** Bleeding due to tamoxifene treatment. Blandulo cystic atrophy with vascularisation

## References

1. Driguez P et al (1993) Aspects hystéroscopiques et histologiques de l'endomètre sous traitements progestatifs. Gynécol, 1(3):133-138
2. David A et al (1993) Long cyclic hormonal cycle therapy in post menopausal women. In: Berg G, Hammar M (eds) The modern management of the menopause. Proceedings of the VII international congress on the menopause, Stockolm, Parthenon Publ
3. Demuylder X et al (1991) Endometrial lesions in patient undergoing tamoxifen therapy. Int J Gynecol Obst, 36:127-130
4. Lahti E et al (1993) Endometrial changes in post menopausal breast cancer patients receiving tamoxifen. Obstet Gynecol 81:660-664
5. Blanc B (1994) Hétérogénéité de l'endomètre au traitement hormonal substitutif combiné administré en continu. In: Sureau Elsevier Stéroïdes Ménopause et endomètre. pp 81-85

# Surgical hysteroscopy: equipment and technique

B. Blanc, R. de Montgolfier

Surgical hysteroscopy requires:
- perfect visibility of the uterine cavity. Visibility afforded by the resectoscope, derived from the urologist's equipment, has been a determining factor;
- miniaturisation of the endoscopic equipment;
- easy assess to all endocavitary lesions.

## 1 Rigid hysteroscopes

### 1.1 The traditional surgical hysteroscope

It has a cylindrical operating sheath with an OD between 7 and 7.5 mm. The optical system has an OD of 4 mm. The ancillary equipment is inserted into the operating channel (flexible scissors, coagulation electrodes, biopsy pliers, ND Yag laser fibers, flexible catheters and intra-tubal equipment for sterilisation). It is a rather brittle kind of equipment because of its small diameter and its structure. Endoscopic procedures need either gas or liquid distension media.

#### Equipment with an optical system

It is a slight variant of the former equipment. It is made up of an exterior sheath which carries an optical system with an OD of 7 mm ending in a pair of rigid scissors or pliers. The optical system is within the sheath. The advantage of this equipment is to have both the optical system and the operative equipment (scissors and pliers) inserted at the tip of the hysteroscope. Indications are resection of uterine septa, synechiae or extraction of osseous patches in case of osteoid metaplasia.

### 1.2 The surgical hysteroscope with an in and out irrigating system

This equipment combines the advantages of traditional operative hysteroscope (operative channel for ancillary equipment) with in and out irrigation flow.

The outside sheath has an OD of 7 mm and 8 mm for the equipment manufactured by Scop Olympus. The operative side channel allows passage of biopsy pliers (OD 5 FR [French]), scissors (OD 7 FR) and laser Yag fibers of 400 to 600 microns. The optical system has an OD of 4 mm at 30 to 70°. The equipment is indicated for treatment of synechiae, uterine septa and pedunculated polyps. It is autoclavable.

### 1.3 The resectoscope

It has been adapted from the urologist's resectoscope (Iglesias resectoscope) (Fig. 1). It is made up of:
- an inside sheath for the in- and out-flow of the fluids;
- an outside sheath with several orifices at its end for draining the fluids;
- a mandrin to insert equipment, which should be used in exceptional circumstances as its blind and forceful introduction can lead to uterine perforation;
- an operative handle to move the optical systems and the wire loops.
  Loops are of different types (Fig. 2):
- cutting loop;
- resection loop at 60 and 90°;
- mobile roller-ball for coagulation, around an axis;
- coagulation loop with a flared fixed part.
  There are three types and two varieties of resectoscopes:
- the small resectoscope with an outside sheath of 20 or 21 charrières (CH) or 7 mm. The loops measure 2 mm. The optical system has an OD of 2.8 mm. Because of its small dimensions, it can be used for the treatment of small intracavitary lesions with OD of 1 to 2 cm, uterine septa and some central and marginal synechiae in nullipara;
- the 26-28 CH resectoscope with an outside sheath of 9 to 9.3 mm, an optical system of 4 mm OD and loops of 4 mm. This resectoscope is indicated for the treatment of more voluminous intracavitary lesions and endometrial resections;

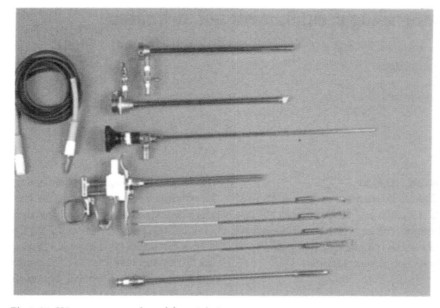

**Fig 1.** 28 CH resectoscope adapted from Iglesias resectoscope

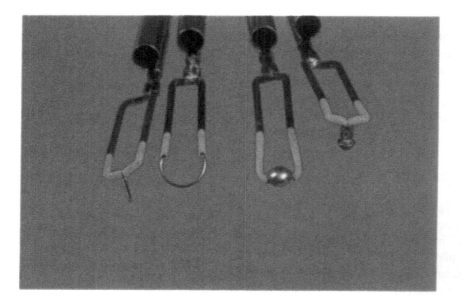

**Fig 2.** Loops of different types

- a smaller model with an outside sheath of 24 CH (8 mm) and an optical system of 3 OD is available for in-between lesions.

Resectoscopes have two different types of handle, the passive model and the active model. In the active system, the loop is moved in the same direction as the handle. When the resectoscope is introduced into the uterine cavity, the handle must be activated to maintain the loop inside the operative sheath. With a passive type, it is the opposite. Traction on the handle lets the loop out of the sheath and it comes back automatically.

Manipulation is less easy but security is higher as the loop is inside its obturator when the resectoscope is introduced.

Visualisation of the uterine cavity is excellent thanks to good irrigation. If the vision is poor, the irrigation system has to be checked; the tip of the outside sheath may be stuck against either the uterine wall or the endocervical cavity, or fluids are not properly drained because the orifices of the outside sheath have been blocked or there is an inflow problem.

The resectoscope allows treatment of benign intracavitary lesions, such as polyps, intracavitary or submucous fibroids, synechiae, uterine septa and benign endometrium pathologies.

## 1.4 Operative techniques

Procedure is identical whatever the type of resectoscope used.

### Installation

*Lithotomy position*
– Perineal and vaginal disinfection with iodine polyvidone;
– drapes are placed on the walls;
– a speculum with a movable valve and prehension of the uterine cervix with Pozzi or Muzeux pliers.

### Dilatation

The cervix is progressively dilated with bougies of 0.5 mm until a workable dilatation is reached. Cervical dilatation can be prepared by traditional or synthetic Laminaria or administration of prostaglandins three hours before the procedure (cytotech®).

### Surgical technique

Introduction of the operative hysteroscope or resectoscope must always be realised under visual control. A full mandrin should not be used to penetrate the uterine cavity blindly except in special cases, as risks of perforation are high. A hollow mandrin into which the optical system of the hysteroscope is inserted allows penetration under visual control and so avoids risks of false passage. In case of cervical stenosis, a diagnostic hysteroscopic procedure is necessary to assess the endocervical stenosis and lesion. In case of difficulty, penetration of the hysteroscope can be mo-

nitored by ultrasonography. As soon as the endoscope is through the cervico-isthmic area, the uterine cavity can be explored to identify the tubal ostia and evaluate the lesions. There are specific surgical modalities for every type of pathology. The length of the surgical procedure should not exceed 50 minutes because of risks of metabolic complications.

## 2 Hysterofibroscopes

### 2.1 Equipment

The hysterofibroscope manufactured by Olympus is 45 cm long with an outside sheath of 5 mm of OD and a co-axial operative channel of 2.2 cm for the passage of biopsy pliers, scissors, resecting loop and laser fiber. Focal distance of the optical system is about 1 mm. The flexible tip can bend up to 90°. Hysterofibroscopy may be performed using both with gas ($CO_2$) and liquid distension media.

### 2.2 Surgical technique

Surgical technique for the hysterofibroscope is the same as for the diagnostic fibroscope with the following phases:
- speculum and vaginal disinfection;
- prehension of the cervix by Pozzi pliers is not necessary;
- introduction of the tip of the endoscope into the endocervical canal;
- passage through the uterine isthmus;
- penetration and observation of the uterine cavity which will be systematically explored. After panoramic vision, a specific observation of the walls, uterus fundus, uterine cornua and uterine edges must be carried out. Intracavitary lesions will be observed on all their surface thanks to the flexible tip.

### 2.3 Incidents

*The isthmus cannot be dilated.* In spite of the small diameter of the operative fibroscope (5 mm), the uterine isthmus is not dilated. The treatment is simple. After one or two minutes, there will be uterine contractions and consequently physiological opening of the cervix. If the cervix is not dilated, use a flexible bougie n° 5 or 6.

*Poor visibility.* Blood, mucous or fibrous operative debris in the uterine cavity. The fibroscope does not have

an in- and outflow. It is necessary to remove all the debris and blood clots:
- through a suction valve;
- by withdrawing the endoscope to let the debris flow out;
- by dilating the cervix with a n°8 flexible bougie.

## 2.4 Realisations

With the surgical hysterofibroscope, it is possible:
– to perform targeted biopsies under visual control with 5 FR pliers;
– to destroy small synechiae by electroresection;
– to perform ND Yag laser treatment of:
- benign pathologies of the endometrium, endometrectomy
- small endometrium polyps
- endocavitary and submucous fibroids
- uterine septa

## 2.5 Advantages and drawbacks

It is a great advantage to have a small diameter surgical hysteroscope (5 mm) to treat young women for sterility and in the case of hypoplastic uterus (syndrome of exposition in utero or DES syndrome).

Drawbacks include loss of luminosity, absence of a double channel for the in- and outflow, high costs of the equipment, and the fact that equipment is easily breakable.

## 3 Fluid distension media and insufflators

### 3.1 Fluid distension media

They should: allow clear visibility and not be miscible with blood; be non-toxic, non-irritating for the endometrium and easy to sterilise; not be changed by any increase of heat, not be conductors if electrical current is used.

**Several fluids are available.** $CO_2$. It is easy to use. There is a theoretical risk of embolism in case of bleeding or vascular wound, but the risk is very small when there is no hyperpressure and the flow is under 80. The field of vision is obscured if there is bleeding thus, procedures must be short.
a. *Saline*. Normal saline is contained in plastic bags. It has excellent optical properties but since the solution easily mixes with blood, there are problems in case of

intra-uterine hyperpressure. It should not be used if electro-surgery is contemplated. It can be used for the mechanical treatment of synechiae and uterine septa.
b. *Glycine.* It is the most commonly used distension medium in France, it is supplied in 3 L plastic containers (URO 3000 1.5%, Laboratory Aguettant). As in urology, it is advisable to use an irrigation set equipped with Y-tubing (Uromatic bladder irrigation set. Travenol) so that per-operative irrigation is never interrupted. There is one theoretical metabolic risk which could be developed further on. Direct cerebral toxicity has been reported.
c. *Dextran*. It has an oncotic pressure comparable to plasma pressure. There are no neurologic or renal hazards but hypersensibility accidents have been reported with important general reactions and risks of severe pulmonary oedema.
d. *Hyskon* (Pharmacia AB). It is a solution of Dextran, thus, it has the same properties, drawbacks and advantages. As it tends to adhere to instruments, it is essential to clean the equipment immediately after a procedure. It is supplied in glass containers and a mechanical device to deliver the fluid is necessary.
e. *Sorbitol and Manitol.* They are viscous fluids and do not provide the same clear visibility. Potential complications include hemodilution, but metabolic complications are limited.
f. *5% Glucose*. It has a similar visibility but deposits may build up inside the irrigation circuits.
g. *Distilled water.* It is forbidden in operative hysteroscopy because of major hazards of hemolysis.

Whatever distension fluid is used, the inflow and outflow of liquid media must be carefully monitored and in case of loss exceeding 500 cc, a perforation should be suspected and a peroperative ultrasonography immediately performed. If liquid effusion is visible (over 50 cc) it should be removed through a punction in Douglas pouch.

### 3.2 Fluid insufflation devices

$CO_2$ requires pumps with constantly controlled flow and pressure to avoid hyperpressure and thus, possible embolisms.
- For liquid distension media, it is essential to avoid intrauterine hyperpressure. The cheapest and simplest way is to have liquid containers hanging 60 cm above the patient and use atmospheric pressure and the weight of the liquid column. We have practised 1500 resections using this device without any severe accident. Pumps are available which deliver liquids under permanent control of

the pressure inside. Amongst them two models are particularly interesting:

- J. Hamou's hysteromat which delivers glycine with variable electronically controlled flow and pressure to maintain a gradient of constant pressure between the positive glycine inflow and the negative glycine outflow, with permanent regulation of intrauterine pressure;
- the Olympus Uteromat, which delivers glycine with variable electronically controlled flow and pressure to maintain a gradient of constant pressure. The quantities of glycine used and lost in each intrauterine operative sequence are monitored on a screen.

## 4 The ND Yag laser

The ND Yag laser used in hysteroscopy requires powerful laser energy (100 W) to achieve satisfying hemostasis (devascularisation) and deep penetration into the myometrium. Its wavelength is 1.064 nanometer (near infrared). Its invisible beam has to be guided by a helium-neon spot (OD 2 MM). It is transmitted through quartz fiberoptics of 400 to 600 micrometers covered with Teflon. Laser power is measured in joules per second at the tip of the laser fibre. The laser beam is activated by a foot-controlled switch.

Its principal effects on biological tissues are vaporization, that is carbonization of a lesion and retraction of the tissues. Vaporization is used to destroy biological tissues and is easily obtained at high powers on a dark tissue by touching the lesion with the contact probe. As it destroys tissues through carbonization, the ND Yag laser has to be used at close range. Vaporization is achieved by the "touch" technique.

The effect of tissue retraction is obtained on pale tissues by using low powers. It can easily be obtained by removing the fiber from the targeted tissue. The ND Yag laser wave penetrates deeply into the tissue and leads to photocoagulation or tissue retraction rather than carbonisation. This effect is achieved by the "non touch" technique.

### Operative techniques

The "non touch" technique achieves in-depth photocoagulation of the tissue by reducing its vascular network without destroying it. Carbonisation should be avoided at the beginning of the cure. The tissue becomes white. The ideal distance to maintain is not constant and has to be found tentatively according to the results of the first waves. Usually the distance is around 4 or 5 cm and the power density is variable according to the lesion. It is about 30 watts for polyps, 20 to 30 watts for visible adenomyosis lesions and may reach 100 watts for voluminous fibroids. In the latter case, it is always preferable to start the cure in the center of the lesion and move in bigger and bigger circles away from the starting point. After each burst, it is necessary to observe the results and accordingly adapt the powers and distance between the tip of the fiber and the targeted tissue.

In the "touch" technique, the tip of the fiber is placed in contact with the tissue to be resected. The choice of the pre-set measures depends on the volume of lesions. In most cases, a pulse of 60 to 70 watts is enough. If there is smoke in great quantities, the power is too high.

The KTP laser has two wavelengths and two modes of emission. It seems theoretically interesting. The two wavelengths 1064 and 532 nanometer and the two delivery modes, continuous beam and super pulse, provide some advantages. The ND Yag laser with a double frequency of 532 mm is an intermediary coagulator and its coagulating effects can be used for highly vascularized superficial lesions. So a swift and controlled destruction of the tissues is possible.

When the laser functions in a continuous wave output, power is rather low (100 watts). As a super pulse, there is a sequence of swift, powerful bursts (300 watts); thus, the ND Yag laser can be used as a highly precise knife whereas the continuous mode is better for photocoagulation of more diffuse lesions.

*Light sources.* Excellent visibility is essential to perform hysteroscopic surgical procedures. Several self-regulated light sources are available for surgical hysteroscopy and coelioscopy. A 250 watts source affords clear visibility for hysteroscopic surgery.

*Video equipment.* It has become a valuable part of hysteroscopic surgery. Surgical procedures have become simpler as the surgeon enjoys a more comfortable position. The video camera must be placed for observation of the lesion to be treated on the monitor in its appropriate anatomic setting. It is invaluable for teaching purposes. The medical staff in the operating room can participate in the procedure.

# Irrigation fluid pumps in operative hysteroscopy

J.L. Mergui

Continuous flow operative hysteroscopy has been part of the daily practice of gynecological surgery for the past twenty years, both in dealing with menorrhagia by resection of fibroids, polyps or endometrium ablation, and in treating the intrauterine causes of infertility such as lysis of synechiae.

Although these endoscopic techniques can be reproduced and are viable, they are subject to a rate of complication which is relatively low but which may nevertheless prove very serious and sometimes even fatal in certain cases [1].

Visualising the uterine cavity requires distending the uterus in order to transform the virtual cavity into a real one, thus allowing visualisation of the surgical site and precise resection surgery appropriate to the lesion.

The distention of uterine cavity can be carried out (usually during the diagnostic period) by using gas ($CO_2$) whose automatically controlled inflow pressure currently permits carrying out hysteroscopic procedure in outpatient surgery in complete safety, thus avoiding gas embolism especially in consultation procedure (without anaesthesia) [2]. However, for operative hysteroscopy it is generally necessary to use distention liquids along with a permanent flow into the uterine cavity to obtain clear vision during the incision of the patient's vasculature. The distention medium used must have low viscosity and be electrolyte-free in order to block the monopolar electric current transmitted by the loops or the electrosurgical instruments (but recently the use of bipolar electrodes allows the use of saline solution: Versapoint). For most operative hysteroscopic surgery currently performed throughout the world and especially in France, the usual distention medium is a 1.5% glycine solution.

Mannitol and Sorbitol solutions are used by some other (often American or British) authors. These three media all have the same properties, namely that they are slightly hypo-osmotic in comparison with blood serum and electrolyte-free to ensure no flow of electric current. In addition to operative hysteroscopic mechanical complications, intravasation of the distention medium (i.e. absorption of the uterine distention fluid into the patient's vasculature) may lead to life-threatening hemodynamic and biological consequences:

- hypervolemia, congestive heart failure and possible pulmonary edema in the event of sudden and large intravasations;
- imbalance in the serum electrolyte level with hyponatremia followed by intercellular hyperhydratation and cerebral edema (hyponatremic encephalopathy);
- possible direct glycine toxicity on the central nervous system.

When this intravasation is large it can significantly influence the functional and vital prognosis of a patient, and strict observance of procedure must be applied because of the consequences on the operative hysteroscopic surgery and on the medico-legal situation. A recent French Ministry of Health circular dated 4 August 1998 (n° 987990) points out the serious risks of using the sterile 1.5% glycine irrigation fluid; because of the serious risks involved in using these products and after notification of the French National Commission of Bio-Technology, the Ministry of Health has asked manufacturers to increase user information with an instruction leaflet and suitable labelling. The leaflet points out that the undesirable effect most often observed, called the reabsorption syndrome or TUP-Syndrome by urologists, is linked to a fluid overload in the systemic circulation and involves simultaneously a certain number of neurological and/or visual symptoms affecting the patient's consciousness and associated with hyponatremia.

While the development of irrigation fluids with lower risk in the event of reabsorption is still on course, the ministry recommends supplementing monitoring by:

- shortening the surgery time;
- controlling the intrauterine irrigation fluid pressures according to the accepted technique;
- monitoring the inflow/outflow fluid rates;
- and finally carrying out an ionogram (the electrolyte level in blood levels) and a hematocrite at the slightest sign of clinical reabsorption syndrome.

The Ministry requests the monitoring of the intra uterine pressures if an automatic instrument (infusion pump) is used and also the communication of any serious accident involving these fluids.

## Different mechanisms of uterine distention

### Hydrostatic pressure

The distention liquid bag (linked to the hysteroscopy operator) is placed above the level of the patient and at this point infusion pressure is that of the water column placed above the surgical site. The resulting pressure is constant and equal to that of the column: The advantage of this system is that there is no hyperpressure risk (increase in the infusion pressure), the flow rate is relatively constant and is equal to that authorised by the operating canal of the operative hysteroscope.

The disadvantage is that when the pressure is insufficient to suitably distend the uterine cavity, it is not possible to increase it so as to allow improved visualisation of a given zone in the uterine cavity, especially in the case of an uncompliant uterus. Besides, there is no monitor of veritable pressure levels.

### Pressure bags surrounding the distention fluid

A counter-pressure band is inserted around the bag in order to give it a higher infusion pressure. The advantages is that it is possible to set a higher pressure than that of the simple use of the water column, and therefore to vary this pressure during the operation when necessary. The disadvantage is that bag pressures are imprecise, very often being lower than the figures shown on the pressure-gauge and it is necessary to add to these figures the pressure created by the height of the bag placed above the patient's level.

### Continuous-flow fluid infusion pump with variable pressure system

These pumps are in fact roller pumps which allow the distention fluid to be injected inside the uterine cavity at a constant rate.

The major disadvantage of these methods is the injection of distention liquid regardless of the intrauterine pressure and the resulting hyperpressures of the uterine cavity, which are incompatible with a safe operative hysteroscopic procedure. The use of such methods should be strictly forbidden in operative hysteroscopy.

## Pressure-controlled fluid infusion pumps

Manufacturers have recently developed uterine cavity distention pumps. These machines consist of a roller pump which drives a low-viscosity distention medium from a reservoir (distention liquid bag) to the endoscope placed in the uterine cavity (Fig. 1). The intrauterine pressure and the maximum flow-rate of the distention medium are electronically controlled and may be pre-set by the operator. When the rate is set at 200 ml/mn for example and the maximum pressure at 80 mmHg, beyond that point the pump automatically stops in order to avoid any hyperpressure in the cavity. Below these pressures, however, the rate may reach the previously set maximum rate.

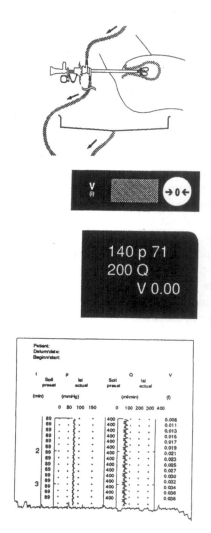

Fig. 1.

More recently, the Uteromat Fluid-Control (Olympus), by using a weighing-based fluid deficit indicator in fluid collection (in the form of a fluid-collection canister placed on scales at the beginning of the operation), allows the calculation of the distention fluid deficit which is equal to the injected quantity of fluid minus the volume of return fluid collected. The canister placed on the scales collects the distention fluid returning from the resection circuit or even from a collection bag positioned under the patients buttocks, and the scales then determine the volume of liquid collected. The difference between this volume and the total volume used is directly shown on the display linked to the endoscopic camera. During the procedure it is therefore possible to visualise on the screen, by using video over-impression:

- the preset nominal pressure;
- the actual pressure during the operation;
- the nominal rate effective throughout the operation;
- the total distention fluid used;
- finally, the distention fluid deficit which indicates the risk of fluid intravasation.

The intrauterine pressure is recorded by a pressure monitor built into the tube which permits changing the infusion rate of the roller pump. This measuring chamber should be set up before beginning fluid filling so that it remains unchanged during insertion. All the different parameters can be connected to a printer in order to supply the operative hysteroscopic monitoring data (Fig. 2).

Of course, these are particularly sophisticated and costly systems which can be rightly seen as currently the very best in monitoring operative hysteroscopy and in the use of distention fluid. It is also possible to set maximum distention liquid deficit limits and indicate the deficit with numerical figures flashing at either 500 or 1000 ml, accompanied by the machine automatically stopping.

Finally, a more recent system makes it possible to set an alarm in all cases of rapid distention fluid deficit, especially if these are above 350 ml/mn. Indeed, if an operative hysteroscopy has been pre-set at a 1000 ml glycine deficit, after 20 minutes of resection there may be a deficit of only 300 ml; conversely if there is a sudden perforation or large cut in the vasculature then an initial 250 ml/mn rate can result in losing 750 ml in the space of 3 minutes and therefore 23 minutes can lead to an intravasation of over a litre of distention liquid. This speed of loss can be indicated by an electronic signal which can interrupt the procedure if the surgeon desires so.

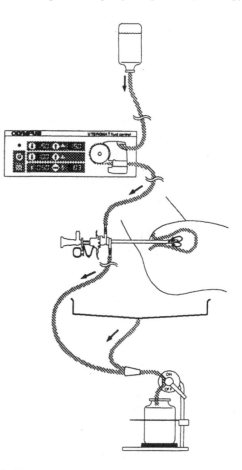

Fig. 2.

These sophisticated systems may be considered as the latest and best in uterine distention monitoring and control during operative hysteroscopy, but the investment cost is often high and whilst they ensure a certain safety, they do not ensure complete safety.

## Electro-mechanical control systems

Some authors have developed infusion pressure control systems by varying the height of the distention liquid bag in relation to the level of the patient. The distention liquid bag is placed on a pole fitted with a motor to heighten or to lower the distention liquid bag level [3] in order to vary the intrauterine pressure (Variflow). Initially developed in the East-European countries, this system has the great advantage of being simple, cheap and relatively effective concerning pressure control. The disadvantage of the system is its lack of reliability due to the absence of control and monitoring of the intrauterine flow, and, of course, of the distention liquid deficits.

## Control criteria of the main indexes

Many authors have become interested in the mechanisms causing intravasation because of the comparatively common occurrence of complications as shown in the recent publication by Castaing in 1999 [1], that is 5.7% of the 352 operative hysteroscopies carried out in the Bichat Hospital ward, also 2 per 1000 in our own operative hysteroscopy experience (carried out by a singly hysteroscopist), and also certain fatal complications described in literature. In 1990, Garry noted that out of 200 patients undergoing a Laser Yag endometrium ablation, randomly assigned into two prospective series of 100 using either a continuous flow pump or a pressure-controlled pump, those with controlled pressure had a glycine distention liquid deficit of less than 85% (1.5).

In 1992, the same author [4] assessed the influence of pressure on a prospective serie studying 26 patients undergoing a Laser Yag endometrium ablation:

- when the pressure was not controlled, the distention liquid deficit was 2027 ml;
- when the pressure was controlled, the distention liquid deficit was 1250 ml with a pre-set 100 mmHg pressure;
- there was no distention liquid deficit when the pre-set pressure was in the region of 70 mmHg [5].

These authors insist therefore on the necessity of controlling the infusion pressure of the distention fluid and of limiting it to pressures lower than 70 mm Hg, giving a clear impression of this control's beneficial character on small series (26 patients).

This impression is again met with in the Shirk and Gimpelson study [6] where operative hysteroscopies were carried out at 60, 80, 90, 100 and 110 mmHg pressures using pressure-controlled pumps. No intravasation occurred when the pressure is lower than 80 mmHg. However, when the pressure rises to 100 mmHg, a distention fluid loss of around 200 ml is noted after ten minutes observation. At 110 mgHg, the distention fluid loss varies between 600 and 800 ml after ten minutes observation. One patient even developed pulmonary edema with distension following a 800 ml distention fluid loss after ten minutes. In 1992, Garry [4] also clearly shows intravasation mechanisms.

Amongst patients having undergone an endometrium ablation by Laser Yag, six patients immediately underwent a postoperative hysterography. This took place using pressures lower than 80 mm of mercury and the hysterography images showed no intravasation absorption. A second hysterography, carried out using a 160 mm mercury pressure, showed a massive intravasation absorption of the contrast medium.

Since then, a study carried out by the operating-room nurses shows that the best intrauterine pressure seems to be the patient's mean arterial pressure. When the intrauterine infusion pressure is set just below or equal to the mean arterial pressure (calculated from the numerical display during the operation given by the arm-band electronic monitoring) on a prospective series of 200 randomly assigned patients, 100% of patients in this experimental group presented a glycocoll loss of less than 500 ml whereas in the control group, whose pressure was not regulated, this rate of loss was found in only 60% of patients, with 15% of patients presenting a glycine distention fluid loss between 500 and 1000 ml; 15% between 1000 and 1500 ml, and 10% above 1500 ml, therefore justifying infusion pressure control during operative hysteroscopy.

## Conclusion

Although relatively rare, the seriousness of the complications associated with distention fluid intravasation into the general circulation system, makes monitoring hysteroscopic procedures a necessity.

It consequently appears indispensable to use infusion pressures lower than the mean arterial pressure, that is from 70 to 80 mmHg.

The infusion pressure must only exceptionally (and for a very short time) go beyond these figures and in the majority of cases it is absolutely unnecessary to use an infusion pressure over 60 mm of mercury. This pressure gives clear uterine cavity vision as long as the cavity is continuously washed. Some authors have even proposed to directly connect the outflow to wall suction in order to reduce the risk of fluid absorption [7]. Other methods, such as the prescription of progestatives, even LH-RH analogues, seem to have shown similar results for some, but there is no real consensus on this [8, 9].

Whatever the situation, it is above all essential when infusion pumps are used to be able to obtain maximum pressures and variable rates of flow. This gives a certain degree of added safety to the procedure.

Finally and moreover, throughout the whole precedure it is also necessary to have a weighing indicator for the fluid inflow and outflow deficit especially at the time of changing a bag. Electronic inflow/outflow monitoring systems with display on a video screen and with the possibility of simultaneous printing have recently appeared on the market. They provide added safety by analysing the irrigation fluid deficit and displaying the main constant operative data. However, sophistication and electronic control are worthless if the infusion pressure levels and the glycine distention fluid deficits are not monitored throughout the procedure in order to avoid a large and, above all, sudden glycocoll intravasation in the general circulatory system. This is something that every operator should keep in mind throughout surgery time.

## References

1. Castaing N, Darai E, Chuong T, *et al.* (1999) Complications mécaniques et métaboliques de l'hystéroscopie opératoire. Contracept Fertil Sex 27(3):210-215
2. Mergui JL, Roassanaly K, Salat-Baroux J (1989) L'hystéroscopie opératoire en 1989. Contracept Fertil Sex, 17: 1059-1078
3. Tomazevic T, Savnik L, Dintinjana M, *et al.* (1998) Safe and effective fluid management by automated gravitation during hysteroscopy. J Soc Laparo-endosc Surg 2(1):51-55
4. Garry R, *et al.* (1992) The effect of pressure on fluid absorption during endometrial ablation. J Gynecol Surg 8:1-10
5. Hasham F, Garry R, Kokri MS, *et al.* (1992) Fluid absorption during laser ablation of the endometrium in the treatment of menorrhagia. Br J Anasth 68(2):151-154
6. Shirk GJ, Gimpelson RT (1994) Control of intra-uterin fluid pressure during operative procedure. Am Assoc Gynecol Laparos, 1(3):229-233
7. Bouli L, Blanc B, Bautrand E (1990) Le risque métabolique de la chirurgie hystéroscopique. J Gynécol Obstét Biol Repro, 19:217-222
8. Baskett TF, Farrell SA, Zilbert AW (1998) Uterine fluid irrigation and absorption in Hysteroscope endometrial ablation. Obstet Gynecol 92:976-978
9. Bennett KL, Ohrmundt C, Maloni J (1996) Preventing intravasation in women undergoing Hysteroscopic procedures AORN J 64(5):792-799

# Various features of each diagnostic and operative fibrohysteroscope

R. MARTY

In the 1960s, at the Yokusuka Clinic in Japan, gynecologists T. Mohri and C. Mohri [1] were working on a method for antenatal diagnosis of fetal malformations. They were the first gynecologists in the world to present a film on fetal movements. The film was fondamental in the arrival of the first hysterofiberscope in endoscopy on November 8, 1963

In 1954, Hirschowitz [2] created the first gastroduodenal fiberscope, which enabled him to reach bulbar lesions. An oesophagoscope was the second flexible fiberscope created on the advice of physicians Philips and Presti. It was not until ten years after the creation of the gastroduodenoscope that this technique was used in gynecology and obstetrics. As mentioned, Mohri [1] recorded fetal images in pregnancies doomed to therapeutic abortion or in post-term pregnancies. The gestational age of these pregnancies ranged from five to ten months.

The flexible method remained unknown in Europe and the United States until 1974. At that time, the Japanese reported on the use of the flexible device and its advantages at a World Congress in Rio de Janeiro (Table 1).

Although rigid hysteroscopy was being widely used between 1975 and 1985, a growing number of gynecologists began to use the flexible device. Studies were published as early as 1988 in Europe [3, 4] and the United States. Over the past eight years, flexible hysteroscopy has expanded again, with France playing a key role [4, 5].

## Fibrohysteroscopes features

Flexible hysteroscope is a generic term for two types of hysterofiberscopes: diagnostic and therapeutic.

Their fundamental features are flexibility, airtightness and optical fibers. Their differences lie in the dimensions and the choice of materials used by the manufacturers: Olympus [6], Fuji, Storz, Leisegang, Machida, Wolf and Circon. The flexible hysteroscope comprises four parts: a *case*, a *sheath* that links it to the *bendable extremity* and a *connection link to the light source* [7].

### The case (proximal extremity)

The case is lightweight and easily held by the operator. A remote control lever for the bendable segment is present on one side of the proximal extremity. The case holds the proximal system, which comprises: the ocular and dioptrical adjustment ring; the entrance orifice of the operative canal which, depending on the devices, is equipped or not with an airtight valve; and the departure of the fiberscope sheath, which is located at the distal part of the case.

### The main sheath

In most of the devices currently available, the main sheath is completely flexible. An exception is the Fuji endoscope which will be discussed later. This pliable segment is relatively resistant to torsion. The movements applied to it are directly transmitted to the distal segment. The main sheath contains the conducting beam of the image, the lighting beams and the operative canal (whose dimensions are detailed later). The sheath is perfectly airtight and is composed of a steel mesh whose pliability depends on the length and thickness of the material.

### The distal extremity

The distal extremity of the flexible fiberscope enables the operator to get an axial view of the uterine cavity. The bendable extremity can be manipulated in at least four directions within the uterine cavity (i.e. up, down, left and right). The ultimate direction of the distal extremity is determined by the movements on the sheath combined with the use of the thumb lever. The distal tip of the endoscope comprises a nontraumatic rim on a transverse section; the objective is located under the operative canal and is surrounded by lighting beams.

Table 1.

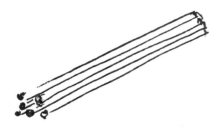

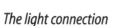

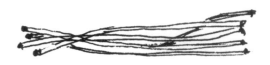

non coherent bundle

### The light connection

The light connection shelters all the optical components in a sheath identical to that of the fiberscope. This part, which most often cannot be dissociated from the case, ends with a plug that is usually specific to the light sources. Adapters connect the endoscope to different types of light sources, but the luminosity decreases by at least 20% with each intermediary.

The operative canal diameter ranges from 1 mm for the diagnostic hysteroscope to 2.2 m for the therapeutic hysteroscope. The canal is used by both the distention medium and supplementary instruments such as biopsy forceps and laser fibers. Thus, it appears that the most effective device should have the smallest possible outer diameter with an operative canal at least 1.2 mm wide (the thinnest diameter for an instrument being 1 mm).

### Microstructure of the optical system

The optical fibers are organized in two categories of bundles: the first, which carries the image to the eyepiece, is coherent and is responsible for the transmission of the image to the eyepiece; the second bundle is noncoherent and conveys the light into the uterine cavity. There are usually two noncoherent bundles per hysteroscope (table 1).

To transmit an image, a fiber beam must be coupled at both extremities with a system of convergent lenses. The image appears on the distal section through a lens system that constitutes the objective and whose focal distance determines the field angle. The image is conveyed to the beam's proximal section, where another system of lenses makes up the ocular and ensures a 10 to 20 fold enlargement. This ocular can be adjusted to the eyesight of the endoscopist.

The information is sent by a coherent beam, which is composed of glass fibers similarly arranged from one extremity to the other. The image is then split up into as many points as optical fibers.

### The optical fiber

It consists of a quartz fiber containing an inner quartz core surrounded by a non refractive outer sheath. The light, after many internal refractions, will exist at the distal end.

The size of each fiber varies from a manufacturer to another and ranges from 6 to 13μ. The optical fibers are organized in two categories of bundles: coherent and noncoherent (Scheme 1).

The number and thinness of the optical fibers do not appear to be a criterion of quality. The thinner and longer fibers are, the more information is lost. Gaps occurring when the fibers are assembled can distort the image. When the refraction index of this component is low, the loss of information is reduced. The obvious advantage of these flexible fibers compared with the conventional rigid optical system is the ability to convey the image no matter what the degree of curvature is (Table 2).

The noncoherent beams are assemblages of optical fibers that are haphazardly arranged. They are coupled with another lens system and extended without interruption from the external light source to the distal extremity of the fiberscope, therefore requiring a good lighting power.

## Comparative study and features of the fibrohysteroscopes

We had the opportunity to evaluate various fibrohysteroscopes from the following factories:
- nine diagnostic fibrohysteroscopes (Circon, Storz, Fuji, Leisegang, Machida, Wolf*, Olympus) (fig. 1-8);
- four operative fibrohysteroscopes (Storz, Fuji, Circon, Olympus) (fig. 9-12).
They are all detailed hereafter.

We have taken into consideration twelve parameters for each fibrohysteroscope. Apart from the dimension, we mention the way of disinfection/sterili-

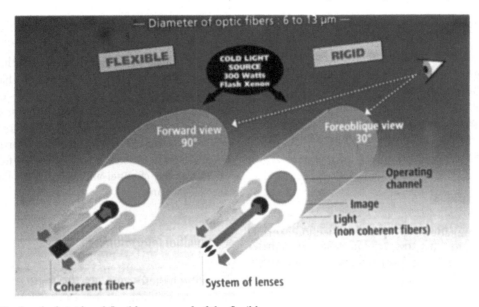

**Scheme 1.** Distal end of rigid and flexible scope and of the flexible scope

zation and the optical facilities (photo-video). A brief comment is made for each endoscope.

\* We did not succeed in our efforts to receive information from Richard Wolf Company.

## Ancillary instrumentation

### Flexible biopsy forceps

Various flexible forceps have been developed by each different company: Fujinon, Circon, Storz, and also Olympus, Cook and Leisegang (Tables 3 and 4). Some of them are disposable. A majority is reusable after a proper careful sterilization. We commonly use, since years, Olympus and Cook forceps for targeted endometrial biopsies, and recently we have also used a 3-French Leisegang flexible biopsy forceps (our equipment is detailed in Tables 3-5).

Since the sample is always small (microbiopsy), it is of great importance to choose the forceps which allows to retain the greatest volume of tissue in one bite. The results regarding the reliability of targeted endometrial biopsy are given in the chapter "Targeted endometrial biopsy" of this book. They have been obtained by using Olympus or Cook instrumentation (3 or 5-French). (Figs. 13-17). We are now evaluating the Leisegang flexible forceps already available. For one biopsy, the pathologist receives 0,47 mm³ more than he usually received with the other forceps. This is a significant improvement of the readibility of the tissue specimen.

Lin's forceps is interesting because allows to increase considerably the volume of tissue sample.

Neverheless, there are two problems: first, the hysteroscope must be pulled out the patient because the shaft has to be introduced inside the operating channel and then the head assembled. The second difficulty is to safely reintroduce the endoscope and push it again through the cervical canal with the head of the forceps protruding from the tip of the hysteroscope [8].

### Flexible grasping forceps

These forceps may be used for the IUD removal. Cook, as well as Olympus, has developed 3 different types (refer to chapters "Office fibrohysteroscopy" and "Hysteroscopy and IUD" of this book).

### Lasso

This type of snare is very useful to perform a polypectomy on small polypes. We use an Olympus lasso (refer to chapter "Office minor operative procedures" of this book).

### Basket

Fujinon has developed a snare designed as a basket. This instrument is about the same as the one used by the urologists and is sometimes very useful, giving better results than the lasso.

## Monopolar electrode

Many companies such as Olympus, Fujinon, Circon or Storz have manufactured a monopolar electrode. This can be used during minor operative procedures (on outpatient basis) (refer to chapter "Office minor operative procedures" of this book). The Nd-Yag laser is the best for surgical procedures but requires a general anesthesia (Fig. 18).

## Katayama catheter

When a cannulation has been scheduled for a cornual obstruction, we use this 2,5 or 3-French catheter (Cook) through the operating channel of the HYF-P Olympus or the HYF-1T.

## A sterile pack

It is opened on the pull out tray of the examination table; it includes one single tooth tenacula, speculum and small plastic sounds, as well as a small plastic container and cotton balls to be used for an antiseptic preparation solution [9].

## Importance of the deflection brake

This device concerns exclusively the Olympus endoscopes family. It is of a great help for the operator when he is alone involved in operative procedures, or when the patient offers a difficult access to the uterine cavity. This brake is situated on one side of the bendable section lever and may be pushed up by the thumb (90°) to progressively stiffen the bendable tip. So, it is possible to adjust the desired stiffness wanted by the endoscopist by pushing up the brake device.

## Effect of stiffness

Some postmenopausal patients presenting bleeding, many nulliparous patients involved on IVF procedures or patients under hormonal replacement therapy have, for different reasons, a small external cervical os and a very narrow cervical canal. In such a circumstance, the use of the brake to stiffen the flexible part of the tip is very helpful to go beyond the difficulty and to introduce successfully the hysteroscope and progress through the cervical canal. In some cases this possibility avoids the need of dilate the cervix before the procedure.

## Maintaining a good position on the tip

Another advantage of the brake is the ability to "freeze" the position of the tip when it has been correctly placed to perform a targeted endometrial biopsy. The handling of the hysteroscope is easier because the operator has no need to push on the deflection lever with the thumb. The operator may use his second hand to push the flexible biopsy forceps inside the operating channel and to perform the biopsy at the selected area.

## Cannulation procedure

The fibrohysteroscopes are the most efficient endoscopes to perform a tubal cannulation, because the operator has always the opportunity to bring the tip of the hysteroscope in front and close to the tubal ostium despite the individual anatomy of each patient. Using the brake allows the operator to introduce easily the catheter inside the selected tube.

## Surgical procedure

The surgical with a fibroscope is performed with a bare quartz fiber of the Nd-Yag laser. The activation of the brake allows to keep the tip in the adequate position and to deliver the laser energy directly and perpendicularly to lesions located laterally in the uterine cavity and in the cornual region. It allows a perfect preciseness during the procedure, avoiding to damage the adjacent endometrium.

## Our instrumentation

The fibrohysteroscope is connected to a cold light source. We use a video camera and perform all our procedures looking to the video monitor screen. All specific or difficult cases are recorded with a magnetoscope (Fig. 19).

## The choice of fibrohysteroscope

Five major parameters have to be taken into consideration: a) the outer diameter of the tip; b) the field angle; c) the deflection brake; d) the quality of the image and e) the diameter of the operating channel.

## The outer diameter of the tip

This means the number of millimeters to be inserted inside the cervical external os and to progress through the cervical canal until the internal cervical os. The easiest possible insertion and tolerance are directly correlated with the size of the hysteroscope. The smallest endoscope is the best.

## The field angle

It is also a very important factor: the best is the widest. It is mandatory for the endoscopist to be able to observe simultaneously both tubal ostia during the panoramic view from the isthmus. This is very important for the orientation before the exploration phase of the procedure.

## The deflection brake

This possibility is useful to ease the insertion phase in case of difficult cervix, to keep the good position of the tip while introducing a flexible biopsy, forceps or tubal catheter. The operator is handling easily the endoscope, because he does not need to push on the deflection lever with the thumb.

## Quality of the image

There are slight differences between the various fibrohysteroscopes available on the market. The quality of the image depends on the quality of the optic fibers, on the global number and on the structure of the coherent bundle delivering the image.

## Diameter of the operating channel

This diameter will determinate the choice of the ancillary instrumentation by its size, 3-French, 5-French or more. The smallest flexible instrumentation available is 3-French ($\pm$ 1 mm). The size of the operating channel is also important to determinate the room left for the normal saline. For example, with a channel of 1.2 mm, the space left by the 3-French instrumentation is 0.2 mm, just enough for a good visualization. With a 2.2 mm operating channel, the space left by the bare Nd-Yag fiber is 1.6 mm, allowing enough space for a good normal saline infusion; when using a 5-French biopsy forceps, the space left available for normal saline is 0.3 mm.

**Table 3.** Various biopsy forceps (3-French): our selected instrumentation

| Company | Shaft (French) | Biopsy head Jaws | Approx vol specimen (mm³) | Disposable (one time use) | Reusable | Sterilization |
|---|---|---|---|---|---|---|
| Cook | 3 | Cup ovale | 0,85 | NO | YES | Steam or ETO |
| Cook | 3 | Cup ovale | 0,85 | YES | NO | NO |
| Olympus | 3 | Cup (rat tooth) | 0,98 | NO | YES | Steam or ETO |
| Leisegang | 3 | Cup | 1,32 | NO | YES | Steam or ETO |

**Table 4.** Various biopsy forceps (5-French): our selected instrumentation

| Company | Shaft (French) | Biopsy head Jaws | Approx vol specimen (mm³) | Disposable (one time use) | Reusable | Sterilization |
|---|---|---|---|---|---|---|
| Cook | 5 | Elongated | 4, 85 | - | YES | Steam or ETO |
| Cook | 5 | Spherical | 2,25 | - | YES | Steam or ETO |
| Olympus | 5 | Cup | 5 | - | YES | Steam or ETO |

**Table 5.** Various retrieval forceps (3 and 5-French): our selected instrumentation -

| Company | Shaft (French) | Biopsy head Jaws | Approx vol specimen (mm³) | Disposable (one time use) | Reusable | Sterilization |
|---|---|---|---|---|---|---|
| Cook | 3 | Rat tooth | | NO | YES | Steam or ETO |
| Cook | 3 | Alligator | | NO | YES | Steam or ETO |
| Cook | 3 | Mouse tooth | | NO | YES | Steam or ETO |
| Cook | 5 | Rat tooth | | NO | YES | Steam or ETO |
| Cook | 5 | Alligator | | NO | YES | Steam or ETO |

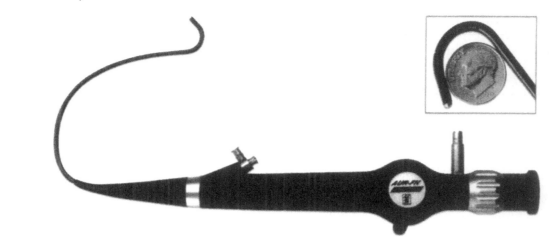

**Fig. 1.** Circon AUR-FH

Circon (AUR-FH): technical data

| Lighting | Field angle (°) | Depth of field (mm) | Bendable section (°) | Deflection brake | Outer diameter (mm) | Working length (mm) | Operating channel diameter | Instruments Admitted ± 1 mm (3-French) | Photo electronic flash | Video camera | Disinfection Sterilization | Light cable |
|---|---|---|---|---|---|---|---|---|---|---|---|---|
| Direct | 85 | 3-50 | 160 | No | 3.25 | 200 | 1.2 | Yes | Yes | Yes | Cold disinfection or ETO | Detachable |

The bendable section with an active deflection of 160° is not useful for gynecological use. The operating channel admits ancillary 3-French instrumentation. There are accessories manufactured by Circon: fulgurating electrode, non retractile grasping forceps and cytology brush. They are disposable. The endoscope has an autoseal protection that eliminates vent valves and caps for disinfection/sterilization. The fiber optic light cable is detachable.
It has no deflection brake. Unfortunately, the field angle is very narrow (85°)

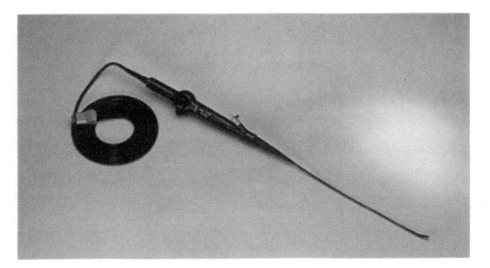

**Fig. 2.** Storz (2.5 mm)

Storz (2.5 mm): technical data

| Lighting | Field angle (°) | Depth of field (mm) | Bendable section (°) | Deflection brake | Outer diameter (mm) | Working length (mm) | Operating channel diameter | Instruments Admitted ± 1 mm (3-French) | Photo electronic flash | Video camera | Disinfection Sterilization | Light cable |
|---|---|---|---|---|---|---|---|---|---|---|---|---|
| Direct | 88 | 1-50 | 110 up 110 down | No | 2.5/2.9 | 250 | 1.2 | Yes | Yes | Yes | Cold disinfection or ETO | Part of the case |

This mini fibrohysteroscope is interesting for the use of diagnostic evaluation in an office procedure for infertility. The field angle is narrow (88°); this means that a panoramic view of both tubal ostia simultaneously from the internal cervical ostium is impossible in a majority of patients. The active bendable section of 110 up and down is correct. The operating channel admits 3-French ancillary instrumentation. There is no deflection brake

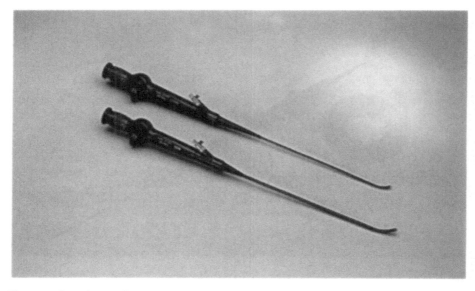

**Figs. 3, 4.** Storz (3.5 mm)

Storz (3.5 mm): technical data

| Lighting | Field angle (°) | Depth of field (mm) | Bendable section (°) | Deflection brake | Outer diameter (mm) | Working length (mm) | Operating channel diameter | Instruments Admitted ± 1 mm (3-French) | Photo electronic flash | Video camera | Disinfection Sterilization | Light cable |
|---|---|---|---|---|---|---|---|---|---|---|---|---|
| Direct | 90 | 1-50 | 110 up 110 down | No | 3.5/3.6 | 250 | 1.3 | Yes | Yes | Yes | Cold disinfection or ETO | Part of the case |

The field angle could be larger and the tip at insertion is relatively large as compared with some others. The bendable capacity of the tip is too large (110 top) and not useful for the uterine cavity. It has no deflection brake. The operating channel admits 3-French flexible instrumentation. Disinfection by soaking (or ETO)

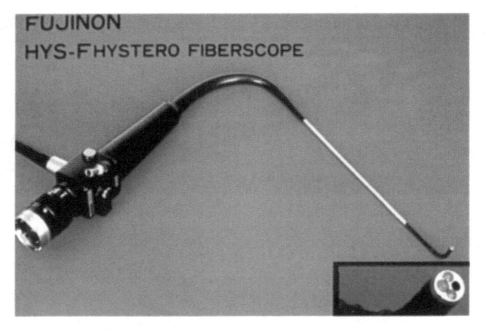

**Fig. 5.** Fujinon HYS-F

Fujinon HYSF: technical data

| Lighting | Field angle (°) | Depth of field (mm) | Bendable section (°) | Deflection brake | Outer diameter (mm) | Working length (mm) | Operating channel diameter | Instruments Admitted ± 1 mm (3-French) | Photo electronic flash | Video camera | Disinfection Sterilization | Light cable |
|---|---|---|---|---|---|---|---|---|---|---|---|---|
| Direct | 90 | 1-50 | 100 top 90 bottom | No | 3.7 | 210 | 1 | No | Yes | Yes | Cold disinfection or ETO | Part of the case |

It is a semi-flexible hysteroscope. The sheath comprises 3 parts: a) the flexible proximal segment which allows the operator to have a comfortable posture; b) the rigid intermediate segment which eases the transition from rigid to completely flexible endoscopes, and c) the flexible distal segment which is common to all other bendable tips. The field angle is narrow and the active deflection is good. It has no deflection brake. The major disadvantage comes from the diameter of the operating channel: 1 mm. This is not enough to admit any instrumentation at all. The disinfection is made by soaking (or ETO)

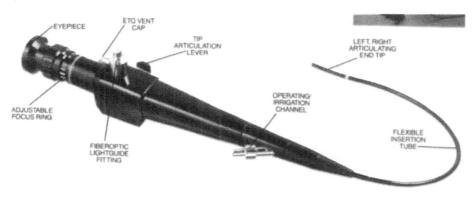

**Fig. 6.** Leisegang (LM-FLEX 7)

Leisegang (LM-FLEX 7): technical data

| Lighting | Field angle (°) | Depth of field (mm) | Bendable section (°) | Deflection brake | Outer diameter (mm) | Working length (mm) | Operating channel diameter | Instruments Admitted ± 1 mm (3-French) | Photo electronic flash | Video camera | Disinfection Sterilization | Light cable |
|---|---|---|---|---|---|---|---|---|---|---|---|---|
| Direct | 95 | 1-50 | 100 right 100 left | No | 3.6 | 250 | 1.2 | Yes | Yes | Yes | Cold disinfection or ETO | Detachable |

This endoscope has a reasonable field angle but not convenient for some nulliparous patients and large uterus. In such a situation, it is not possible to see from the internal cervical os both tubal ostia simultaneously. It has no deflection brake and the diameter at the insertion part is large. It has a detachable fiberoptic light cable and sterilization can be made by ETO or soaking. The operating channel admits ancillary instrumentation (3-French)

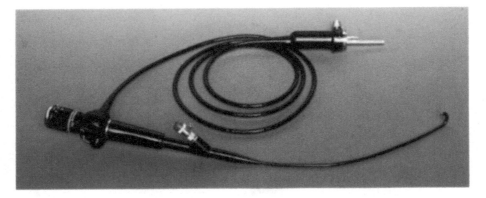

**Fig. 7.** Olympus (HYF-P)

Olympus (HYF-P): technical data

| Lighting | Field angle (°) | Depth of field (mm) | Bendable section (°) | Deflection brake | Outer diameter (mm) | Working length (mm) | Operating channel diameter | Instruments Admitted ± 1 mm (3-French) | Photo electronic flash | Video camera | Disinfection Sterilization | Light cable |
|---|---|---|---|---|---|---|---|---|---|---|---|---|
| Direct | 90 | 1-50 | 100 top 100 bottom | Yes | 3,6 | 160 | 1.2 | Yes | Yes | Yes | Cold disinfection or ETO | Part of the case |

The field angle should be larger to be able to see simultaneously both tubal ostia when observing from the internal cervical os. The diameter of the tip at insertion is convenient, but it is too large for some difficult patients. The bending capacity is adequate and the operating channel admits the 3-French flexible instrumentation. The disinfection is made by soaking. The existence of a brake for the active deflection of the tip is very useful. This type of fibrohysteroscope is the one we are using since years with excellent results

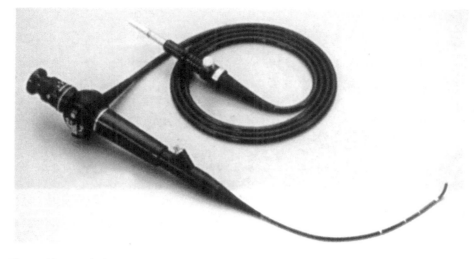

**Fig. 8.** Olympus (mini HYF-XP)

Olympus (mini HYF-XP): technical data

| Lighting | Field angle (°) | Depth of field (mm) | Bendable section (°) | Deflection brake | Outer diameter (mm) | Working length (mm) | Operating channel diameter | Instruments Admitted ± 1 mm (3-French) | Photo electronic flash | Video camera | Disinfection Sterilization | Light cable |
|---|---|---|---|---|---|---|---|---|---|---|---|---|
| Direct | 100 | 1-50 | 100 top 100 bottom | Yes | 3 | 160 | 1.2 | Yes | Yes | Yes | Cold disinfection or ETO | Part of the case |

The field angle 100° is appropriate for the simultaneous observation of both tubal ostia from the isthmus. The ultra slim diameter 3 mm allows to easily negociate the introduction of the tip through a great majority of cervix. As compared with the HYF-P, the optical system is more powerful: it has nearly the double number of glass fibers and advanced new lenses systems. It delivers sharp detailed images that are brighter and more natural looking. This new minifibroscope is going to replace progressively the HYF-P. The operating channel allows to introduce all the 3-French flexible instrumentation. The deflection brake is very useful to facilitate targeted endometrial biopsies, or cytobrushing or tubal cannulation. The disinfection is made by soaking (or ETO). We have evaluated successfully this minifibrohysteroscope for two years in our University Hospital, private Hospital and Office practice

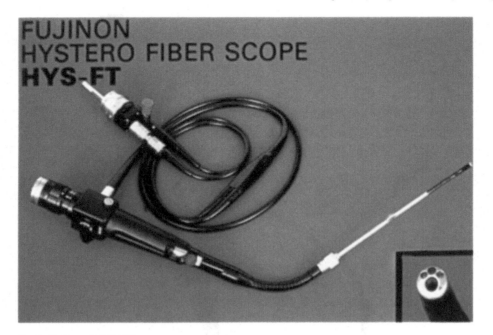

**Fig. 9.** Fujinon (HYS-FT)

Fujinon HYS-FT/HYS-RT: technical data

| Lighting | Field angle (°) | Depth of field (mm) | Bendable section (°) | Deflection brake | Outer diameter (mm) | Working length (mm) | Operating channel diameter | Instruments Admitted ± 1 mm (3-French) | Photo electronic flash | Video camera | Disinfection Sterilization | Light cable |
|---|---|---|---|---|---|---|---|---|---|---|---|---|
| Direct | 90 | 1-50 | 100 top 90 bottom | No | 4.8 | 205 | 2 | Yes | Yes | Yes | Cold disinfection or ETO | Part of the case |

This endoscope is semi-flexible. The sheath comprises 3 parts: a) the flexible proximal segment which allows the operator to have a comfortable posture; b) the rigid intermediate segment which eases the transition from rigid to completely flexible, and c) the flexible distal segment which is common to all other bendable tips.

A special characteristic of this operative hysteroscope is the presence of a ring inserted at the initial part of the rigid segment, giving a 140° axis rotation. It has no deflection brake. The field angle is narrow for a surgical use with the Nd-Yag laser.

The active deflection is adequate, but the diameter of the operating channel is narrow as compared with others. One may use 5-French ancillary instrumentation. The disinfection is obtained by soaking (or ETO)

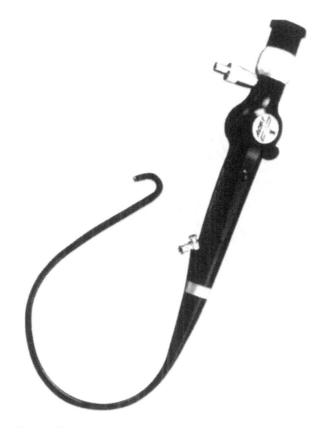

**Fig. 10.** Circon (ACN 1-50)

Circon (ACN 1-50): technical note

| Lighting | Field angle (°) | Depth of field (mm) | Bendable section (°) | Deflection brake | Outer diameter (mm) | Working length (mm) | Operating channel diameter | Instruments Admitted ± 1 mm (3-French) | Photo electronic flash | Video camera | Disinfection Sterilization | Light cable |
|---|---|---|---|---|---|---|---|---|---|---|---|---|
| Direct | 110 | 5-50 | 180 top 170 bottom | No | 4.8 | 370 | 2.1 | Yes | Yes | Yes | Cold disinfection or ETO | Detachable Autoclave |

It has a good field angle. The bending section has too much deflection (180-170), which is good for urology but not necessary for a gynecological practice. Rotating light part and rotating biopsy/irrigating part. The operating channel is suitable for 5-French ancillary instrumentation. It has a detachable light carrier cable (autoclavable). It has no deflection brake. Disinfection is made by soaking (or ETO)

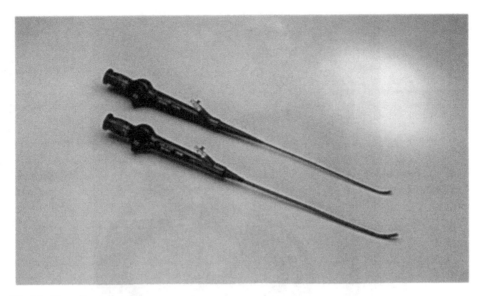

**Fig. 11.** Storz (5 mm)

Storz (5 mm): technical note

| Lighting | Field angle (°) | Depth of field (mm) | Bendable section (°) | Deflection brake | Outer diameter (mm) | Working length (mm) | Operating channel diameter | Instruments Admitted ± 1 mm (3-French) | Photo electronic flash | Video camera | Disinfection Sterilization | Light cable |
|---|---|---|---|---|---|---|---|---|---|---|---|---|
| Direct | 120 | 1-50 | 120 top 120 bottom | No | 5/5.3 | 280 | 2.3 | Yes | Yes | Yes | Cold disinfection or ETO | Part of the case |

The active deflection 120 up and down is good for operative cases. The operating channel admits easily 5-French instrumentation or a bare Nd-Yag laser fiber. The space left for normal saline infusion is enough. It has no deflection brake. Disinfection can be made soaking or sterilization by ETO

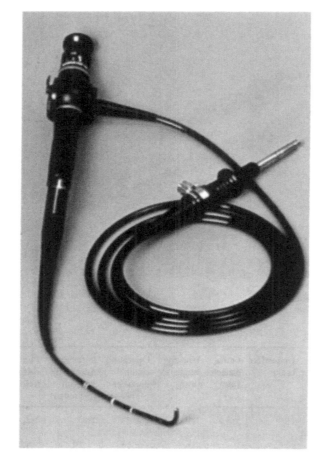

**Fig. 12.** Olympus HYF-IT

Olympus HYF-IT: technical note

| Lighting | Field angle (°) | Depth of field (mm) | Bendable section (°) | Deflection brake | Outer diameter (mm) | Working length (mm) | Operating channel diameter | Instruments Admitted ± 1 mm (3-French) | Photo electronic flash | Video camera | Disinfection Sterilization | Light cable |
|---|---|---|---|---|---|---|---|---|---|---|---|---|
| Direct | 120 | 2-50 | 120 top 120 bottom | Yes | 4.9 | 290 | 2.2 | Yes | Yes | Yes | Cold disinfection or ETO | Part of the case |

The field of view is suitable for surgical procedures. The operating channel has a diameter allowing the introduction of 5-French flexible instrumentation or of a bare fiber of Nd-Yag laser. The space left for the normal saline insufflation is respectively 0,55 mm and 1,6 mm. A deflective brake for the active deflection is present. Disinfection is made by soaking or ETO. We choose this type of fibroscope for all our operative procedures with the Nd-Yag laser. The space left inside the operating channel after the introduction of the bare fiber provides enough volume of normal saline for an adequate uterine distention. The activation of the deflective brake gives a great security and preciseness when firing in a difficult position

## Machida (FS-HYS)

| Lighting | Field angle (°) | Depth of field (mm) | Bendable section (°) | Deflection brake | Outer diameter (mm) | Working length (mm) | Operating channel diameter | Instruments Admitted ± 1 mm (3-French) | Photo electronic flash | Video camera | Disinfection Sterilization | Light cable |
|---|---|---|---|---|---|---|---|---|---|---|---|---|
| Direct | 80 | 3-50 | 100 top 90 bottom | No | 3.6 | 215 | 1 | No | Yes | Yes | Cold disinfection or ETO | Part of the case |

We never evaluated this hysteroscope, but we must point out that the field angle is very narrow (80°) and the diameter of the operating channel does not allow to pass any kind of instrumentation. It has no deflection brake. Disinfection by soaking (or ETO)

## Wolf

| Lighting | Field angle (°) | Depth of field (mm) | Bendable section (°) | Deflection brake | Outer diameter (mm) | Working length (mm) | Operating channel diameter | Instruments Admitted ± 1 mm (3-French) | Photo electronic flash | Video camera | Disinfection Sterilization | Light cable |
|---|---|---|---|---|---|---|---|---|---|---|---|---|

We never received the required infection from the factory

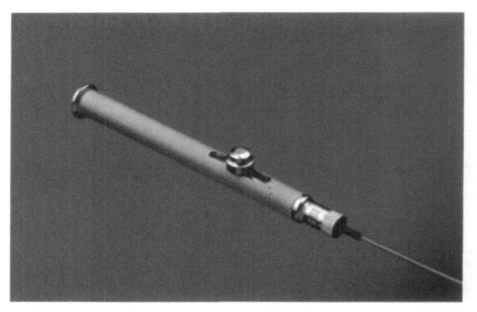

**Fig. 13.** handle of a (3 french forceps)

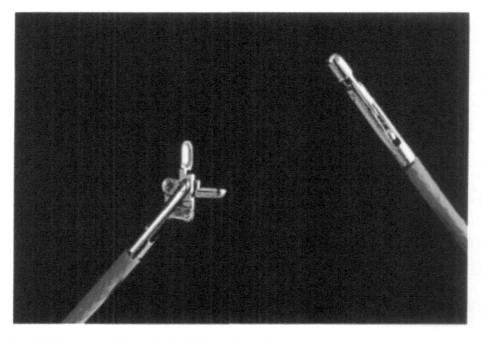

**Fig. 14.** Saws open and closed (3 French biopsy forceps)

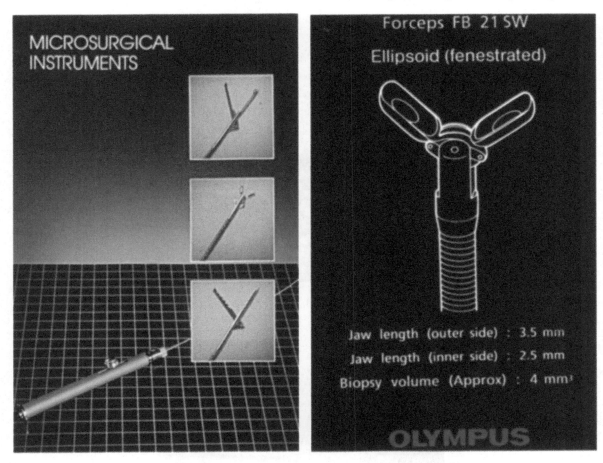

**Fig. 15.** 3 French biopsy forceps and retrieval

**Fig. 16.** Biopsy forceps 5 French

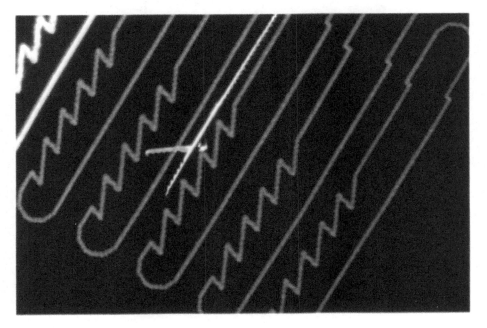

**Fig. 17.** Jaws of alligator forceps

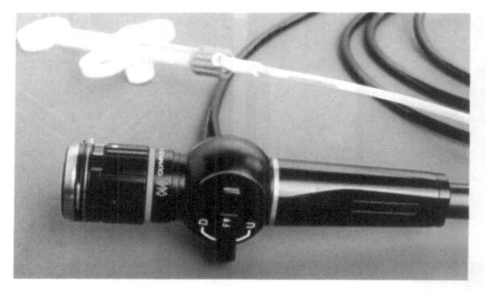

**Fig. 18.** Monopolar electrode

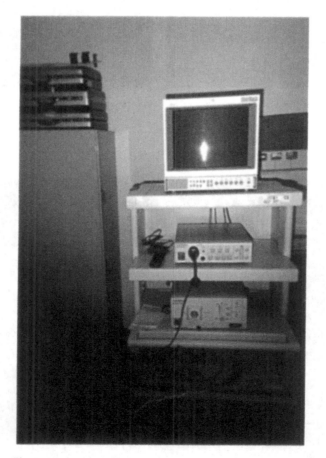

**Fig. 19.** Instrumentation set

## Our choice

After a two years evaluation of the prototype, we have selected the new mini fibrohysteroscope HYF-XP to perform ambulatory and office procedures [10]. The new technical improvements of this fibroscope have obvious practical benefits (Table 6) (Figs. 20-22).

Table 6. HYF-XP new technical improvements: practical benefits

**Step by step procedure**

| | |
|---|---|
| External os | • easier insertion<br>• lower failure rate |
| Cervical canal | • smoother progression<br>• better patient tolerance |
| Internal os | • excellent panoramic view<br>• simultaneous observation of both tubal ostia |
| Uterine | • better resolution for accurate cavity observation of coloured vascular pattern<br>• increased preciseness for directed biopsies or tubal cannulation |

**During the full procedure**

• easier observation
• faithful image on the screen

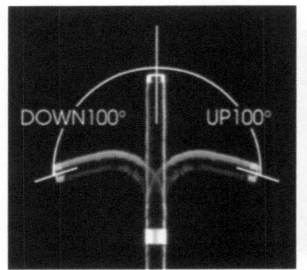

Fig. 20. Bending capacity of the tip

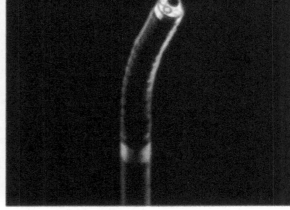

Fig. 21. Detail of the tip

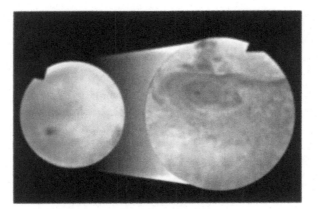

Fig. 22. Clearer and larger picture than previous models

## References

1. Mohri C, Yamadori F (1968) Problem of observing the human ovum descending in the fallopian tube by a tubaloscope. In: Mohri T, Mohri C (eds) Our 25 years experience with endoscope. Japan
2. Hirschowitz (1954) Endoscopic examination of the stomach and duodenal cup with the fiberscope. Lancet 1: 1074-1078
3. Marty R (1987) A propos de la fibrohysteroscopie souple diagnostique et opératoire. Contracept Fertil Sex V(15): 593
4. Marty R (1988) Experience with a new flexible hysteroscope. Int J Gynecol Obstet, 27: 97
5. Marty R (1988) Présentation d'un hystéroscope de la troisième génération: le Fujinon flexible système 2000. Congrès de la Fédération des Gynécologues Obstétriciens Français, 17:54
6. Mussuto P (1993) Les Défis de la flexibilité en hystéroscopie. Ses apports diagnostiques et thérapeutiques en gynécologie obstétrique: des perspectives d'avenir. Thèse pour le Doctorat en Médecine. Faculté de Médecine Broussais-Hôtel-Dieu, PA 060032, p 22
7. Marty R (1996) Flexible Hysteroscopy Instrumentation. In: Isaacson KB (ed) Office Hysteroscopy. Mosby-Year Book, St-Louis (MO), pp 31-33
8. Lin BL, Iwata Y, Valle RF (1994) Clinical application of Lin's forceps in flexible hysteroscopy. J Am Assoc Gynecol Laparosc 1:383-388
9. Marty R (1995) Flexible Hysteroscopy and Targeted Endometrial Biopsies. Syllabus Postgraduate Course 7. AAGL 24th Annual Meeting, Orlando, Florida, pp 24-30
10. Marty R, Uzan M, Carbillon L (1998) A new mini fibrohysteroscope for diagnostic evaluation. International Congress of Gynecologic Endoscopy. Atlanta, Book of Abstracts pp 29-104

# Principles of high frequency surgery

B. Blanc, R. de Montgolfier

## Endogenous effects of the electrical current in biological tissues

Living tissues are electrical conductors. Three endogenous effects can be observed:

- electrolytic effects with continuous current and low frequency alternative currents;
- stimulation of nerves and muscles with low frequency alternative or pulsed currents;
- thermal effects with high frequency alternative currents (HF).

## Thermal effects in HF surgery

### Cutting

Biological tissues can only be cut if tension between the cutting electrode and the selected tissue is high enough so that electrical arcs are produced by concentrating high frequency current on specific areas in the tissues. The temperature produced by the electrical arcs through the tissues is so high that the tissues are immediately destroyed or burnt. A tension crest (Ip) of about 200 Vp is needed to produce an electrical arc between the metallic electrode and the living tissues. Under 200 Vp, no electrical arcs are produced and the tissues cannot be cut. Over 200 Vp, electrical arcs increase proportionally to tension.

High frequency surgical equipments made from semi-conductors have been manufactured since 1970. The only difference in the cutting properties is that the variation of the depth of coagulation is no longer modified by blending a non modulated HF current produced by a vacuum tube and a modulated HF current produced by the discharger, but by adjusting the amplitude and the degree of modulation of the HF current. The traditional technique of applied high frequency surgery implies that the depth of coagulation should not only depend on adjusting the power and degree of modulation but also on the thickness of the electrode and the cutting depth and speed.

The HF surgical units with automatic control circuits have been available since 1985. Control circuits maintain the intensity of electrical arcs and/or the crest value Ip of the outgoing HF tension. Thus, the depth of hemostasis is relatively independent from the frequency and cutting depth.

Cutting biological tissues with a high frequency knife equipped with automatic tension regulation includes the following advantages:

- according to the setting, the cut borders are coagulated at a constant depth;
- adapted electrical cutting electrodes allow the best quality of incision depth and direction;
- with modern electric knives, a constant mode of cutting is provided by automatically controlled electrical arc intensity and/or tension amplitude between the cutting electrode and the tissue. Hemostasis is constant whatever the speed and/or depth of the cutting.

### Coagulation

Biological tissues can only be thermally coagulated if a 70° C temperature is reached. It is impossible to bring thermal energy to tissues so that only the volume to be coagulated will be brought to the required temperature as evenly as possible, without harming the surrounding tissues.

If the electrode is in contact with the selected tissues, tensions over 200 Vp must only be used in exceptional cases that is:

- with relatively small electrodes;
- during a relatively short period of time;
- if important areas have to be coagulated;
- if there are tolerable risks of carbonisation of the tissues to be coagulated.

### Modes of coagulation

Soft coagulation is characterised by the absence of electrical arcs between the electrodes and tissues during all the coagulation process to avoid carbonisation of the surrounding tissues. Soft coagulation is prescribed for all cases for which mono or bipolar electrodes are maintained in contact with the selected sites.

The possibility of regulating and reproducing the depth of soft coagulation increases with the decrease of impedance of the HF generator. An automatic HF generator of tension control is ideal for such uses. Soft coagulation can only be used with optimal efficiency if the process of coagulation is interrupted as soon as steam appears. The same method is used to avoid adhesion effects.

Reinforced coagulation is characterised by the fact that electrical arcs are intentionally generated between the coagulation electrodes and the tissues to obtain a deeper coagulation, rather than soft coagulation produced by using thinner or smaller electrodes. There are risks of carbonisation of the tissues, since tension used for forced coagulation is at least 500 Vp; therefore, this coagulation is only recommended when thin or small electrodes are used to obtain deeper coagulation.

Spray coagulation is characterised by the fact that long enough electronical arcs are intentionally generated, thus making direct contact between the electrode and tissues no longer necessary. Highly modulated HF tensions with crest value of a few KV are used for spray coagulation.

## New developments in hysteroscopy

According to recent literature, endometrial ablation has many advantages over hysterectomy, though hysterectomy rates remain high. Most of the new developments in hysteroscopy tend to improve the safety of current procedures. Excessive intravasation of electrolyte and electrolyte-free solutions are the causes of life-threatening complications. Bipolar systems allowing the use of saline solution, in the different operative treatment modalities for vaginal bleedings due to intracavitary uterine pathological structures, have brought great improvements in avoiding traumatic complications. The saline solution eliminates risks of hyponatremia.

**Gynecare Versapoint,** a bipolar electrosurgical system, is one of such innovative procedures (Fig. 1).

## Gynecare Versapoint 5 Fr bipolar hysteroscopic electrode

It is a single use bipolar microelectrode (1.6 mm OD) connected to a generator by a cable. It can fit into diagnostic hysteroscopes (5 Fr channel).

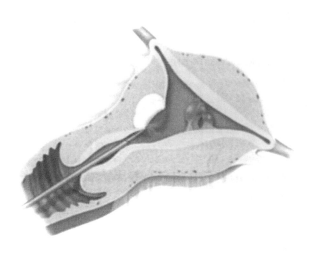

Fig. 1. Versapoint bipolar surgery

The Versapoint electrode is particularly powerful. It combines the resection capabilities of monopolar output with the safety of bipolar energy. Perforation and burning trauma are usually avoided with bipolar electrosurgery.

There are three modes of operation: 1) the vaporization mode with the creation of a "vapor pocket"; the desiccation mode, and the section mode.

Vaporization of tissue allows good visualization and better control, speed and safety of the procedure, as it eliminates resected "chips".

Differently-shaped electrodes are available:
- twizzle electrode for vaporization and needle-like cutting;
- spring electrode for rapid tissue vaporization and desiccation;
- ball electrode for precise tissue vaporization and desiccation.

These electrodes only activate by touching tissues.

As the electrodes are small, dilatation of the cervix and then general anesthesia are no longer required. A local anesthesia or only just premedication may be necessary. The use of isotonic saline eliminates risks of hyponatremia, thus making the procedure applicable to an outpatient department. This technology allows cost-effective diagnosis followed in the same session, if needed, by treatment of benign intrauterine pathologies such as uterine fibroids, polyps, synechia and septa. The procedure is simple and does not rely on the same surgical skills as hysteroscopic procedures.

## Gynecare Versapoint bipolar resectoscopic system

This new instrumentation operates in isotonic solutions. A vaporizing tip electrode can be used in the treatment of intrauterine myomas, polyps, septa and benign conditions requiring endometrial ablation. It uses 24 Fr bipolar resectoscopic vaporizing electrode. With its bipolar energy it can vaporize, cut and desiccate tissues. Instantaneous tissue vaporization eliminates resected chips.

Therefore, this is a new, cheap, easy and safe approach to remove submucous fibroids, polyps and resect intrauterine adhesions and septa.

## References

1. ERBE Principes de la chirurgie haute fréquence. ERBE Elecktromedizin GnbH D-72072 T Bingen, Germany
2. Chin KAJ, Penketh RJA (1998) Clinical evaluation of the Versapoint Bipolar Diathermy for Operative Hysteroscopy. 28th British Congress of Gynaecology, Harrogate, UK, Abstr 330
3. Loffer FD (1998) New developments in Hysteroscopy. ISGE Meeting, Sun City, South Africa, Abstr 112
4. Millan LC, Kerkar R, O'Riordan J, Smith B (1998) Operative outpatient hysteroscopy using the Versapoint system: a preliminary feasibility study of 25 cases. ESGE Meeting, Lausanne, Switzerland
5. Miller CE (1998) Versapoint Bipolar Vaporization System: a Bipolar Micro electrode for Hysteroscopic Surgery using normal Saline as a distension medium. ISGE Meeting, Sun City, South Africa, Abstr 143
6. Miller CE, Davies S, Johnston M (1998) Application of the Versapoint Bipolar Vaporization System for Hysteroscopic Surgery in an Office Setting. AAGL Meeting, Atlanta, USA, Abstr 113
7. Nico JT, Vleugels MPH (1998) Economical outcome of Ambulatory Hysteroscopic Treatment of Myomas with Versapoint. ISGE Meeting, Amsterdam, Netherlands, Abstr 108
8. O'Donovan PJ (1998) Versapoint: Bipolar Diathermy in a saline medium; an overview. ISGE Meeting, Sun City, South Africa, Abstr 26
9. Vleugels MPH (1998) Hysteroscopic Surgery moves from Theatre to Office Procedure by the normal saline field Bipolar Electrosurgery. ISGE Meeting, Sun City, South Africa, Abstr 162
10. Vleugels MPH (1998) A new Bipolar Technology in hysteroscopic treatment of uterine fibroids. ISGE Meeting, Amsterdam, Netherlands

# Office minor operative procedures with the fibrohysteroscope

R. MARTY

Diagnostic hysteroscopy is now the gold standard for the uterine evaluation and office diagnostic hysteroscopy is accepted by the majority of gynecologists. More recently, many physicians all over the world have been practising the techniques of operative office hysteroscopy.

This last step enables the physician to diagnose and treat various pathologies, such as polyps, synechia or small pediculated myomas, to remove foreign bodies and to confirm tubal patency or to discover fallopian tubal blockage (proximal obstruction or polyp).

The numerous advantages of the fibrohysteroscope vs. conventional rigid hysteroscope are related with its four major characteristics: narrowness, bending tip, frontal view and flexibility. These major features make the fibrohysteroscope the most appropriate endoscope for diagnostic evaluation and minor operative procedures performed in office or ambulatory settings.

The gynecologist is looking for the smallest possible instrumentation, which means the lower rate of cervical dilatation, pain and local anesthesia. The physician is also looking for the easiest and most atraumatic progression through the cervical canal, which means the <u>necessity of a permanent adaptation of the hysteroscope to each individual anatomy</u>. The fact that the fibrohysteroscope is always able to be placed in the optimal position for the surgical procedure represents a major advantage over the rigid hysteroscope. In addition, the frontal view of the flexible scope does not require any experience unlike the 30° for oblique view of conventional scopes [1].

It is possible to perform successfully and without risk minor operative procedures in an office setting or on an outpatient basis outside the operating room of a private or public hospital. Apart from targeted endometrial biopsies, the major indications are IUD removal, polypectomy, some synechiolysis, retrieval of product of conception, some small submucous pediculated myoma and fallopian tubal cannulation.

## General protocol

The reader must refer to chapter "Diagnostic evaluation" of this book.

For instrumentation, the fibrohysteroscope has a $\pm$ 5 mm outer diameter with an operating channel of 2.2 or 2.3 mm (Olympus, Fuji, Storz and Circon). The distending media is normal saline 0,9% administered by gravity (refer to chapter "Uterine distention" of this book).

If the decision is taken during a diagnostic evaluation performed with a minifibrohysteroscope (3 mm), it is suitable to switch to an operative fibrohysteroscope (5 mm). Sometimes, it will be necessary to slightly dilate the cervical canal up to 5 mm by plastic sound. This must be explained to the patient and, if she complains, one must proceed to a paracervical block.

There are two eventualities:

– *surgical procedure decided prior to introduce the fibrohysteroscope:* all these patients have already had a vaginal sonography or hysteroscopy. The indications are:

- troublesome IUD;
- suspected polyp;
- suspected myoma;
- suspected synechia;
- retained products of conception;
- tubal proximal blockage.

The choice of the instrumentation must be an operative 5 mm fibrohysteroscope;

– *surgical procedure decided during a diagnostic evaluation:* apart from targeted endometrial biopsy and the removal of very small polyp, it is necessary to use the operative fibrohysteroscope 5 mm, because the ancillary instrumentation is 5-French diameter requiring an operating channel of 2.2 mm. The use of this type of instrumentation allows to perform all the following procedures:

- IUD removal;
- polypectomy;

- some small submucous myomectomy (pediculated);
- synechiolysis;
- removal of retained product of conception;
- tubal exploration and blockage removal.

## Ancillary instrumentation

### Grasping or biopsy forceps (Figs. 1, 2)

There is a great choice of grasping or biopsy forceps manufactured by several factories (Olympus, Fuji, Storz, Wolf and Circon) with a 3-French or a 5-French diameter (refer to chapter "Endometrial biopsy" of this book).

### Snare: Lasso or Basket (Fig. 3)

Various lasso, snare or basket are manufactured by Olympus, Fuji or Circon (5-French diameter).

### Monopolar electrode (Fig. 4)

They can be used with the operative fibrohysteroscope (channel $\geq 2$ mm) and are indicated for electrocoagulation. They are available from Olympus, Storz or Circon. If electrocoagulation is chosen, this is a definite contraindication for the use of an electrolyte containing liquid medium such as saline or lactated Ringer's. One must use $CO_2$ as a distending medium.

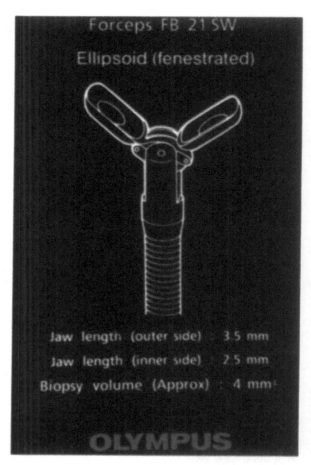

Fig. 1. French biopsy forceps (Olympus)

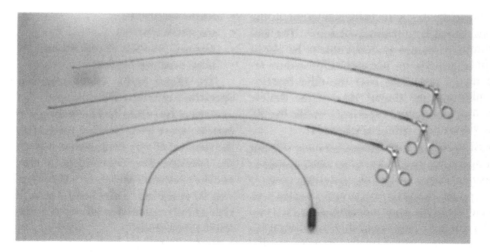

**Fig. 2.** Various flexible biopsy forceps (Storz)

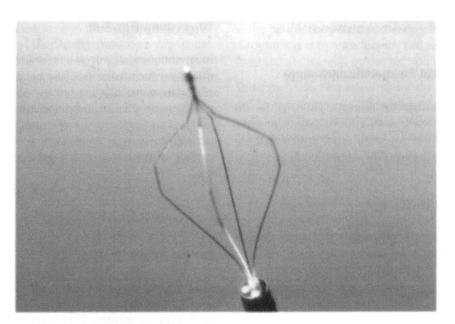

**Fig. 3.** Basket snare 5-French (Olympus)

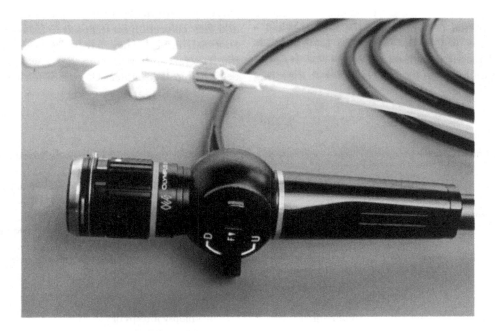

**Fig. 4.** HYF-1T and monopolar electrode

## Bipolar electrode

Circon has recently presented a new instrumentation allowing to perform electrocoagulation in a normal saline distention. This is promising and could be used with the flexible operative hysteroscope [2].

## Specific protocol for specific pathology

It is essential to make the judicious choice of the instrument to be used for each different pathology. Seven different procedures can easily be performed with a fibrohysteroscope in the office (Table 1).

## Targeted endometrial biopsy

This minor operative procedure is easy to perform will all the fibrohysteroscopes having an operating channel greater than 1 mm. The results are good if a protocol is strictly followed (refer to this chapter of this book).

## Removal of IUD

When the IUD is localized, a close investigation of the uterine cavity and walls must be made, looking for a tear or a partial perforation of the uterus. When a perforation is diagnosed, the ablation must be made during a laparoscopic monitoring on a one-day basis hospitalization. When the IUD is localized, the string may be pulled by the surgeon, and if the string is lost, the removal is usually made with a grasping forceps (refer to this special chapter of this book).

## Polypectomy (Figs. 5-8)

Most endometrial polyps are located at the fundus, often near the tubal ostia. They are usually single but, when numerous, may be confused with a diffuse polypoid hypertrophia of the endometrium. Endometrial polyps show various types of histology partly correlated with the surface appearance. A thorough understanding of the histology is helpful in identifying polyps.

There are two kinds of polyps: functional or non functional.

### Functional polyps (mucous)

Most of these patients have no significant symptoms. Some of them have menorrhagia. They represent 36% of all intra outgrowths. They are generally quite small with a 2-10 mm diameter and can have a large pedicule. They grow in various shapes, hemispheric, conical or irregular. The colour depends on the date of the cycle. Sometimes, it is not easy to discover them, because they are made from the glandular epithelium and their coloration corresponds to that of the nearby endometrium [3]. They may be discovered only when the hysteroscopist performs the "low pressure test" described in the chapter "Uterine distention".

Table 1. Minor operative procedures (office hysteroscopy). Protocol average duration: 15 minutes; complication: none

| Procedure | | Instrumentation | Remarks |
|---|---|---|---|
| Polypectomy | • Pediculated<br>• Sessile | Lasso or basket<br>Monopolar electrode | $CO_2$ required |
| IUD removal | • Lost thread<br>• Embedded<br>• Troublesome | Grasping forceps | |
| Synechiolysis | Filmy-mild | Biopsy forceps or<br>monopolar electrode | $CO_2$ required |
| Fallopian tubal cannulation | Intramural portion | Katayama catheter | |
| Submucous myomectomy | Small pediculated | Lasso or basket | |

## Non functional polyps

Most of these patients have abnormal uterine bleeding. They are the most common polyps and their frequency increases between age 35 and 50. Their shapes and sizes are various. Sometimes, when palpated with the tip of the fibrohysteroscope, their consistency looks like fibroma [4]. A vascular pattern may be observed through the thick endometrial surface. Some of them may be very large and may occlude the entire endometrial cavity.

## Cystic Type

They have a short pedicule and a milky appearance contrasting with nearby endometrium. Blood vessels may be seen on the surface. They are fragile and easily broken.

## Glandular hyperplasic Type

They are the most common endometrial polyps. If not large, they have a yellowish red colour, they are smooth and the glandular ostia are clearly seen on the surface. If they grow larger, the ostia become invisible. No blood vessels are present. At the top they often bleed because of the shedding of the epithelium. Surrounding endometrium may be either of hyperplasia pattern or normal. It is the difficult to differentiate them from pediculated myoma, because they are covered with a thin endometrium with a diluted blood vessels network. Sometimes it is also difficult to differentiate the type of polyp (functional or non). They often occur during the menopause.

## Adenomyomatous Type

They are partially composed by myomatous tissue and endometrial elements. They can be as large as 30 mm and usually have a long pedicle; they are yellowish. One can observe in some areas of the surface a yellowish red colour without blood vessels and nearby a yellowish white colour with dilated blood vessels overlying the elevated myomatous area as a submucous myoma. Some of these polyps have abnormal uterine bleeding.

## Various techniques of polypectomy

The removal of polyps requires different techniques, depending on their size, shape and localization.

**Long pedicule.** They are easily removable. The easiest way is the use of a snare. When the fibrohysteroscope is close to the polyp, the snare is withdrawn in the operating channel and pushed until the tip is situated close to the polyp. Then the loop is opened and placed at the base of the polyp, and the pedicule is cut [5, 6]. Another way is to use a forceps and separate the polyp from the uterine wall by pulling and cutting [7].

**Short pedicule.** One must choose the forceps introduced in the operating channel towards the base of the pedicule of the polyp. As soon as in good position, the jaws are closed and the polyp is extracted.

**Sessile polyp.** The best way is to destroy it with a monopolar electrode.

**Large polyp.** The ablation of such a polyp requires the use of a morcellation technique performed through a biopsy forceps. Another way is the coagulation.

**Small polyp located at the cornual area or close to the tubal ostia.** These polyps must be removed because they are often responsible of infertility. They are generally tiny and are easily removed with a biopsy forceps.

**Polypoid endometrial hypertrophia.** In such a case, the patient must have a one-day hospitalization and a curettage must be made under general anesthesia.

After a polypectomy, in all cases it is of major importance to check if the base was totally removed, specially after a morcellation. To avoid recurrencies, it is necessary to make sure of the total destruction of the polyp and eventually to coagulate the base to avoid recurrence [8, 9].

## Submucous myomectomy (Figs. 9, 10)

Some small, pediculated submucous myoma may be removed during office hysteroscopic procedure. They may be less than 1 cm. They are not frequent and may be removed in the same way as a polyp with a forceps, or destroyed by electrocoagulation.

## Synechiolysis

We use the classification of intrauterine adhesions divided in three types: mild, moderate and severe. The grade I is thin and filmy; the grade II is thick, fibromuscular [10], (Fig. 11). Synechiolysis is easy to perform on grade I; one can use an alligator forceps or a biopsy forceps to break the adhesion. For grade II the endoscopist has the choice between a biopsy forceps or monopolar electrode, but this is possible only with

# HYSIOLOGICAL ASPECTS

These photos were made with the 3.5 mm fibrohysteroscope (HYF type P)
The « weft » aspect (« moiré » effect) does not exist anymore with the new 3 mm fibrohysteroscope
(HYF type XP), because the number of optic fibers is increased by 1.6 and they have a smaller diameter.

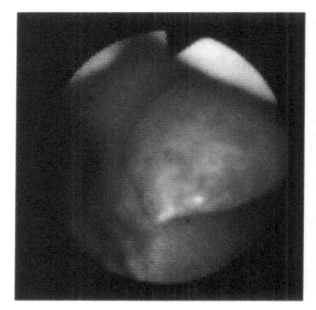

Fig. 5.  Small pediculated endometrial polyp

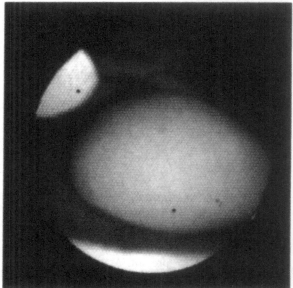

Fig. 6.  Grasping forceps on pediculated polyp

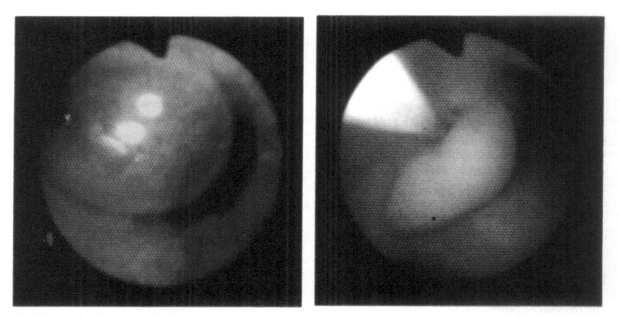

Fig. 7.  Cornual polyp, pediculated

Fig. 8.  Grasping forceps on base of pediculated polyp

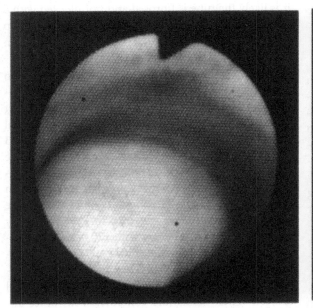

**Fig. 9.** Removable myoma

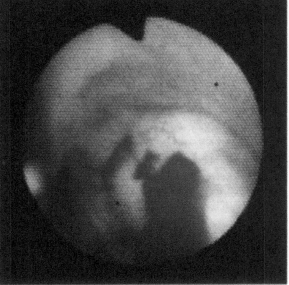

**Fig. 10.** Morcellation of small myoma

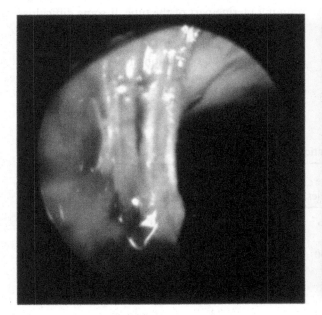

**Fig. 11.** Synechia early grade II

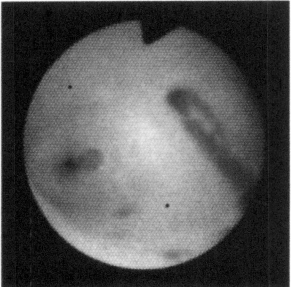

**Fig. 12.** Approach of right tubal ostium

small or focal adhesions. A majority of grade II requires a one-day hospitalization with general anesthesia. The prognosis is good when adhesions are filmy or focal and the reproductive outcome is over 90%.

## Residual tissue after delivery

If it remains a small or focal amount of placental tissue, it is easy to remove it like a polyp, using a grasping forceps or biopsy forceps.

## Tubal cannulation (Figs. 12, 13)

A proximal tubal cornual obstruction may be often suggested by a hysterosalpingography or after the failure of a laparoscopic tubal cannulation. If a fluoroscopic tubal cannulation is unsuccessful, it leads to perform a hysteroscopic cannulation. If a hysterosalpingography shows a blockage of one or two tubal ostia, the gynecologist must eliminate a temporary spasm; for that purpose, he must administer during the procedure an antispasmodic or Trinitrin 4% per os. It is also recommended to perform a second hysterosalpingography to confirm the obstruction. If this fails, the patient must be referred for a hysteroscopic cannulation, and in case the hysteroscopic repermeabilization is also unsuccessful, the patient must have microsurgery for tubal reconstruction or may be referred for IVF.

## Protocol

Such a patient must receive antibiotherapy per os the day before and after the procedure, which never requires local anesthesia. The ideal endoscope is the HYF-1T (4.9 mm), because it has a 2.2 mm outer diameter operating channel admitting easily a coaxial system to be inserted. When the tip of the fibroscope is correctly placed in front and close to the tubal ostia, the brake is activated to freeze this ideal position. The Katamaya 3-French catheter (Cook) (Fig. 14) with its guidewire is introduced directly into the 2.2 mm operating channel; when the catheter is on the outside of the tip of the fibroscope, it is easily advanced into the fallopian tube. Then, the Katayama catheter is introduced into the interstitial portion of the tube. If the guidewire cannot be advanced into the fallopian tube, it is likely the tube is fibrosed and not blocked with a plug. In such a circumstance, the procedure must stop and the patient should be referred to a microsurgeon for IVF.

As usual, we monitor all the procedures on a video screen which helps the assistant to follow the operation and acts as a diversion for the patient. In a short personal serie of 13 patients, with a bilateral cornual obstruction (10 after a hysterosalpingography and 3 after a fluoroscopic tubal cannulation), the procedure never required any local anesthesia and was well tolerated. No complication occurred. We succeeded in reopening the tube in 11 patients (rate 84,6%). These results are close to those obtained by Valle [11] or by Gimpelson [12]. In a review with 120 cases with a bilateral cornual obstruction, Burke obtained 96 postoperative patencies (80%). They had one complication: a single cornual perforation with the tubal catheter. Their results are compared with other authors in Table 2.

This procedure is very useful to eliminate a plug or for the lysis of some very proximal tubal adhesions; however, the gynecologist must work only in the intramural uterine part of the tube. If some difficulties happen, it is possible to perform a falloposcopy (refer to the chapter in this book).

To conclude, the evolution of the treatment of tubal cornual occlusion may be resumed in the decisional chart (Table 3).

**Table 2.** Comparative results of hysteroscopic tubal cannulation (%)

| Marty (Flexible) | Gimpelson (Flexible) | Valle (Rigid & Flexible) | Burker (Flexible) | |
|---|---|---|---|---|
| 84.6 | 87 | 70.9 | 80 | Recanalization rate |
| 46.4 | – | 45-50 | 50 | Pregnancy rate |
| 0 | – | 8 | 4 | Ectopic pregnancy |
| 18.1 | 40 | 20-30 | 13 | Reocclusion |

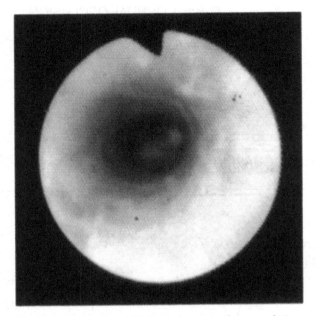

**Fig. 13.** Interstitial part of left tubal ostium after cannulation

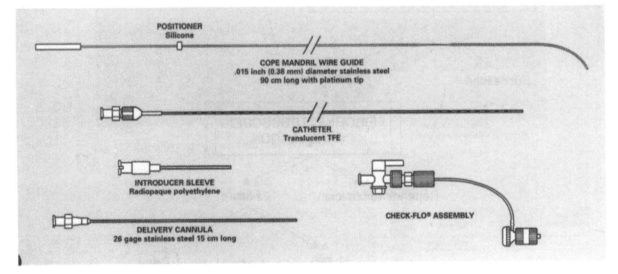

**Fig. 14.** Katayama catheter (3-French, Cook)

**Table** 3. Decisional chart for managing tubal cornual occlusion

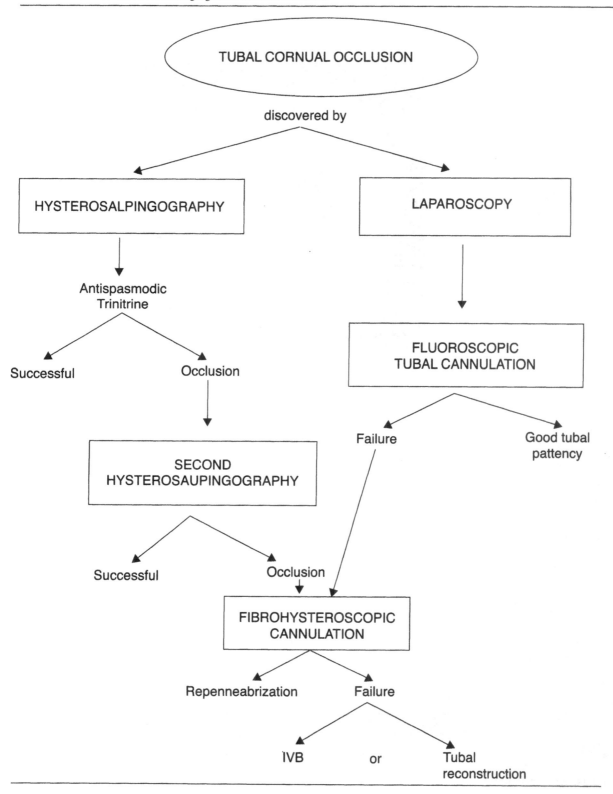

## Personal data

Among our private patients during the past two years we have selected N = 125 patients who had a minor operative procedure on an outpatient basis without anesthesia. One third had a polypectomy, another third had IUD removal and the last third had synechiolysis, fallopian tubal cannulation or submucous myomectomy [13].

The average duration of these procedures was fifteen minutes. We did not observe any complication and the procedure was well tolerated (Table 4).

**Table 4.** Minor operative procedures (outpatient basis; average duration: 15 min; complication: none)

| Procedure | Patients | % |
|---|---|---|
| Polypectomy | 47 | 37.60 |
| IUD removal | 39 | 31.20 |
| Synechiolysis (mild) | 18 | 14.40 |
| Fallopian tube cannulation | 13 | 10.40 |
| Submucous myomectomy (small pediculated) | 8 | 6.40 |
| Total | 125 | |

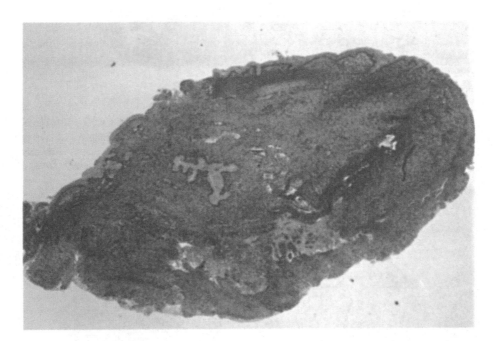

**Fig. 15.** Pathology of endocervical polypectomy

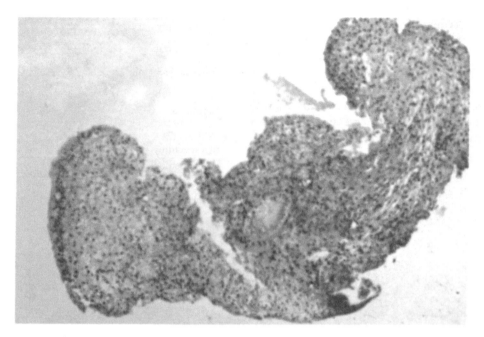

Fig. 16.  Pathology of endometrial polypectomy

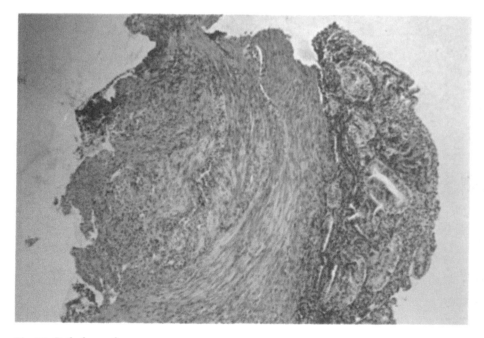

Fig. 17.  Pathology of myoma

## Conclusion

Minor operative procedures in an office setting can be performed only when the surgeon is an experienced hysteroscopist. The physician must have a good practice of therapeutic hysteroscopy in the operating room. The protocol must be adjusted to each individual pathology and these procedures are performed under videomonitoring. The patient is involved, observing the screen and listening to the surgeon's explanations. A complete selection of ancillary instrumentation must be available and perfect sterile conditions must be respected. A judicious selection of the patients is made in order to decide if a paracervical block is necessary.

In our extensive French experience of such operative office hysteroscopy, we never had any major complication, but sometimes a slight bleeding may occur or mild cramps are reported by the patient during the procedure.

If the gynecologist avoids to be too much self confident, this type of surgery is safe for the patient and is time and cost saving for both of them.

## References

1. Marty R (1993) Flexible Office Hysteroscopy. Book of Memories, pp 11-12, Congreso Multidisciplinario de Endoscopia, Mexico
2. O'Donovan PJ (1998) Versapoint: Bipolar diathermy in a saline medium: an overview. Book of Abstracts, 7th Annual Meeting of the International Society for Gynecologic Endoscopy, Sun City, South Africa, pp 0-026
3. Sugimoto O (1978) Endometrial polyp. In: Sugimoto O (ed) Diagnostic and Therapeutic Hysteroscopy. Igaku-Shoin, Tokyo, pp 114-115
4. Marty R (1996) Nine Years of Experience with Flexible Hysteroscopy. In: Isaacson KB (ed) Office Hysteroscopy. Mosby-Year Book, St-Louis, Missouri, p 63
5. Lin BL, Iwada Y, Mizuhara H, Ebihara T, Miyamoto N, Sakakura K, Soyama Y, Seki K, Makino T (1991) Trial Study on Endometrial polypectomy by newly developed snare under flexible hysteroscopy. Acta Obst Gynecol Jap 43(12):1728-1730
6. Lin BL, Iwata Y, Liu KH, Valle RF (1990) Clinical applications of a new Fujinon operating fiberoptic hysteroscope. J Gynecol Surg 6:81
7. Valle RF (1997) Therapeutic Hysteroscopy. In: Valle RF (ed) A Manual of Clinical Hysteroscopy. Parthenon Publishing Group, New York, London, p 56
8. Gimpelson RJ (1996) Techniques for operative office hysteroscopy. In: Isaacson KB (ed) Office Hysteroscopy. Mosby-Year Book, St-Louis, Missouri, p 104
9. Marty R, Valle RF (1995) Eight Years' Experience performing procedures with flexible hysteroscopes. J Am Assoc Gynecol Laparosc 3(1)
10. Valle RF, Sciarra JJ (1984) Hysteroscopic Treatment of Intrauterine Adhesions. In: Siegler AM, Lindemann HJ (eds) Hysteroscopy Principles and Practice. Lippincott, Philadelphia, p 195
11. Valle RF (1997) Therapeutic Hysteroscopy. In: Valle RF (ed) A Manual of Clinical Hysteroscopy. Parthenon Publishing Group, New York, London, p 73
12. Gimpelson RJ (1996) Techniques for operative office hysteroscopy. In: (see ref 8) Office Hysteroscopy. Mosby-Year Book, St-Louis, Missouri, p 107
13. Marty R (1998) A French Experience of 10 Years practising Fibrohysteroscopy Diagnostic and Therapeutic. Book of Abstracts, 7th Annual Meeting of the International Society for Gynecologic Endoscopy, Sun City, South Africa, pp 0-048

# Hysteroscopy and IUD

R. Marty

Normally IUD deserves a regular six months checking by the gynecologist. When it becomes troublesome, the most efficient way to treat the complications is to performa hysteroscopic evaluation. In patients complaining with pelvic pain, menorrhagia or metrorrhagia, sometimes amenorrhea, the hysteroscope is the best tool to detect an endometritis, to reveal a coexistant uterine pregnancy or to suspect an extrauterine pregnancy. Hysteroscopy is also the best way to look for an occult IUD, to locate the device and eventually to remove it safely when the tail or threads are invisible or not palpable.

Ultrasound and hysterography can be performed to aid in the search of the occult IUD, but hysteroscopy enables to detect and remove simultaneously the device; sometimes, it is necessary to associate a laparoscopy.

A small chapter will be dedicated to the opportunity of performing systematically a hysteroscopy prior to the insertion of an IUD.

## IUD removal after hysteroscopic surgery

After specific intrauterine surgery performed hysteroscopically, it is necessary to have a second look. After synechiolysis, many authors deliver oestrogen postoperatively to promote endometrial regeneration and insert an IUD to avoid the formation of secondary adhesion [1]. After some large myomectomy or sometimes after hysteroscopic metroplasty, authors recommend to insert an IUD to be removed after healing in order to avoid formation of postoperative adhesions.

Hysteroscopy must be performed to remove the IUD left in place, but also to check the uterine cavity shape and scars and to evaluate the endometrial lining. This can be easy performed during an office procedure without anesthesia.

## Disappearance of the threads or tail

This happens when the thread has raised inside the cervical canal and may be retracted inside the uterine cavity. The tail may also be lost from the device when pulling for ablation (Table 1). In such a circumstance, a vaginal ultrasound must be performed to check the presence of the IUD and to see if it remains in a correct position to be effective. If so, the IUD may be left in place and removed only when its time duration is over. Furthermore, sonography allows to see if the device is not fractured and if it has not penetrated the uterine wall or perfored it. The risk of a perforation varies, according to the different authors, from 0.1 to 8.7% [2].

## Various protocols

### First protocol: forceps

It can be used a Novak cannula a Bengolea or a grasping forceps, or a specially designed forceps for retrieval. This is a half-blind procedure.

### Second protocol: brush

The use of a cylindrical brush is sometimes indicated when the firt protocol has failed. A trial was conducted on N = 27 patients referred after a failed attempt of IUD removal using either a hook or a clamp. The brush was introduced in the cervical canal until the device was extracted by a rotating movement. Twenty-seven women whose IUD could not be removed from the uterine cavity because of an indiscernible string, were referred for a trial of IUD removal. All patients had used a plastic, copper-releasing IUD. Before admission, they had undergone an attempt of IUD removal by their physician using either a hook or clamp.

In N = 24 patients the removal was possible using the cylindrical brush to view the string. In three cases it was necessary to perform a hysteroscopy in which two no-string were founded. The cylindrical brush can be used safely as an adjunct to remove an IUD

**Table 1.** hysteroscopic procedure for last or torn IUD thread

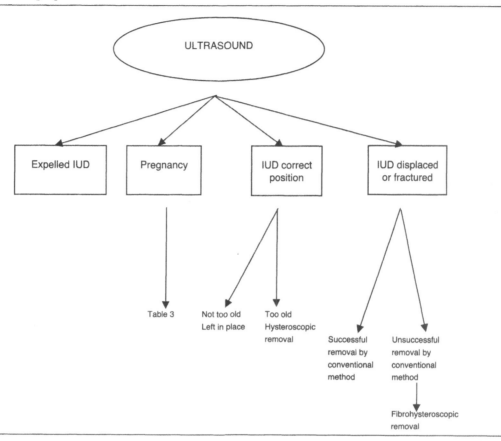

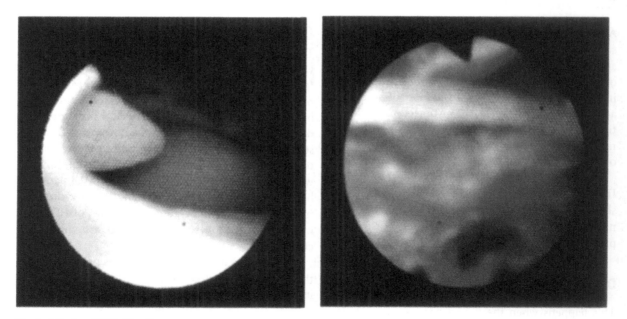

**Fig. 1.** Misplaced IUD (detail)          **Fig. 2.** Thread inside uterine cavity

and is a simple method that may be performed before another invasive procedure is attempted [3].

## Third protocol: hysteroscopic removal

The best period is during the proliferative phase of the cycle because the cervical canal is open and the endometrium is thin. This is an office procedure performed without anesthesia. The endoscope approach is atraumatic and safe [4, 5]. The close investigation of the uterine walls seeks for their possible tearing or perforation and/or inflammatory reaction limited to the presence of the foreign body [6]. The hysteroscope allows to check the whole surface of the device and eventually to evaluate the degree of embedding in the depth of endometrium.

When this assessment is achieved, the removal is generally easy to perform. Sometimes, the fibrohysteroscope is used for the bending capacity of the tip to hook the device. Sometimes, it is necessary to use a biopsy forceps introduced through the operating channel to pull the threads out or to grasp the device and extract it. If the IUD is embedded in the endometrium, the procedure requires a local anesthesia to have a painless removal. An hysteroscopy must also be performed when excessive resistance exists to the removal of an IUD, because this could be caused by a partial uterine perforation. In such a condition, a decision may be made concerning the need for a laparoscopic control (Table 2).

In a series of N = 45 patients with misplaced intrauterine devices (30 extrauterine and 15 intrauterine), only those patients with intrauterine misplacements, in whom conventional blind removal was not possible, were included in the study. All of the 15 misplaced IUD could be removed hysteroscopically. Twenty-two of the 30 extrauterine misplaced devices (73%) could be removed laparoscopically. One patient required both laparoscopy and hysteroscopy. Only 7 (15,5%) of 45 patients required laparotomy for safe removal of misplaced devices. Considerable comfort and minimal hospital stay associated with endoscopic procedures should make these as the first line attempt to remove a misplaced intrauterine or extrauterine translocated device [7].

## IUD associated with pain or menometrorrhagia

For these symptomatic patients it is mandatory to perform an endoscopic control of the uterine cavity and to look for an inflammatory reaction, particularly in the endometrial bed of the device and close to it (refer to the chapter "Endometrial Biopsy" of this book); the rest of the endometrial lining remains normal.

**Table 2.** Hysteroscopic procedure for excessive resistance to IUD removal

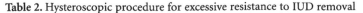
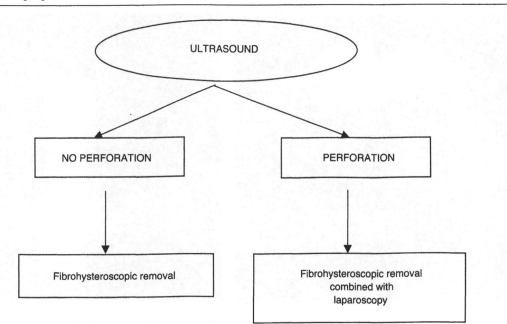

# HYSTEROSCOPY AND IUD

These photos were made with the 3.5 mm fibrohysteroscope (HYF type P)
The « weft » aspect (« moiré » effect) does not exist anymore with the new 3 mm fibrohysteroscope (HYF type XP), because the number of optic fibers is increased by 1.6 and they have a smaller diameter.
Figures des pages 4, 5 et 10

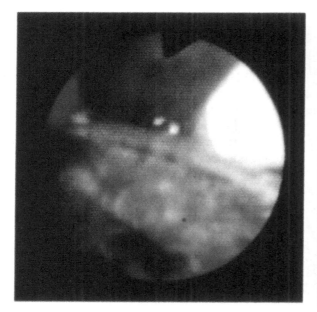

**Fig. 3.** Misplaced IUD + thread inside uterine cavity

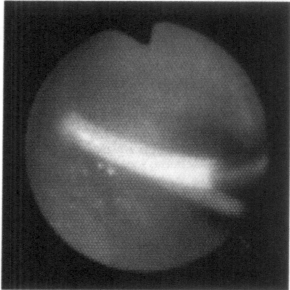

**Fig. 4.** Misplaced gravigarde with tip inside the left tubal ostium

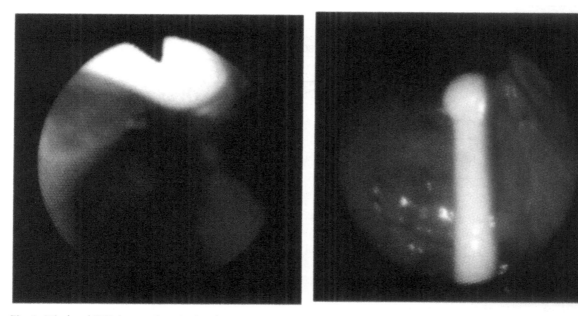

**Fig. 5.** Misplaced IUD (copper junction) + clots

**Fig. 6.** Tip of IUD inserted in left tubal ostium

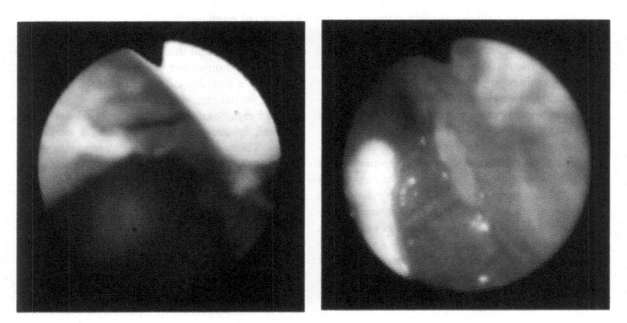

**Fig. 6, 7.** IUD and endometritis

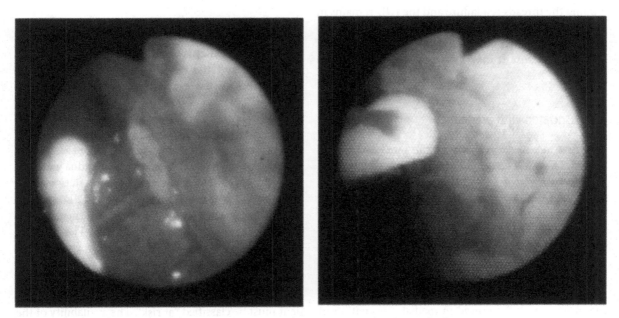

**Fig. 8.** IUD and vascular network reaction

**Fig. 9.** Misplaced IUD tilted

Another complication is acute endometritis [8] early after the placement or later. In such a case, the IUD is removed by hysteroscopy. At the same time, the endoscopist observes a red endometrial lining with hypervascularization. A culture of the device must be made looking for the responsible germ.

In the chronical endometritis the basal layer is infected and reinfects the functional layer each month. In the biopsy, the pathologist often observes a high rate of plasmocyte. Sometimes he may detect Actinomyce, which are usually found in the normal flora of digestive tract. The local action of the IUD allows this colonisation of the endometrium. The macroscopic hysteroscopic aspect shows a red endometrial lining with hypervascularization and subechelial vessels and sometimes small cystic elevation.

Because of these possible infectious complications, IUD have sometimes a negative reputation, but various authors spoke in favour of the choice of this method of contraception [9, 10]. In the patient with abnormal uterine bleeding, the reason may be the presence of a pathological growth, such as a myoma, a polyp or an endometrial hyperplasia. This means that a hysteroscopic evaluation of the uterine cavity must always be performed to look for a possible coexistant pathology with the IUD.

## Excessive resistance for removal with visible thread

Sometimes the threads are visible and when the gynecologist trys to remove the IUD by pulling the threads, he detects an excessive resistance; sometimes, pulling the threads is a failure and the IUD remains in place (Table 2). In all these circumstances, it is necessary to perform an ultrasound before the removal of the IUD, because it may have perforated the uterine wall.

## IUD associated with pregnancy

The first manifestation may be the retraction of the thread. In such a circumstance, IUD extraction is advisable to avoid a septic abortion. Few series have been published. Wagner [11] reported the results after the removal of IUDs from 18 pregnant women under hysteroscopic control, and in 14 patients the pregnancies remained intact (77%). Valle [12] described 12 patients undergoing this procedure: 8 carried the pregnancy uneventfully to term (67%); 2 aborted spontaneously, and 2; developed significant bleeding during the procedure and required immediate evacuation of the products of conception [12].

Martenne-Duplan [13] reported a short series of N = 8 patients with a desired pregnancy. In 6 patients, the IUD was removed with one abortion and 5 made term deliveries. In 2 patients the IUD was left in place, the pregnancy was normal and the patient had a normal term delivery (rate 87%).

In a large serie of 310 patients [14] having troublesome IUD, 52 out of 115 presenting tail retraction had the tail eased out through the cervix and the IUD left in place. In the other 63 patients discrepancies between the size and shape of the uterus and the IUD were observed only rarely when the displacement was caused by a pathological modification or malformation. In 96 patients, the tail was torn off during attempted extraction and in 42 patients the device was removed, hysteroscopically followed by a suction curettage. Thirty-seven persons had several side effects from the IUD. The remaining patients of the group had stringle uterine devices.

Our French experience is a short serie of N = 11 pregnant women with an IUD [15]. In all the cases we used a fibrohysteroscope (4.9 mm) Olympus and a flexible grasping forceps. In 7 (64%) patients we succeeded to remove the device and they all had a normal term delivery. In 2 patients it was not possible to remove the IUD, but both patients delivered at term after a normal pregnancy. In 2 patients the ablation of the IUD was followed by a subsequent spontaneous abortion (19%).

## Protocol

As a first step, an ultrasound must be performed. (Table 3).

a) If the pregnancy is not desired, an abortion is performed and the device is removed at the same time before the evacuation by suction curettage [16].

b) The pregnancy is desired, or induced abortion refused: the patient must be aware of a possible immediate or delayed abortion. In some cases, when the IUD is located beneath the decidua near the nidation or if it is covered by the gestational sac, abortion is unavoidable. After the IUD ablation with pregnancy left in place, the subsequent abortion rate varies between 20 to 30%. The rate of a subsequent abortion when the IUD cannot be removed varies between 45 to 65%.

If the pregnancy goes on, the obstetrician must look for a possible intrauterine infection and this patient must be classified "at risk". The availability of the new minifibrohysteroscope (3 mms) to perform these

**Table 3.** Hysteroscopic procedure during pregnancy

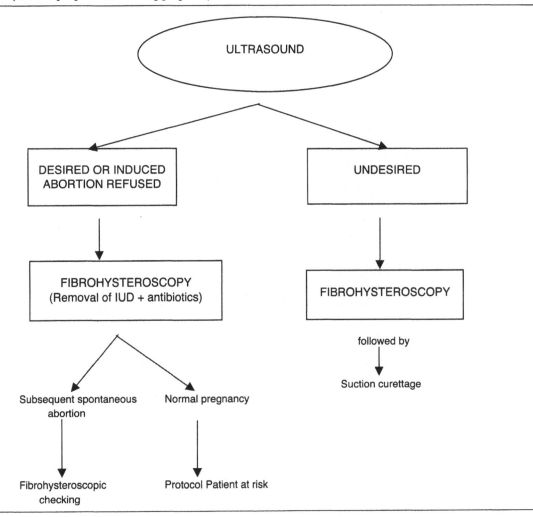

delicate ablations during pregnancy leads us to believe that the prognosis will be better.

## Indications of hysteroscopy before inserting IUD

### Systematic indications

The following indications are obvious:
- previous recent gynecologic infections;
- previous uterine surgery such as:
  • cesarean section
  • myomectomy
  • synechiolysis
  • Uteroplasty
- previous unexplained spotting or menometror-rhagia;

- existence of a myoma;
- previous ablation of a troublesome IUD.

## Is routine hysteroscopy justified before IUD insertion?

We have published in 1984 [17] a data N = 202 in which we observed that at least 6% of the IUD complications were predictable as a consequence of a pre-existing uterine disease. We also demonstrated (N = 80) that the uterine cavity, after 30 months of exposure to an IUD showed no significant changes in the endometrium and did not affect the basal endometrial rayer.

More recently, in our University Hospital, we have conducted 2 new studies [18]. In a first serie (A) N =

# SERIE A

Table 4.

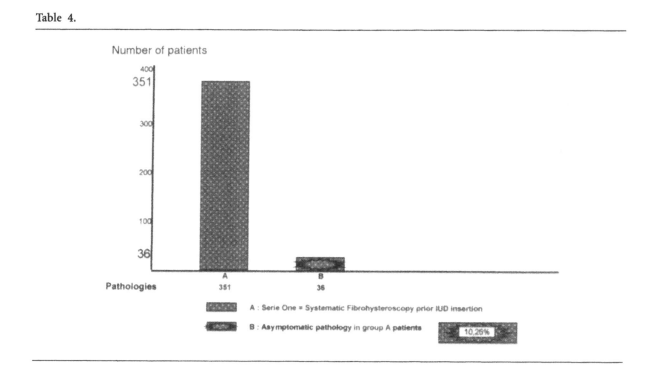

Number of patients

A : Serie One = Systematic Fibrohysteroscopy prior IUD insertion

B : Asymptomatic pathology in group A patients    10,26%

Table 5.

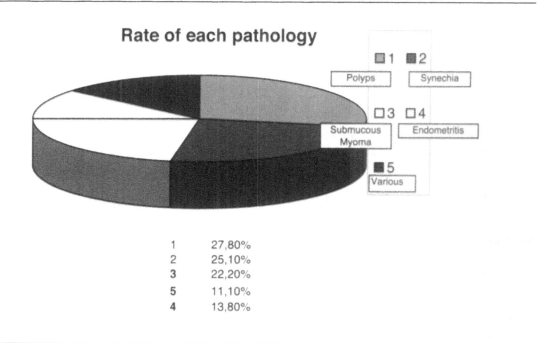

## Rate of each pathology

| ■1 | ■2 |
| Polyps | Synechia |

| □3 | □4 |
| Submucous Myoma | Endometritis |

| ■5 |
| Various |

| 1 | 27,80% |
| 2 | 25,10% |
| 3 | 22,20% |
| 5 | 11,10% |
| 4 | 13,80% |

**Table 6.**

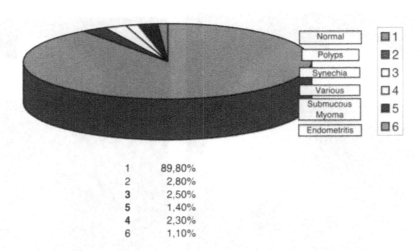

## Repartition on overall patients

| | |
|---|---|
| 1 | 89,80% |
| 2 | 2,80% |
| 3 | 2,50% |
| 5 | 1,40% |
| 4 | 2,30% |
| 6 | 1,10% |

# SERIE C

**Table 7.**

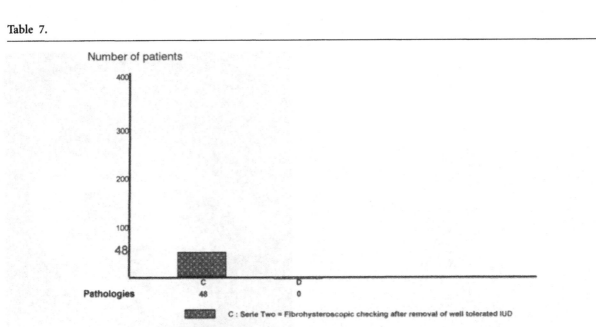

Number of patients

Pathologies    48    0

C : Serie Two = Fibrohysteroscopic checking after removal of well tolerated IUD

D : Pathological findings in C patients (0%)

# HYSTEROSCOPY AND IUD

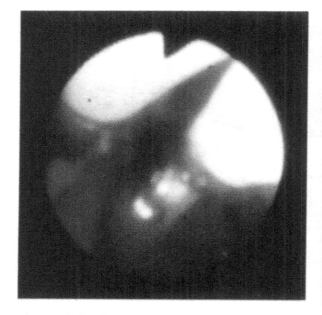

**Fig. 10.** Misplaced IUD + grasping forceps

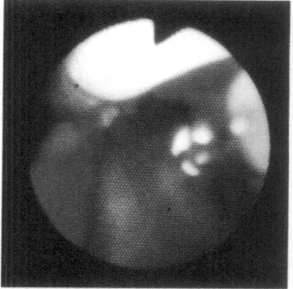

**Fig. 11.** Misplaced IUD (retrieval forceps)

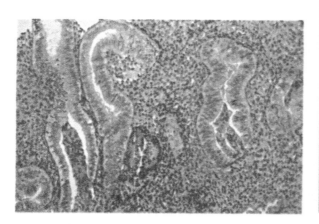

**Fig. 12.** Endometrial reaction over IUD

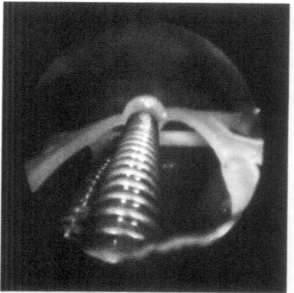

**Fig. 13.** Two IUDs in one uterine cavity

351, these symptomatic patients had a systematic fibrohysteroscopy prior to IUD insertion (Table 4). We have founded a pathology in 36 cases (B) (rate 10,26%). Tables 5 and 6 show the detailed pathology: the most frequent findings were respectively polyps, synechia and submucous myoma.

In a second serie (C) we have performed a hysteroscopic diagnostic evaluation of the uterine cavity (N = 48) during the scheduled removal of well tolerated IUD. In this series, we did not find any pathology (0%) (Table 7).

These results can be correlated with our previous findings; they suggest that a majority of troublesome IUD comes from an asymptomatic pathology. Following this prevention procedure, we have observed a significant decrease of complications with the IUDs as compared with our previous rate before the preventive protocol.

Hysteroscopy is the ideal instrumentation to be used for the treatment of IUDs complications. The first step must generally be an ultrasound examination to confirm the presence of the device, to look for a possible pregnancy, to diagnose fractional IUD and to detect a partial uterine perforation. The second step is therapeutic in the removal of the IUD by hysteroscopy. This approach is atraumatic and safe. Most of the time, this can be done during an office procedure without anesthesia with a flexible hysteroscope; sometimes the ablation will require a local or general anesthesia if combined with a laparoscopic monitoring. If a pregnancy is discovered, the IUD must be removed hysteroscopically if possible. In such a condition, it seems very appropriate to preview a one day hospitalization in order to face an immediate abortion or significant bleeding. Since minihysteroscopes now available permit a good observation of the pregnancy and easy removal of the device with a minimal trauma, we prefer the use of a fibrohysteroscope.

## References

1. March CH, Israël R (1987) Hysteroscopic Management of recurrent abortion caused by septuate uterus. Am J Obstet Gynecol 156:834

2. Blanc B, Boubli L (1996) Endoscopie Uterine. Pradel, p 64

3. Ben Rafael Z, Bilder D (1996) A New Procedure for removal of a «lost» intrauterine device. Obstet Gynecol 87:785-786

4. Valle RF, Freeman DW (1975) Hysteroscopy in the management of the "lost" intrauterine device. Advances Planned Parenthood 10:164

5. Valle RF, Sciarra JJ, Freeman DW (1977) Hysteroscopic removal of intrauterine devices with missing filaments. Obstet Gynecol 49:55

6. Mussuto P (1993) Les défis de la flexibilité en hystéroscopie. Ses apports diagnostiques et thérapeutiques en gynécologie obstétrique: des perspectives d'avenir. Thèse pour le Doctorat en Medecine, Faculté de Médecine Broussais-Hôtel-Dieu, 4.1.2.12 pp 50-51, 060032

7. Mittal S, Kumar S, Roy KK (1996) Role of endoscopy in retrieval of misplaced intrauterine device. Aust NZ J Obstet Gynecol 36:49-51

8. Parent B (1996) Endomètre sous contraception orale et DIU. Gynécologie Obstétrique Pratique 76:1

9. David A, Grimes MD (1992) The intrauterine device, pelvic inflammatory disease and fertility: the confusion between hypothesia and knowledge. Fertil Steril 58:670-673

10. Bernard-Huynh (1993) Abstract Gynecol 105:7

11. Wagner H (1983) Diagnosis and Treatment of complications of intrauterine devices. In: van der Pas H, Herendael BJ, Lith DAF, Keith LG (eds) Hysteroscopy. MTP Press Ltd, Boston, p 185

12. Valle RF, Siegler AM (1988) Therapeutic Hysteroscopic Procedures. Fertility and Sterility, p 692

13. Martenne-Duplan J (1993) Hystéroscopie diagnostique et contraception par DIU. Gynécologie 1(7-8):388-390

14. Lueken RP (1984) Management of the lost Intrauterine Device with hysteroscopy. In: Siegler AM, Lindemann HJ (eds) Hysteroscopy Principles and Practice. JB Lippincott, Philadelphia, pp 227-228

15. Marty R (1996) Our French experience in a short serie of N = 11. (unpublished)

16. Lueken RP, Lindemann HJ (1979) Problems with IUD's. Use of Hysteroscopy. Proceedings of the First National Congress in Gynecology and Obstetrics, (14):16

17. Marty R (1984) Carbon dioxide hysteroscopy without anesthesia in 478 patients. In: Siegler AM, Lindemann HJ (eds) Hysteroscopy Principles and Practice. JB Lippincott, Philadelphia pp 48-49

18. Marty R (1997) Unpublished data

# Office and operative hysteroscopy on one day basis

B.-L. LIN

The most difficult procedure to perform during a hysteroscopy is the insertion of the hysteroscope through the narrow cervical cannel and into the uterine cavity for the diagnosis or treatment of intrauterine lesions. As the uterine cavity is curved, instead of using a straight rigid hysteroscope, it is more reasonable to introduce a flexible hysteroscope for intrauterine manipulations [1]. From 1983 to October 1999, 10149 cases of diagnostic hysteroscopy (8328 cases with flexible hysteroscopy and 1821 cases with rigid hysteroscopy) were performed in our hospital. I performed approximately 98% of these cases. From 1985 to October 1999, I carried out 1517 cases of resectoscopic operations, including 1020 resectoscopic myomectomy and 121 cases of resectoscopic metroplasty. Here I will introduce flexible hysteroscopy, a procedure now commonly performed in Japanese offices.

## Instrumentation

### Flexible diagnostic hysteroscope

The following two scopes can be used without tenaculum, cervical dilation and analgesia or anesthesia.
1) *Fujinon Soft and Rigid Flexible Diagnostic Hysteroscope* (outer diameter 3.7 mm) [2].
   This scope which I developed with the support of Fuji Photo Optical company in 1985 is composed of three sections in its functional portion: a soft, flexible front; a rigid middle, and a soft rear. The scope has a panoramic visual angle of 90° in air, 65° in 10% glucose, and an irrigation channel of 1 mm. The bending capacity is 100° up and 90° down. Because of the rigid middle section, the scope can be manipulated and inserted easily into the uterine cavity.
2) *Olympus New Flexible Diagnostic Hysteroscope* (outer diameter 3.1 mm)
   In 1998, I developed this new scope with Olympus Optical company. Its working portion is composed of soft material only. However, the consistency of the soft portion is firm enough to allow for an easy insertion of the scope. The scope has a panoramic visual angle of 100° and an irrigation channel of 1.2 mm. The bending capacity is 100° up and down. The resolution of the image is sharper due to the increased number of optic fibers. The scope can be changed into a continuous flow system when equipped with Lin's Outer Sheath.

### Flexible operating hysteroscope

If it is necessary to perform a direct intrauterine manipulation after using the aforementioned scopes, the following flexible operating hysteroscopes are generally used without tenaculum, cervical dilation and anesthesia.

### Fujinon soft and rigid operating flexible hysteroscope (outer diameter 4.9 mm) [3]

I developed this scope with Fuji Photo Optical company in 1987 and it was remodelled in 1995 to increase its functions. The functional part of the telescope consists of three sections: a soft, flexible, front section; a rigid rotating middle section, and a semirigid, self-retaining rear section. The scope has a 2.2 mm operating channel, a panoramic visual angle of 120° and its tip has the ability to be flexed 100° upward and downward. All these features, together with the 180° rotational ability of the rigid section, allow for easy maneuvering in all directions inside the uterine cavity.

### Olympus operating flexible hysteroscope (outer diameter 4.9 mm)

The scope has a soft working portion, a panoramic visual angle of 120°, a 2.2 mm operating channel and a bending capacity of 120° upwards and downwards. Lin's giant forceps were designed for this scope, significantly increasing its operating ability.

## Lin's giant forceps [4]

The conventional flexible biopsy forceps is too small to obtain a sufficient specimen for establishing an exact pathologic diagnosis. The grasping forceps, which is also very small, sometimes cannot directly hold a lost intrauterine device (IUD) whose thread is not present or is broken. To solve these problems and to increase the operating ability of the small caliber flexible operating hysteroscope, I developed Lin's giant biopsy forceps, grasping forceps and scissors forceps with the support of Olympus Optical company. Their clinical applications include: 1) directed biopsies, 2) the removal of lost IUDs, and 3) the cutting of intrauterine adhesions. These procedures can be usually performed without tenaculum, cervical dilation, anesthesia and/or analgesia.

## Lin's outer sheaths for a continuous flow system and easy operation of the scope [5]

In addition to the problem of insertion, another problem the hysteroscopist often encounters is the unclear visual field caused by intrauterine bleeding or other floating materials. This can lead to a failed hysteroscopic diagnosis. A continuous flow system, which is already available for rigid hysteroscope, is the only solution to this problem. With Olympus Optical Company I designed in 1997, several kinds of Lin's outer sheath (Fig. 1) for a continuous flow system of either flexible

diagnostic hysteroscopy or operating hysteroscopy. There are two functions which caracterize outer sheaths: first, they allow for a continuous flow system, and second, they increase the rigidity of the shaft in a soft hysteroscope for easy insertion, holding and controlling of the scope. The sheaths can be divided into two types according to their consistency. One is a soft outer sheath, which I often use, and the other is a hard outer sheath. When equipped with a hard outer sheath, the flexible hysteroscope acts like a rigid scope that can be forced to approach an intrauterine target. If needed, the scope can be advanced further through the outer sheath for observation. With a continuous flow system, hysteroscopic intrauterine diagnoses are possible during intrauterine bleeding, but not with heavy bleeding. From 1997 to 1998, I experienced more than 1000 cases of flexible diagnostic hysteroscopy of continuous flow system also without using tenaculum, cervical dilation and analgesia or anesthesia.

## Media

Most doctors in Japan use a fluid medium instead of carbon dioxide for hysteroscopies. I prefer using a 10% glucose solution for uterine distention. Its 500 ml plastic bag is suspended approximately 80 cm above the patient. The pressure cuff is applied if the pressure is required. When bleeding was encountered in our study of blood dilution tests [6], the visual clarity of the scopes with 10% glucose was greater than that of scopes with normal saline. Intrauterine cytological examination immediately after hysteroscopic procedure should be avoided because cell chromatin can be changed by the high osmolarity of the 10% glucose solution. However, this will not affect tissue pathology.

## Techniques

### Flexible diagnostic hysteroscopy

From March 1997, all diagnostic hysteroscopic procedures have been performed in continuous flow systems. Prior to insertion, Lin's soft outer sheath (outer diameter 4.1 mm) is used with the scope. The tip of the sheath is fixed to 2 cm behind the tip of the flexible scope. Thus, the irrigating fluid flows out of the uterine cavity through the space between the scope and the sheath.

The hysteroscopic procedure is as follows. The pelvic examination is carried out to confirm the size

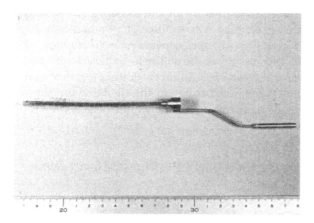

Fig. 1. Lin's outer sheath (outer diameter 4.1 mm)

and position of the uterus. A speculum is used to expose the cervix; cervical mucous is removed with a 2 ml syringe for the study of ferning. In most cases the tenaculum is not necessary. Cervical dilation, anesthesia and analgesia are not required. While using the angled lever to manipulate the flexible front tip up and down, a scope is introduced into the cervical canal within the operator's field of vision. The operator advanced the scope into the uterine cavity to perform an atraumatic, simple and well-tolerated hysteroscopy. The intrauterine cavity, as well as the tubal ostia, can be observed easily and closely by moving the front tip. In case of submucous myoma, the soft outer sheath can be replaced by a hard outer sheath to perform a forced examination of the pedicle.

### Flexible operating hysteroscopy

**Directed biopsy.** If directed intrauterine biopsy after diagnostic flexible hysteroscopy is needed, an operating flexible hysteroscope, assembled with Lin's biopsy forceps, is introduced into the uterine cavity. This is performed step by step under direct vision, without cervical dilation and anesthesia. Because the large biopsy cap is assembled outside the tip of the scope, care is taken to prevent injury of the cervix with the biopsy cap. When the target area is reached, the biopsy cap is opened to remove the tissue. Then, the specimen is obtained and the scope is removed.

**Removal of lost IUDs.** Diagnostic flexible hysteroscopy is performed to confirm the type, status and location of the IUD. An operating flexible hysteroscope equipped with Lin's grasping forceps is introduced into the uterine cavity according to the aforementioned procedure with the Lin's biopsy forceps. The end or the body of the IUD is grasped directly and removed while withdrawing the scope.

**Cutting of intrauterine adhesions.** The location and type of the intrauterine adhesions are first confirmed by a flexible diagnostic hysteroscopy. A flexible operating hysteroscope equipped with Lin's scissors forceps is introduced into the uterine cavity to cut the adhesions. Severe adhesions cannot be removed by this method.

## Summary

By using the flexible hysteroscopes which we developed, office hysteroscopy can be easily performed without using tenaculum, cervical dilation and analgesia or anesthesia. Lin's outer sheath allows for a continuous flow of the flexible hysteroscopy, making intrauterine examinations possible even during intrauterine bleeding. The operating ability of the small caliber flexible hysteroscope is undoubtedly enhanced by the applications of Lin's giant forceps.

## References

1. Marty R, Valle RF (1995) Eight years' experience performing procedures with flexible hysteroscopes. J Am Assoc Gynecol Laparosc 3(1):113-118
2. Lin BL, Iwata Y, Liu KH, Valle RF (1990) The Fujinon diagnostic fiber optic hysteroscope. Experience with 1503 patients. J Reprod Med 35(7):685-689
3. Lin BL, Iwata Y, Liu KH, Valle RF (1990) Clinical applications of a new Funon operating fiberoptic hysteroscope. J Gynecol Surg 6(2):81-87
4. Lin BL, Iwata, Y, Valle RF (1994) Clinical applications of Lin's forceps in flexible hysteroscopy. J Am Assoc Gynecol Laparosc 1(4):383-387
5. Lin BL, Ishigawa MY, Komiyama MK, Akiba YO et al (1997) The development of outer sheath for hysterofiberscope. Japn J Gynecol Obstet Endosc 13:69-72
6. Lin BL, Miyamoto M, Tomomatu M, Saito JI et al (1988) The development of a new hysteroscopic resectoscope and its clinical applications on Transcervical Resection (TCR) and Endometrial Ablation (EA). Japn J Gynecol Obstet Endosc 4:56-61

# Endouterine resection: surgical procedure

B. Blanc

## Definition

Uterine resection is the hysteroscopical resection of large benign intrauterine lesions such as fibroids and polyps.

## Installation

After local or general anesthesia, the patient is placed in the lithotomy position and properly grounded. Parietal desinfection of the perineum is realised with Betadine. Shaving is generally not necessary and Betadine is also used for the vagina. When the wall fields are in position, a speculum is introduced and Pozzi prehension forceps or double prehension pliers (Muzeux Palmer) are placed on the cervix. Dilation of the cervix, if necessary, is achieved cautiously and progressively with soft bougies (N°7, 21CH or N° 9-10, 27CH). Laminaria either traditional or synthetic can also be inserted beforehand. The resulting dilation is rapid but sometimes painful. Further conditions depend on the kind of equipment in use.

## Hysteroscopical surgical techniques with resector

The resectoscope with its optical unit, an electrode, the cold light cord and a camera are linked up to the high frequency generator. After checking the equipment and camera, the inflow and outflow irrigation channels are turned on and the equipment is progressively introduced under visual control to avoid risks of perforation or false passages. If the insertion of the resectoscope is impossible as in the case of cervical stenosis, the resectoscope is pulled out of the irrigation sheaths and replaced by a mandrin. Blind insertion has to be very carefully monitored as risks of perforation are high. With some types of mandrin, the optic system can be inserted into a central channel. The risk of false passages is reduced as the insertion of the equipment is realized under visual control. When the sheath has been inserted, the mandrin is pulled out and replaced by the operating system (the resectoscope with its optical unit, an electrode, the cold light cord and a camera linked up to a high frequency generator).

The following stage is the exploration of the uterine cavity with identification of the tubal ostia, visualization of the lesions which can include polyps of the endometrium and/or intracavitary fibroids. The angle formed by the lesion and the endometrium wall is assessed as well as the pedicular or sessile nature of the base, the volume of the myoma, the number of fibroids and the troncular vascularisation on the surface and pedicle.

## Surgical technology

Resection is performed under visual control from back to front. The troncular vessels on the surface of the myoma and the pedicle vessels are coagulated preventively. When the resectoscope is active, the resector is introduced with its handle folded so as to protect the tissues from the blade. Inside the uterine cavity, the handle will be carefully unfolded under visual control. The resection loop will be released and placed behind the tissue to be resected. By pulling in the handle and thus the hand, the loop is moved from back to front under strict visual control. The motion will not simply entail flexing the fingers but also flexing the forearm on the arm. The double motion makes for larger debris. When the resectoscope is passive, the movement is reversed. The introduction of the resector into the uterine cavity implies that the handle is delivered, and its articulation releases the outside loop of the resector. Resection is performed according to the same procedure from back to front under strict visual control. The resection of the fibroid can start from the free side of the myoma or from the middle part. The place from which resection starts depends on the position of the fibroid and particularly on its volume.

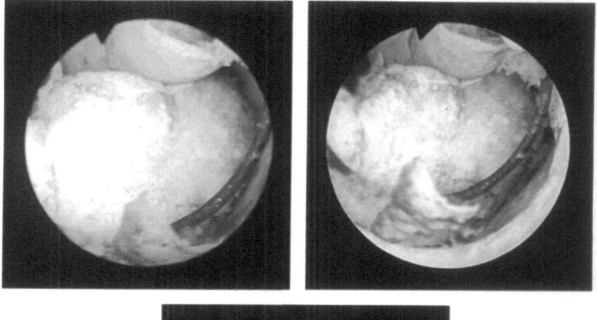

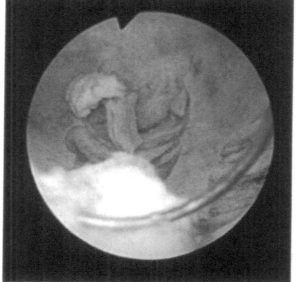

**Figs. 1, 2, 3.** Different phases of the resection of an intracavitary fibroid

For big myomas, it is often preferable to perform a middle section.

For strict endocavitary myomas (type 0), resection is usually simple, for myomas do not have an interstitial basis.

With a sub-mucous fibroid of the dominating type (type 1), the procedure occurs in two phases: the resection of the endocavitary portion and then the resection of the interstitial section. The latter resection is usually simple if the volume of the fibroid is small.

When the interstitial fibroids have jutting domes (Type 2), the procedure is far longer and difficult. The first phase is to resect the jutting dome. The resection of the interstitial base has to be progressive and careful so as to avoid uterine perforation. The resecting loop should not sink into the thick wall of the fibroid for its limits with the myometrium are not always clearly marked. The risks of vascular wounds (and vascular passage of fluids) and uterine perforation are high. A contraction of the uterine muscle has to be obtained since it will project the interstitial base towards the inside of the uterine cavity. A contraction can be obtained in several ways either with Syntocinon perfusion, abdominal massage, or massages of the operating limits with the resecting loop. The latter manoeuvre is the best way. The resecting loop, which is passive, is placed against the outside limit of the resected zone. This movement, if repeated several times, produces a reflex contraction of the myoma which projects the basis of the fibroid toward the uterine cavity on a few millimeters. The jutting dome can then be resected and the manoeuvre can be repeated several times.

As for initial submucous fibroids (Type 3) without real jutting domes, the indication of endouterine resection is not traditional. It can be performed as a complement to resection of another submucous myoma during endometrectomy. The ablation of the endometrium may reveal the presence of an unseen myoma, and can only be used for small fibroids for the risks of vascular wounds and uterine perforation are particularly high. The procedure is the same as the preceding one and the uterine massage has to be particularly careful and repeated.

The preoperative diagnosis includes an endovaginal ultrasonography to check the limits of the fibroid in relation with the uterine walls. If the myometrial wall is less than 10 mm thick the risk of perforation is particularly high. The disposal of the debris entails a problem: when the fibroid is small and the uterine cavity large, it is better to push the debris to the bottom of the cavity and finish the resection first. The debris will be taken out later. When the fibroid is large and the uterine cavity small, it is sometimes necessary to interrupt the procedure to clear out the resected debris which might impede the remaining resection. A large blunt curette or a pair of blunt pliers can be used. No efficient extractors are available.

## Incidents

The video image has to be consistently clear to allow the endouterine resection under permanent visual control. Video images of inferior quality may have several causes: the camera may not be correctly set; there may be vapor between the optics and the camera or debris may be present on the optical system. However, the most frequent cause is an irrigation problem:

- poor permeability of the channels which should be checked before the procedure by injecting a small quantity of fluid before the equipment is inserted;
- obturation of the irrigation and drainage orifices by blood or mucous debris in the course of the procedure;
- the orifices may be too close to the uterine wall or inside the cervical canal. The resector has to be moved and irrigation is resumed.

## Accidents

### Uterine perforation

It can be caused by the blind introduction of the equipment at the beginning of the hysteroscopy. The procedure has to be stopped. It is usually a mechanically-caused perforation which is easily solved. The patient has to be monitored for 24 hours in a hospital. If the perforation is caused by the resection loop, the chances of wounding an intra-abdominal organ (intestines, bladder, rectum) or blood vessels cannot be underestimated. In any case, the procedure has to be stopped and the electrolyte composition of the blood has to be measured (hematocrit FN). If the diagnosis is carried out during the procedure, it may not be necessary to perform a diagnostic coelioscopy. A pelvic ultrasonography will allow the operator to look for an important intra-abdominal passage of fluids which will have to be aspired by a cathether at the level of the Douglas. If the diagnosis of perforation cannot be established or if there is any doubt, a colposcopy is preferable for an objective assessment of the pelvic-abdominal situation.

### Pre-surgery hemorrhage

The endouterine resection of a myoma or polyp is not generally hemorrhagic. In case of hemorrhage the vessels have to be coagulated under visual control. In case of diffuse bleeding, coagulation has to be performed quickly, selectively or by surface effect as the risks of intravascular passage is high in the case of a wound of the uterine muscle. It is always necessary to ask for tests so as to assess the metabolic complications.

# Hysteroscopic metroplasty

B. BLANC, R. de MONTGOLFIER

Knowledge of the organogenesis of the feminine genital and urinary tracts is essential to understand uterine anomalies. Kidney anomalies associated to urinary tract anomalies are closely related to the different stages of the organogenesis. Frequency of uterine anomalies is around 1.5% amongst patients. Anomalies usually impair gestation.

## 1 Embryology

The genital tract develops in close relationship with the urinary tract, which evolves very early during the third week of the embryo life. The kidneys, after their formation, find the definitive location in the ninth week. The feminine genital tract develops from the two müllerian ducts. At first, the two canals migrate towards each other, then from the tenth to the thirteenth week, the caudal parts of each canal fuse, ultimately forming the uterovaginal canal. The upper portions, the future fallopian tubes, remain separate. From the thirteenth to the eighteenth week, the median septum separating the two müllerian ducts progressively disappears.

The severity and type of the malformations of the genital tract depend on the time of their appearance in the course of the embryo development.

When the anomaly takes place between the sixth and ninth week, a bilateral or unilateral aplasia associated to urinary defects is nearly always constant.

Between the tenth and the thirteenth week, if the two müllerian ducts do not fuse properly, the uterus becomes bicornuate. Defects of the urinary tract are frequent.

Between the thirteenth and the eighteenth week, resorption of the septum may be incomplete but with no concomitant effects on the urinary tract, which therefore does not need further examinations.

## 2 Diagnosis

In a clinical study, diagnosis may be reached in different ways.

### Outside pregnancy

- Discovery of an anomaly during a pelvic examination:
  - sagital septum of the vagina;
  - cervical bifidity or, on the contrary, absence of the cervix;
  - no perception of a uterus in the pelvic examination;
  - renitent convexity of the vagina lateral wall;
  - more or less complete vaginal aplasia.
- Discovery of an anomaly, during a complete assessment of a patient's situation, because of:
  - repeated abortions;
  - repeated premature deliveries;
  - sterility;
  - primary dysmenorrhea;
  - dyspareunia.

### During pregnancy

- Recurrent abortions or a very premature delivery may lead to a diagnosis. They may occur after iterative pregnancies because of:
  - the presence of a lateral uterine mass;
  - repeated dystocic presentations;
  - rare but severe accidents, such as rupture of a rudimentary uterine cornu linked to the development of a pregnancy in an immature uterus in which the blind cavity only communicates with the corresponding tube (a pseudo-unicornuate uterus);
  - torsion of a gravid uterus (by congenital absence of ligaments);
  - a pravia obstacle made up of the non-gravid tube.

### During delivery

Hemorrhages are frequent (inertia or retention) and need manual exploration of the uterine cavity which sometimes reveals the anomaly.

## In the immediate post-partum phase

Diagnosis may be done by ultrasonography after a premature delivery or a dystocic presentation.

## Nosology

Musset's classification is routinely used as it takes embryological, clinical and radiological problems into account [1].

There are four families. In each variety, the volume of the uterus may be either normal or hypoplastic. The frequency of hypoplasia amongst anomalies is high and should be stressed. Their diagnosis remains unclear. It essentially rests on hysterography and hysterometry below 70 mm and a fundus width under 40 mm. The endovaginal ultrasonography with a velocimetry by color Doppler may reveal the hypoplastic vascularization in the uterus. Hypoplasia is of unfavorable prognosis in case of pregnancy and is as important as the anomaly itself in case of an interrupted pregnancy.

## Musset's four varieties are:

-   uterine aplasia;
-   didelphus uterus;
-   septate uterus;
-   communicating uterus.

## Complete assessment of the anomaly

It should include a pelvic and endovaginal ultratomosonography associated to a color-coding Doppler to be prescribed first.

The ultrasonographic diagnosis of uterine anomalies relies on the differentiation of septate uterus from didelphus uterus. The diagnosis may be reached by chance particularly during the first trimester ultrasonographic investigation of pregnancy.

When a uterine anomaly is suspected, a few simple rules should be followed for the best ultrasonographic performance.

The examination should take place in the second part of the cycle for a patient without any estroprogestative treatment, or during the menstrual period so as to define the axis of the uterine cavity.

Vaginal and abdominal ultrasonographic exams should be combined.

There are two possibilities, both the analysis of the cavities and the color Doppler cartography.

The abdominal ultrasonography with a full bladder is useful in transverse sections, to define the anterior outline of the uterus :

-   a regular convex image towards the bladder can only be a septate uterus. The septum appears as a central hypogenous zone, though a discreet fundic inflexion does not change the diagnosis;

-   a clear corner image of the bladder is in favor of a didelphus uterus.

The study of the endometrium is already possible. Tiers of transverse sections show two separate echogenous formations progressively moving towards each other as the sections move from top to bottom.

The vaginal ultrasonography is more valuable to analyse the endometrium on condition; strictly transverse sections of the uterus can be realised, which is the most difficult as the uterus is in an intermediate position. The best time for exploration and definition of an anomalous uterus is near ovulation and during the secretory phase because of the significant thickness of the endometrium.

In the rare cases of a didelphus uterus with blind hemivagina, the ultrasonography reveals a lower pelvic collection, moderately echogenous corresponding to the hematocolpos and facilitating the visualisation of the genital tract above.

Hysterosonography discloses two separate cavitary collections seen transversally. It may be useful if the time within the cycle is not favorable for the exploration or if the patient is under a mini-dosed estroprogestative, with a moderate atrophy of the endometrium which is less echogenous.

Hysterosalpingography is better than hysteroscopy to evaluate tubal permeability, but it does not disclose the nature of the anomaly.

Laparoscopy still has a few indications when a diagnosis cannot be reached, and IVP is no longer useful since kidney ectopia can be diagnosed during abdominal ultrasonographic exploration. In case of aplasia IVP is still necessary to assess the anatomy and function of the remaining kidney.

In the case of primary amenorrhea, clinical exploration of the outside genital tract and a subpelvic ultrasonographic examination may lead to the diagnosis of an incomplete bilateral aplasia by absence of any uterine image, in a lengthways section, with a full bladder.

## Musset's classification

### Uterine aplasia

It is due to the absence or the anomalous migration of one or two müllerian ducts with inhibition of the underlying part of the genital tract. There are uni or bilateral, complete or incomplete uterine aplasia.

### Incomplete bilateral aplasia or the Rokitanski Kuster-Hauser Muller syndrome

Hysterography cannot be performed since there are no uterus and no vagina. Ultratomosonography shows the absence of a uterine cavity behind the bladder, the absence of a vagina and sometimes the presence of a retrovesical fibrous residue representing the uterus. Ovaries are visible. Ultrasonography sometimes shows a unilateral renal agenesia or an ectopy.

Laparoscopy allows an exact classification but does not seem useful in such cases when fertility is impossible. Treatment should aim at installing sexual activity. Frank's method of creating a cutaneous vagina is the best. When it is impossible to do so, a neo-vagina can be created after vesico-rectal dissection but there are risks of atresia and stenosis if sexual activity stops. Creation of a neo-vagina from a sigmoid loop should be exceptional.

### Unilateral complete or incomplete uterine aplasia

There are two varieties: the unicornuate and the pseudo-unicornuate uterus. In the latter, the uterus may be represented as either a full or a hollow nodule, or a nodule communicating with a tube. It is important to recognize this cavity as a pregnancy may develop in the rudimentary uterus.

HSG, which is identical for both varieties, shows an image as an acute accent. The uterine tube is pushed towards one side and the two symmetrical convex edges join at the opening of the tube.

Hysteroscopy shows a stretched out cavity with a tubal orifice in the middle.

With ultrasonography, the transverse sections show a nearly median cervix, a slanting isthmus and a uterine cavity on the side. The lateral deviation is always more important for the true unicornuate uterus than for the pseudo-unicornuate one (a crescent-shaped image) and the kidney defect is nearly always associated to the true unicornuate uterus. The presence of a uterine nodule can be suspected in the ultrasonographic investigation in case of a pseudo-unicornuate uterus.

Laparoscopy is necessary to complete a correct diagnosis. When there is a pseudo-unicornuate uterus whose nodule communicates with the tube, it is preferable to resect it. When the pseudo-unicornuate uterus is in relation with a tube, it may be necessary to resect the uterine stump to prevent a pregnancy and also in the presence of invalidating dysmenorrhea. The ablation can be performed by laparoscopy.

### Bicornuate uterus

It is a defect of the organogenesis which takes place between the tenth and thirteenth week with more or less complete persistence of the müllerian ducts. The two varieties are the bicervical didelphus uterus (with unilateral menstrual retention and a permeable variety) and the unicervical didelphus uterus.

### Bicervical didelphus uterus with unilateral menstrual retention

The existence of a primary dysmenorrhea and the distortion of the vaginal cavity point at the diagnosis.

Hysterography and hysteroscopy reveal a uterine cavity similar to the cavity of the unicornuate uterus. The uterine cavity is stretched out and one tubal orifice situated in the central part of the uterine fundus is present.

On the blind side, ultrasonography shows a big retentional unicornuate uterus whose liquidian cavity is slightly echogenous over a liquid pocket corresponding to the blind hemivagina. On the other side, ultrasonography reveals a unicornuate uterus whose size and structure are normal. On the retentional side, the ultrasonography reveals an aplasia or an ectopy of the upper urinary tract.

Laparoscopy discloses a voluminous median pelvi-abdominal tumor, the hematocolpos described by Musset with the following words: "a big head, with two small ears which are the uterine tubes". The lesions of pelvic endometriosis are frequent because of tubal reflux. They condition the reproductive implications. The treatment of menstrual retention should be limited to draining the hematocolpos by a lateral vaginal incision. When there is no hematocolpos, a hematometry and hematosalpinx are to be found. It is necessary to perform a hemi-hysterectomy by laparoscopy which is extremely easy as there is no urethra on the retentional side.

## The permeable bicornuate bicervical uterus

Hysterography discloses two cervixes, two isthmi and two different cornua, at a right angle with the isthmus.

Hysteroscopy shows two unicornuate-like uterine cavities with only one central tubal orifice, while ultrasonography reveals a double uterine structure on all the transverse sections with the bladder sunk in the middle of the two hemi-uteri. Unfortunately, the latter sign is not constant and it is all the more visible as there is a vesico-rectal ligament. There is also a divergence between the two great axes of the hemi-cavities. This ultrasonographic aspect is characteristic of the post-partum phase, and the hemi-uterus which was previously gravid is more voluminous. There is no endoscopical treatment of this malformation. Obstetrical accidents are not frequent. Surgical indications are exceptional and linked to antecedents of repeated late abortions. The treatment is surgical plasty of the two hemi-uteri.

## The unicervical didelphus uterus

Hysterography reveals several types, the unicervical didelphus uterus complete with one cervix, two isthmi, two cornua, and the unicervical didelphus uterus with irregular cornua. In this exceptional case, the renal anomalies are constant on the hypoplastic side.

Hysteroscopy reveals two uterine cavities with one tubal lateral orifice. The ultrasonography shows the aspect of the two hemi-uteri at the level of the uterine body, with sometimes a sign of the bladder, two diverging major axes, the presence of one cervix and one or two isthmoi according to the type of anomaly. The intestine peristaltism is useful to observe the dense mobile images corresponding to the loops of the small intestine pushing through the two uterine masses, which is a characteristic extra-sign.

Laparoscopy confirms the diagnosis. It is not essential, however, as there is no usual treatment for this anomaly. In case of repetitive late abortions, an abdominal hysteroplasty may reshape the uterus. It is a difficult intervention with an unfavorable obstetrical prognosis.

## Septate uterus

Septa are the most frequent uterine malformations (40% of the cases) and are due to an anomaly of late organogenesis (between the thirteenth and the eighteenth week). There are no associated renal lesions. It is a defect concerning the resorption of the middle septum separating the two hemi-uteri which have joined in the middle line. The septum resorption usually begins at the cervix and extends towards the uterus fundus. The resorption anomaly may begin at any time between the thirteenth and eighteenth week, which explains the existence of complete septate uteri (with one or two cervixes), a partial septum and a simple fundic indentation.

### Circumstances of discovery

Outside pregnancy, septate uterus may be discovered while investigating:
- a secondary infertility (late abortions);
- pre-term deliveries;
- dystocic presentations;
- sterility;
- more rarely, dispareuny in case of vaginal septa;
- cervical bifidity.

During pregnancy, a uterine septum may be diagnosed in the following circumstances:
- a premature interruption of pregnancy;
- a dystocic presentation;
- a delivery accident (hemorrhage or retention).

### Paraclinical evaluation

As there are no clinical signs, it is essential to carry out paraclinical investigations [1]. Hysterosalpingography discloses a bifid uterus. No criteria exist to differentiate it from a didelphus uterus except in the case of a total septate uterus. In that case, there is a very special T-like aspect. The uterine cornu is at a right angle with the bottom of the septum, perpendicular to this, and has its opening at the level of the uterine isthmus. In case of a bifid uterus, there is usually an obtuse angle of divergence between the two hemi-uteri. When the uterus is septate, the angle is more often acute.

Hysterography discloses the thickness of septa, the degree of uterine hypoplasia and leads to a correct evaluation of the gains of uterine surface to be obtained after the section of septa. Decherney [2] thinks that septa can be operated on if they are one centime-

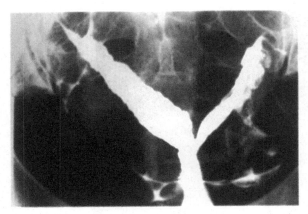

**Fig. 1.** Hysterosalpingography of a septate uterus (note the acute angle)

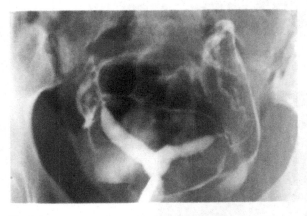

**Fig. 2.** Septate uterus (note the obtuse angle). The contrast product shows the uterine fundus thus confirming the septate uterus

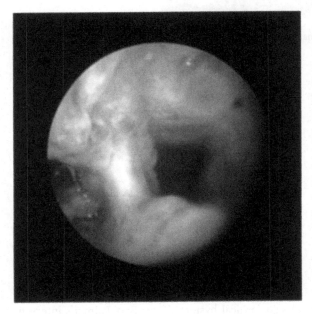

**Fig. 3.** Septate uterus

ter thick at their base. Associated lesions such as polyps and synechiae can be diagnosed with hysterography. Their frequency is usually high because of previous curettages. The investigation also reveals the existence of an anatomically incompetent cervix which may be responsible for obstetrical accidents. It also reveals the degree of tubal permeability.

## Hysteroscopy

It is an outpatient procedure performed either with a rigid hysteroscope or a flexible hysterofibroscope in a liquid medium or with $CO_2$. It provides data on the uterine bifidity but it cannot produce the diagnosis of the septate quality of the malformation. It reveals:

- the level of the septum either complete, partial or fundic;
- the thickness of the septum and the importance of the uterine hypoplasia;
- the existence of associated lesions, polyps or synechiae, though it does not reveal tubal permeability.

These two investigations are complementary but cannot by themselves reach a diagnosis of a septate anomaly.

Pelvic ultrasonography is the investigation which differentiates a septate uterus from a didelphus uterus or from a double uterus. The abdominal pelvic ultrasonography is usually enough. In a transverse section, it shows the two cavities separated by a median septum which is little echogenous and whose separate axes shape the classical image of a double-barrel gun.

With several transverse sections it is possible to evaluate the level of the septum and its maximum thickness. Diagnosis of the type of anomaly can be approached by the study of the posterior face of the bladder. If there is no interposition of a corner of the bladder, this is a possible sign of septate uterus. With a bicornuate uterus, it is possible to observe a posterior part of the bladder sunk between the two hemi-uteri. It is to be found in 30% of bicornuate uteri, particularly when there is a vesico-rectal ligament which pulls the distended bladder behind. It cannot be considered as specific. In a frontal section, the aspect of the septum, its thickness and its height in relation with the cavity can be well observed.

In transvaginal ultrasonography, the thickness of the septum and its height can be easily measured. Ultrasonography allows a sure diagnosis of the septate uterus in most cases, though there is an exceptional category of septate uteri presenting with a concave aspect of the uterine fundus at the level of serosa emer-

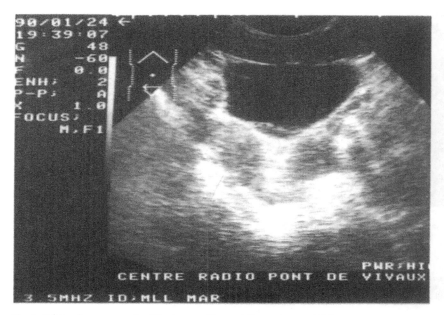

**Fig. 4.** Pelvic ultrasonography. The two cavities and the septa are visible

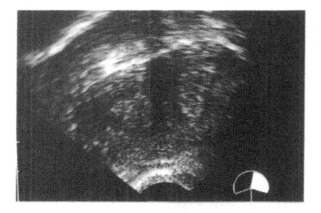

**Fig. 5.** Same patient: transvaginal ultrasonography (septate uterus)

gence zone of the septa. This aspect may lead to the diagnosis of a bicornuate uterus, so laparoscopy is necessary when the diagnosis is doubtful.

### Color coding Doppler

This method was first used to assess myometrial vascularisation. Energy Doppler is now the best method to identify vascularisation because of its much higher sensibility. Doppler low velocity flow mapping of myometrial vessels is very useful to bring out the differences between two crowns which are characteristic of a bicornuate uterus and one crown characteristic of

a septuate uterus. The septum is usually avascular, but a very high sensibility may reveal a few vessels.

### Laparoscopy

It confirms the diagnosis of septate uterus and shows a practically normal uterine fundus. It is however stretched out transversally and its median portion has a depression corresponding to the inserted septum. It is the place where the incision was realised during classic surgical hysteroplasty (Bret-Palmer's intervention).

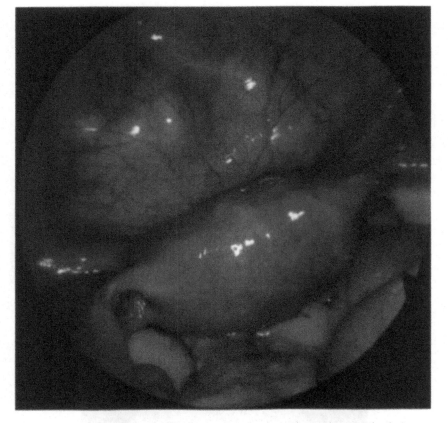

**Fig. 6.** Laparoscopy confirms the diagnostic of septate uterus (normal uterine fundus)

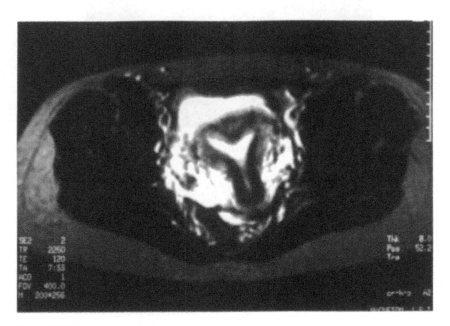

**Fig. 7.** MRI shows septa

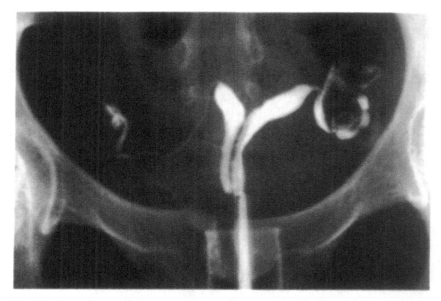

**Fig. 8.** Patient prior surgery

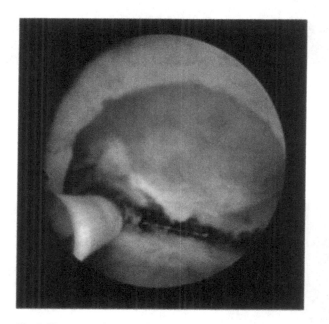

**Fig. 9.** Hysteroscopic metroplasty

## IRM exploration

It allows a diagnosis of uterine anomaly and its variety. It is useful in case of doubt, to avoid a laparoscopy.

## Communicating uterus

It is rare. The origin is an embryonic defect at the twelfth week when resorption of the septum begins at the level of the isthmus and moves on towards the top, while the sub-isthmic resorption takes place during the thirteenth week.

## Hysterosalpingography

The diagnosis is hysterographic and shows a lengthened X-shaped image. There are four varieties:
- Type I: a communicating total septate uterus;
- Type II: a communicating bicornuate, bicervical total uterus with or without a blind hemivagina;
- Type III: a communicating corporeal cervical septate uterus;
- Type IV: a communicating bicornuate and cervical septate uterus of T Linde.

Ultrasonography shows nothing about the communication.

## Hierarchy of explorations [3]

When assessing a genital anomaly, ultrasonography should always be realised as it is the only precise endo- and exouterine exploration. Its sensibility, however, is low (30 to 40%) and depends on the operator's experience. In the investigations about fertility, it reveals the presence of a septum. In this case hysteroscopy should be preferred to hysterography as direct vision is more revealing than a radiographic screen to assess the level, thickness and vascularisation of the uterine septum and associated lesions. Laparoscopy should be performed exceptionally, and only if the diagnosis of septate or bicornuate uterus is not clear.

## Treatment

Authors express divided opinions about complications of uterine septa as they are usually asymptomatic. However, two points can be made. The importance of the anomaly is not correlated to the frequency and severity of obstetrical accidents. The same type of anomaly may cause obstetrical accidents in one woman while another woman may have a perfectly normal pregnancy, or may alternatively present a normal pregnancy and obstetrical accidents. So it is difficult to assess the role of an anomaly in the genesis of obstetrical accidents.

Amongst the causes to explain the physiopathology of reproductive failures we find:
- the narrowness of the uterine cavity;
- an incompetent cervix;
- a poor endometrial decidualisation;
- an inefficient vascularisation of the uterine septum.

The endoscopic treatment of uterine septa is a widely accepted approach implying little invasiveness and short hospitalisation time. Some teams practice it as an ambulatory procedure. Its results compare favourably with the results of abdominal hysteroplasty.

## Indications are modified

The surgical endoscopical indication seems to be more rapidly offered and sometimes even when there is no history of obstetrical complications. Teams involved in Medically-Assisted Procreation are in favor of a systematic treatment of all septa, even "indentation" before trying out MAP, IVF or other procedures.

Endoscopical hysteroplasty should not be applied to every case of septate uterus for the following reasons [4]:
- even with a septate uterus a pregnancy may be quite normal, and such cases are numerous;
- hysteroplasty may have iatrogenous consequences such as destruction of a tubal ostium by an excessively lateral electrosection, a fragile uterus fundus with risks of rupture during a further pregnancy;
- pregnancies are usually normal when the septum is complete, so section of the septum does not seem in order except in the case of late abortions or premature deliveries.

Indications of endoscopical hysteroplasty are guided by obstetrical antecedents and anatomic conditions:
- antecedents of late or semi-late spontaneous abortions (after the twelfth week);
- antecedents of spontaneous first-term abortions barring those caused by chromosomic or hormonal troubles;
- persistent sterility when no other factors can explain the sterility;
- dystocic presentation with C-section;
- partial uterine septum.

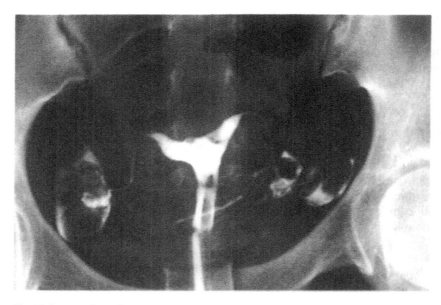

**Fig. 10.** Same patient after surgery

Personal series. (5 Tables)

**Table 1.** Obstetrical and gynecological antecedents

| | |
|---|---|
| No. of pregnancies | 146 |
| Repeated abortions | 102 |
| Preterm deliveries | 9 |
| < 28 weeks of amenorrhea | 1 |
| between 28 and 35 weeks of amenorrhea | 8 |
| In utero death | 0 |
| Late abortions | 27 |
| Full-term pregnancies | 4 |
| Elective abortions | 3 |
| Medical abortions | 1 |
| Primary sterility | 30 |
| Secondary sterility | 63 |
| Viability | 13 |
| Premature births | 9 |

**Table 2.** Associated sterility factors

| Type of sterility | 1 | 2 |
|---|---|---|
| Tubal obstruction | 5 | 4 |
| DES syndrome | 4 | 1 |
| Dysovulation | 3 | 4 |
| Endometriosis | 1 | 2 |
| Synechiae | 1 | 1 |
| Masculine sterility | 13 | 2 |
| Total | 28 | 16 |

**Table 3.** Functional results amongst all the patients for sterility I and II

| | |
|---|---|
| No. of followed-up patients | 84 |
| No. of viable children | 46 (54,8%) |
| No. of pregnancies | 63 (75%) |
| No. of full-term deliveries | 44 (52.3%) |
| Premature miscarriages | 12 |
| Late miscarriages | 2 |
| Pre-term deliveries | 3 |
| In utero death | 1 |
| Extrauterine pregnancy | 3 |
| C-section | 10 |
| Vaginal delivery | 36 |
| Elective abortions | 2 |
| No desire for fertility | 2 |
| Ongoing pregnancy | 1 |

**Table 4.** Functional results in sterile patients

| | |
|---|---|
| No. of patients | 30 |
| Lost to follow-up | 2 |
| No. of pregnancies | 18 (64.1%) |
| • spontaneous | 9 |
| • MAP | 9 |
| Full-term deliveries | 14 |
| Elective abortions | 1 |
| Miscarriages | 1 |
| Preterm deliveries | 1 |
| In utero death (abruptio placentae) | 1 |

**Table 5.** Functional results amongst patients with a history of obstetrical complications

| | |
|---|---|
| No. of patients | 63 |
| Lost to follow-up | 7 |
| Number of pregnancies | 45 (80.3%) |
| • spontaneous | 43 |
| • MAP | 2 |
| Term delivery | 25 |
| Preterm delivery | 2 |
| Vaginal delivery | 20 |
| C-section | 8 |
| Ongoing pregnancies | 1 |
| Extrauterine pregnancy | 3 |
| Elective abortions | 1 |
| Miscarriages | 13 |
| • early | 11 |
| • late | 2 |

# References

1. Musset R, Belaish J (1964) Les anomalies morphologiques congénitales le l'utérus. 22ème assises gynécologiques. Strasbourg, Masson ed, p.257-319

2. Decherney AH, Russel JB, Crache RA and al. (1986) Hysteroscopic management of mullerian fusion defects. Fert Steril, 5, 726-728

3. Blanc B (1990) Hiérarchie des explorations paracliniques dans l'exploration d'une malformation utérovaginale, Gynécologie, 41, 236-238

4. Blanc B, Cravello L, Porcu G and al. (1998) Surgical hysteroscopy in treatment of septate uterus. Systematic treatment of selected indications. Bull Acad Natle Med, 182, pp 251-261

# Endometrium polyps

B. Blanc

Endometrium polyps are localised growths in the uterine mucosa made up of glands and stroma around a vascular axis of one or several spiral arteries. They are caused by an anomaly of hormonal receptivity with persistence of estrogenous receptors and the decrease or disappearance of progesterone receptors. The stroma and particularly the endometrial glands go on growing to allow the development of the polyp. They are to be found with hormonal disorders such as dysovulation, luteal insufficiency or hyperestrogeny. Their frequency is about 5% [1].

They appear at any time in the course of genital life, being exceptional before puberty, and can develop during menopause, even in late menopause (80 years). The average age is between 30 and 60and there is usually only one in 80% of the cases. The average volume varies and the average size is usually 2.5 cm. They are usually to be found in the fundus but can develop in any location of the uterine cavity. A polyp usually has a thin pedicle so hysteroscopical excision is easy though blind curettage has generally no efficacy.

Histologically polyps have an endometrial structure with dense stroma and glands in the proliferative phase. In the pedicle, there is always a vascular axis made up of one or two small spiral arteries with thickened walls. The endometrium around the polyp usually has a normal proliferative aspect. In the postmenopausal period, the endometrium of the glandular cystic type is usually inactive. Patients on Tamoxifen for breast cancer may develop endometrial polyps [2-4]. Tamoxifen has an ambivalent action on the endometrium, both agonist and anti-agonist to the action of oestradiol. The histological structure combines both a glandular-cystic aspect and a leyomyomatous factor. These patients must be closely monitored as endometrium cancers have been described in the literature. It is, however, unnecessary to do so if there are no bleeding problems. Association with endometrium cancers is rare (0.55%) [5]. Endometrium polyps are no risk factors for an endometrium carcinoma if there is no anti-estrogen treatment.

## Circumstances of discovery

Uterine polyps are discovered during investigation of the menstrual cycle disorders such as metrorrhagia, menorrhagia, anomalies of the menstrual cycle or postmenopausal metrorrhagia or when a case of sterility is evaluated (with hysterography and pelvic, abdominal and vaginal ultrasonographies). Clinical examination is normal except for polyps coming through the cervix.

## Paraclinical evaluation [6, 7]

### Hysterography

Polyps appear as regular lacunar images, clear on clichés of the mucosa as the uterus starts filling or emptying. When the uterine cavity is full, images pale. Contrary to intracavitary fibrous polyps, they do not distort the uterus because of their mucous structure. On a profile cliché the thin pedicle is sometimes visible.

### Pelvian and endovaginal ultrasonography (Fig. 1)

A polyp is a round, echogenous image in the middle of the uterine cavity. It is better observed at the beginning of the cycle when the endometrium is thin. In the pre-menstrual period it is more difficult to see individual polyps because the endometrium is thick (8 to 15 mm).

### Hysteroscopy (Figs. 2, 3)

When there is a pink-coloured lesion showing the aspect of a poorly vascularized endometrium, the diagnosis is confirmed by hysteroscopy. There may be one or several polyps of variable volume. The end of the endoscope can be used to lift the polyp and disclose the pedicle. In postmenopausal women, they are

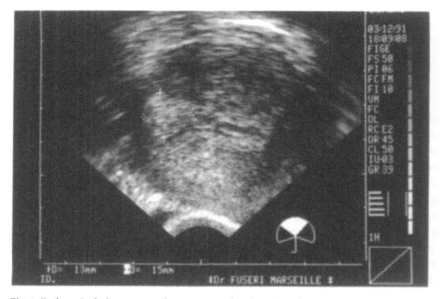

Fig. 1. Endovaginal ultrasonography. Mucous polyp distorting the uterine cavity

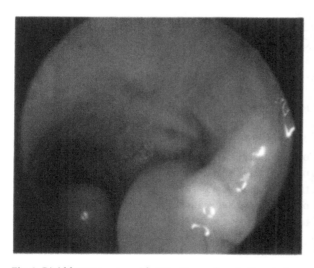

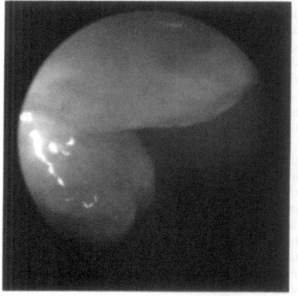

Fig. 2. Rigid hysteroscopy with $CO_2$. Two polyps in the uterine cavity

Fig. 3. Hysteroscopy: mucous polyp

often more voluminous and are to be found either in the uterus fundus or in the cornua region. They are pedunculated and mobile inside the uterine cavity. They are usually soft but in the case of fibro-mucous polyps, their consistency is denser.

## Endoscopic treatment: surgical technique

Hysteroscopical treatment is preferred to curettage which leaves fragments of the pedicle in situ and sometimes even misses the whole polyp. As early as 1958, Word, Gravel and Wideman [8] showed that 10% of the polyps were left in situ (49 cases out of 512 of total hysterectomies). Englund and Ingelman Sundberg [9] had already reported the fact in 1957 (33 remaining polyps out of 124 total hysterectomies with previous biopsy curettage). The risk of missing a lesion in utero is particularly high when the polyp is located in the precornual region [10]. The endoscopic treatment should be carried out in a liquid medium as the polyp floats in the uterine cavity. When the medium is $CO_2$, the polyp is often flattened against the endometrium by gas pressure and may not be identified.

There are three surgical endoscopic methods to treat a pedunculated polyp:

- section of the pedicle base with a surgical hysteroscope made up of a 4 mm optical system and an operating channel into which scissors can be introduced. With an Albarran system, the ancillary material can be oriented to facilitate resection. The distending medium is a saline solution. Flexible scissors are used and resection is not hemorrhagic. The polyp will be removed in a second phase of the procedure under visual control by introducing the prehension pliers into the side channel;
- resection of the polyp base is carried out with the diathermic loop in a glycine perfusion and the resector is introduced after cervical dilation. When the polyps are small in a woman who has never been pregnant or a woman with desire for a pregnancy, it is preferable to use a small-size resector (21CH) as a bigger one might result in an incom-

petent cervix. First all the faces of the polyp are observed. The base of the pedicle can be coagulated and then it is resected with the loop placed behind the base of the pedicle and pushed from back to the front to lessen the risks of uterine perforations. One or several passages are necessary according to the volume of the pedicle base. If it is a bigsize polyp it is sometimes preferable to cut it into two or three fragments before cutting the base of the pedicle to remove it;

- Laser resection. The Nd-Yag laser can also be used for coagulating the pedicle with the non-touch technique followed by resection of the pedicle with the touch technique. So the surrounding endometrium is not hurt.

## References

1. Philippe E, Charpin C (1992) Pathologie gynécologique et obstétricale. Masson, Paris p 94
2. Nuovo MA (1989) Endometrial polyps in post menopausal patients receiving Tamoxifen. Int J Gynecol Pathol 8:125-131
3. Corley D, Rowe J, Curtis MT et al (1992) Post menopausal bleeding from unusual endometrial polyps in women with chronic Tamoxifen therapy. Obstet Gynecol 79:11-6
4. Uziely B, Lewin A, Brufmang et al (1993) The effect of Tamoxifen on the endometrium. Breast Cancer Research Treatment 261-271
5. Salm R (1972) The incidence and significance of early carcinome in endometrial polyps. J Pathol 108: 47-53
6. Blanc B (1983) Atlas d'hystérosalpingographie comparée. Sandoz, Rueil Malmaison, pp 144-155
7. Blanc B, Boubli L (1991) Manuel d'hystéroscopie opératoire. Vigot, Paris, pp 65-66
8. Word B, Gravel LC, Wideman GL (1958) The fallacy of simple uterine curetage. Obst Gyn 12(6):642-648
9. Englund SE, Ingelman Sundberg A, Westin B, Hysteroscopy in diagnostic and treatment of uterine bleeding
10. Gribb JT (1960) Hysteroscopy: an aid in Gynecologic diagnostic. Obst Gyn 15:593
11. Blanc B (1996) Endoscopie utérine. Pradel, Paris pp 125-132

# Adenomyosis

B. Blanc

Adenomyosis is an important uterine pathology. Its frequency is not well-known, and severe cases do not respond well to hormonal treatments. To avoid hysterectomy which seems inevitable, several authors have envisaged a conservative endoscopic alternative. However, as long as following fundamental questions remain unanswered, this alternative cannot be considered.

How pertinent is diagnostic hysteroscopy in the evaluation of adenomyosis?

How curative is surgical hysteroscope?

How can a conservative treatment be reconciled with a menopause substitutive hormonal therapy afterwards?

Adenomyosis is an intramyometrial, endometrial diverticulosis. The diverticula are connected to the myometrium and lead to the development of zones of localised (15%) or diffuse (85%) hypertrophy. Strictly speaking, the term "adenomyosis" should be used for areas located in the myometrium at a depth superior to the thickness of the endometrium or when the distance between the basal endometrium and the adenomyosis area is over 2.5 mm. Adenomyosis may be isolated or associated with other pathologies such as fibroids, the endometrial proliferative disease or external endometriosis.

From a clinical point of view, adenomyosis may cause bleeding (menorrhagia or menometrorrhagia), or be painful with secondary dysmenorrhea or an aggravation of a previous dysmenorrhea and an increase in the volume of the uterus. Some clinical forms are asymptomatic so it is difficult to assess its frequency in the general population. Adenomyosis is discovered in 25 to 70% of hysterectomies performed for other reasons.

## Paraclinical diagnosis [1]

### Hysterography

It is still the most informative technique associating both direct signs such as more or less diverticular images and indirect signs such as rigid edges, or preostial dilatation. If adenomyosis is suspected, hysterosalpingography is indicated, as the exploration seems more successful than hysteroscopy to reach a diagnosis. In case of diverticular images, it is possible to assess their volume and particularly their depth.

### Endovaginal ultrasonography

Endovaginal ultrasonography may reveal unechogenous intra-myometrial images.

### NMR

NMR provides interesting data (about the thickened junctional layers and intramyometrial hypersignals) but it is too expensive for current practice.

### Diagnostic hysteroscopy

Diagnostic hysteroscopy should take place in the immediate post-menstrual phase before the changes in the mucosa conceal the modifications of the uterine walls. It shows both direct signs such as diverticular orifices or blue cysts, and indirect signs left by the changes around adenomyosic diverticula. They may be mucous reactions (pseudo-endometritis with hypervascularization, or myometrial distortions such as widening of the pre-ostial region, or rigidity).

Diagnostic hysteroscopy cannot confirm or infirm the adenomyosis diagnosis. Yet, it is necessary for a reliable evaluation of the uterine cavity and a correct therapeutic decision. A diagnostic myometrial biopsy may be indicated.

Mac Causland [2] reported signs of adenomyosis in 66% biopsies of patients for whom diagnostic hysteroscopy had revealed no adenomyosis. He also noticed correlations between the depth of the diverticulosis and the severity of the bleeding symptoms. The biopsy can be performed at the end of the intervention by resecting the bottom of a furrow to find out residual adenomyosis.

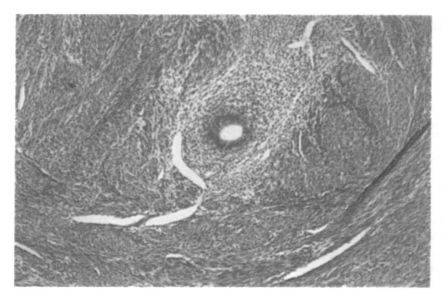

**Fig. 1.** Pathology view. Adenomyosis: diverticula connected to the myometrium

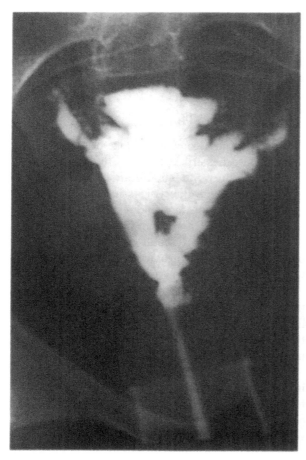

**Fig. 2.** Hysterography: enlarged uterine cavity. Big fundus diverticula (note the synechiae)

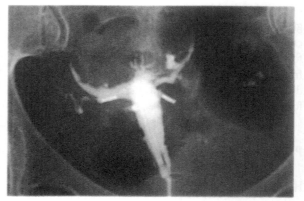

**Fig. 3.** Hysterography: fundus diverticula with erecta tubes (note the IUD)

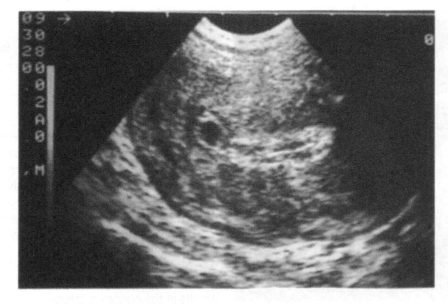

**Fig. 4.** Endovaginal ultrasonography (unechogenous image near the cavity)

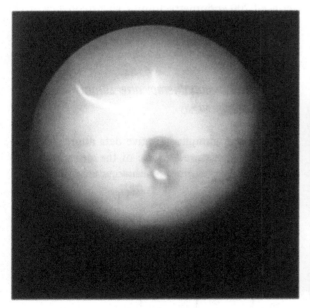

**Fig. 5.** Hysteroscopy with fluid: adenomyosic diverticula

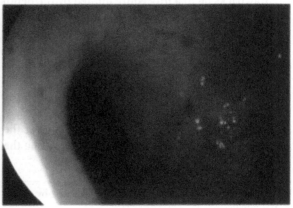

**Fig. 6.** Rigid hysteroscopy: with erecta tubes

## Surgical hysteroscopy

It is the only alternative to hysterectomy. A preoperative treatment of the endometrium by atrophying progestatives or LH-RH agonists can help the procedure and perhaps improve the prognosis by thinning down the endometrium, making it ready for a deeper treatment.

Two types of procedures are available:

- the interventions [3] aiming at resecting the endometrium and the superficial myometrium. The ablation may be total or subtotal, preserving a short isthmic zone. Their advantages include ha-

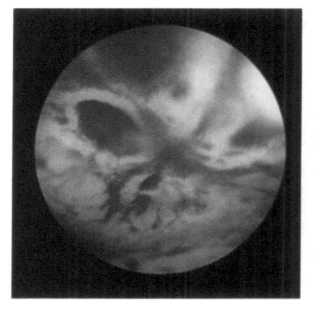

**Fig. 7.** Rigid hysteroscopy: adenomysis mucous reaction. Pseudo-endometriosis aspect

ving a complete histologic control, while their drawbacks lie in a procedure limited by the depth of the resected area (4 mm). So there is no efficacy when adenomyosis is deep as the diverticul are more than 4 mm long into the myometrium;
- the destructive interventions aim at an in-depth treatment;
- the laser Yag, particularly the non-touch technique;
- coagulation as a complementary technique at the bottom of the furrows or electively by treating the fundic and pericornual areas.

Frequency of adenomyosis in the patients treated by endometrial ablation

| Authors | Year | % |
|---|---|---|
| Magos | 1991 | 12 |
| Mergui | 1991 | 31 |
| Hellen | 1993 | 12.5 |
| Blanc-Boubli | 1993 | 29 |

In a personal series of 113 patients, 36 of whom presented adenomyosis with a mean follow-up period of 20 months, the success rate was 58.3% amongst the adenomyosis cases as against 76% when there was no adenomyosis.

Characteristics of the population

|  | Adenomyosis | No adenomyosis |
|---|---|---|
| Age (years) | 44.8 ± 0.6 | 46.5 ± 0.6 |
| Gestation | 3.2 ± 0.5 | 2.8 ± 0.31 |
| Parity | 2.2 ± 0.3 | 2.14 ± 0.23 |
| Length of the disease | 3.17 ± 0.8 | 1.5 ± 0.32 |

Two factors are determining:
- uterine volume. When hysterometry is over 10 cm and is associated with adenomyosis, the prognosis is bad with 51% of good results;
- time. Results of the endometrectomy seem to deteriorate postoperatively in the presence of adenomyosis.

## Results of the endometrectomy

Finally, the endometrial ablation may reveal or even create adenomyosis. Hellen [4] reported two cases in a series of 200 endometrectomies, so a frequency of 1% but two times, amongst the 25 cases of adenoyosis revealed by histological tests.

## *Substitutive hormonotherapy after surgical hysteroscopy for adenomyosis*

There are not enough objective data about the question in the literature because of the short follow-up time. Experimental physiopathologic models are rare.

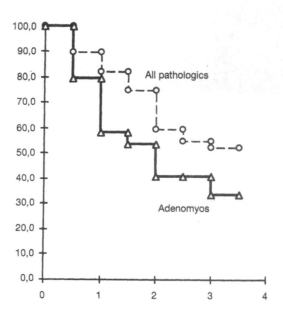

As a spontaneous evolution, the postmenopausal involution is not predetermined. It begins with the disappearance of the glands, as the stroma is preserved for a longer period. Observations of severe postmonopausal endometriosis and adenomyosis as reported in the literature show the following facts:

|  | Endometriosis | Adenomyosis |
|---|---|---|
| Age of diagnosis | 58.8 | 57.2 |
| Years after menopause | 9 | 11 |
| Signs of persistent hormone impregnation | 54% | 33% |
| Substitutive Hormonotherapy | 27% | 41% |

Surgical hysteroscopy is a recent technique and its long-terms effects are not known. So, it is only possible to put forward propositions in the matter of substitutive treatments of the menopause after endometrectomy for adenomyosis.

It seems reasonable to wait for a one-year delay.

Any treatment should have a progestative component with a strong antiestrogen action; the most logical plan should be a continuous treatment (the so-called no-menses treatment).

A clinical and paraclinical surveillance based on vaginal ultrasonography seems to legitimate as long as we have no long term follow-up data for the treatment.

Endoscopic endocavitary explorations are indispensable in case of bleeding recurrences and patients should be informed about the precautions before beginning the treatment.

So, as a conclusion, surgical hysteroscopy can reduce the indications of hysterectomy for adenomyosis. This technique, however, has no efficacy when the uterus volume is over 10 cm. Results may be improved by the laser Yag or by combining techniques, but the treatment of deep adenomyosis areas increases the morbidity of the method. The action of LH-RH agonists is being assessed. The hormonal substitutive treatment in those patients will be carefully considered, never begun too early and in any case with a progestative component.

## References

1. Blanc B (1983) Atlas d'hystérosalpingographie comparée. Sandoz, pp 144-155
3. McCausland (1992) Myometrial biopsy. Am JOG, 166: 1619-1628
3. Lewis BV, Magos AL Endometrial ablation. Churchill Livingstone
4. Hellen EA (1993) The histopathology of transcervical resection of the endometrium: an analysis of 200 cases. Pathology 22:361-365

# Abnormal benign endometrial proliferative states

B. Blanc

According to its histological definition, hyperplasia of the endometrium or abnormal endometrial proliferation includes several pathological states caused by excessive growth of the uterine mucosa. This abnormal growth is due either to a functional anomaly of the hormonal response or to an organic pathology which may indicate the onset of an invasive carcinoma (hyperplasia with or without atypia).

These states of the endometrium are characterized by one morphological anomaly of the uterine mucosa, either homogeneous or heterogeneous, diffuse or localised, and most often by an increase in the thickness of the endometrium. Hysteroscopy associated with biopsies is a determining diagnostic feature. Therapeutic hysteroscopy may help to avoid hysterectomy when medical treatment has failed and if a thorough evaluation of the condition has been performed.

## Epidemiology: risk factors

The most common cause is inappropriate estrogenic stimulation. The Stein Levanthal syndrome is to be found in young women suffering from hyperplasia of the endometrium. Chamlian [1] reported that out of 97 young women presenting with endometrial hyperplasia, 24 had a Stein Levanthal syndrome. Other factors include an insufficient luteal phase particularly in the anovulatory cycles of the premenopausal period, or estrogen-producing ovarian tumors or estrogenotherapy inadequately challenged by progesterone. Personal factors such as obesity (androstenedione turning into estone in the fat tissues), nulliparity, hypertension and diabetes are also relevant.

## Histopathology

Hendrickson and Kempson's [2] classification includes:
- hyperplasia without atypia;
- endometrial hyperplasia with atypia (slight, medium, severe).

IGSP and WHO classifications are very similar:
- simple hyperplasia (SH) with densification of the glands and a higher ratio glands/stroma;
- complex hyperplasia (CH) with densification of the glands, a higher ratio glands/stroma and heterogeneity of the glandular structures;
- simple hyperplasia with atypia (SHA) combining simple hyperplasia and cellular atypia (Fig. 1);
- complex hyperplasia with atypia (CHA) combining complex hyperplasia and cytonuclear atypias.

Whatever the type of classification, there are some important points:
- atypia is a major prognosis factor [3];
- cystisation is a mode of spontaneous cure but the definition "cystic glandular" hyperplasia is inappropriate since it is only a case of cystic glandular atrophy;
- the difference between a simple and a complex pathology lies in heterogeneity, which is a key element in the endoscopic observation;
- generally speaking, biopsies provide the most important findings concerning carcinoma risks.

Table 1. Hyperplasia/nb/patients

| Simple | Regression (%) | Persistence (%) |
|---|---|---|
| Adenocarcinome (%) | simple 93 80 1 91 | complex 29 80 17 3 |
| atypy | simple 13 69 23 8 | complex 35 57 14 29 |

(according to [3])

## Clinical aspects

The risks of developing atypical hyperplasia and cancer increase after menopause. The most common feature is abnormal bleeding, liquid secretions are rarer. However, the patient may be asymptomatic. In a

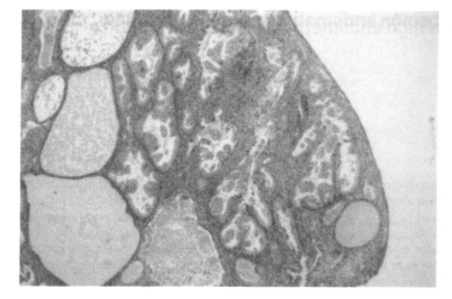

**Fig. 1.** Simple hyperplasia with atypy

study reported by Archer [4] concerning 801 asymptomatic menopaused patients, he noted 41 cases of endometrial hyperplasia and 4 cases of atypical hyperplasia.

For a long time, hysteroscopy has been the only imaging technique. Round, regular, polylobed images are the most common aspect. The persistence of the mucous line is of good prognosis.

Endovaginal ultrasonography (Fig. 2) is used to collect information. The thickness of the endometrium is only informative in postmenopausal women or in the first part of the cycle. According to Osmers [5] when the endometrium is more than 4 mm thick after menopause, and if the woman does not receive any substitutive treatment, a diagnosis can be established for all hyperplastic states and endometrial cancers (sensibility 100%, specificity 52%, VPP 26.9%, VPN 100%). For Grandberg [6], when the endometrium is 5 mm thick, it is possible to identify 87% of all endometrial anomalies. In endometrial hyperplasia, the average thickness as measured by ultrasonography is 9.7 ± 2.5 mm for Grandberg, and 13 mm for Bourne [7]. Echostructure, homogeneity and regularity of the images can also be studied by ultrasonography, but the most unusual aspects are to be found in cases of cystic glandular hyperplasia.

These aspects associated with pathologies such as myomas can simulate heterogeneity. With ultrasonography, it is possible to assess the volume and structure of the uterus and the adnexa (ovaries). The Doppler exam, even with a colour code, has not proved useful, pulsatility index being 1,05 (difference 0,31-1,8) according to Bourne.

## Non endoscopic endouterine evaluation

Routine cervix cytology is of little interest. Endouterine cytological tests are on the whole less efficient in hyperplasia than in cancer reports (Ferenczy [8] 19.5% false negatives). Histological samples collected with cannula, pipette or by aspiration are more satisfactory but less informative than in the endometrium cancers.

Table 2.

|  | Correct collection (%) | Precision cancer (%) | Precision hyperplasia (%) |
|---|---|---|---|
| Biopsy | 91 | 81 | 68 |
| Aspiration | 90 | 97.5 | 91.7 |

Blind insertion of the different equipment may be painful for menopaused patients so hysteroscopy under visual control yields better results in assessing this type of pathology.

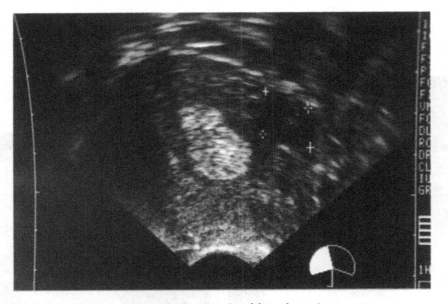

Fig. 2. Endovaginal ultrasonography: hypertrophy of the endometrium

## Hysteroscopy

For menstruating women, the appropriate date is the beginning of the cycle. Hysteroscopy is performed in the office, with either $CO_2$ or a fluid perfusion. The general aspect of the endometrium has to be evaluated. The state of the vascularization has to be assessed quickly at the beginning of the procedure by looking closely at the mucosa without touching it. Localised changes of regular hypervascularization are only informative at the beginning of the examination, since they tend to appear as the investigation proceeds or after contact with the tip of the endoscope. It is necessary to evaluate the homogeneity of the endometrium or on the contrary, the lack of homogeneity marked by cystic zones or proliferating zones. The thickness of the uterine mucosa is appreciated by pressing the endoscope against the wall of the uterus and measuring the furrow thus produced. This furrow only appears if the walls of the uterus are resilient enough. It may be missing in some cystic glandular cases and complex hyperplasia.

Hystological material is collected during the hysteroscopic procedure. The manner of collecting tissues depends on endoscopic observations. When the mucosa is regular and thick, with no anarchic hypervascularization and homogeneous, different modes of collection are possible, Novak's cannula, Cornier's pipette or N°4 "vacurette" or syringe aspiration. For the collection to be qualitatively and quantitatively sufficient, the uterus has to be empty. But when the mucosa seems heterogeneous with irregular hypervascularization or in certain rare cases with localised pathologies, the collection has to be performed under visual control. Pliers need to be introduced into the side channel. A small calibre resector may be more useful. Local anesthesia by paracervical block affords good comfort to the patient while all the necessary biopsies for reliable results are performed.

## Hysteroscopic aspects

Here are a few reported endoscopical aspects with no intention of establishing a histological diagnosis from macroscopical aspects.

Hysteroscopical semiological aspects include:
- simple proliferative states comparable to an endometrium during the secreting period with a regular, thick mucosa, with no anarchic hypervascularisation (Fig. 3);
- cystic-glandular states with poor vascularization, a heterogeneous, rigid structure, with cystic dilations in which the endoscope leaves no furrows (Fig. 4);
- polypoid proliferations, usually normally vascularized, with different proliferations which are homogeneous and resilient (Fig. 5);

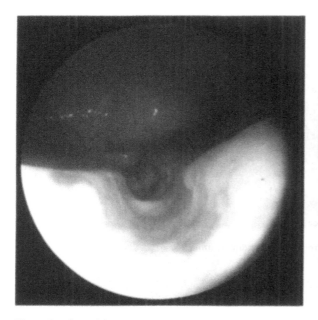

**Fig. 3.** Simple proliferative state

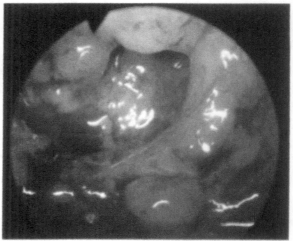

**Fig. 4.** Cystic-glandular states

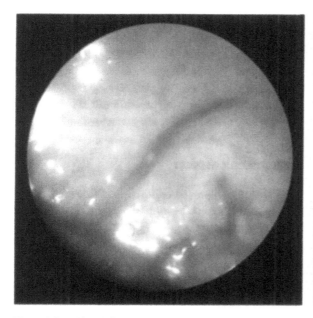

**Fig. 5.** Polypoid proliferations

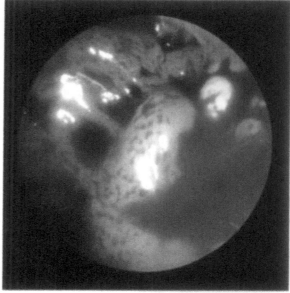

**Fig. 6.** Endometrium hypertrophy with vascularisation and heterogeneous zone

- complex proliferations associated with heterogenous zones of highly developed vascularization (Fig. 6).

### Reliability of the endometrial hysteroscopical assessment

Gimpelson [9] shows that hysteroscopy yields the same results as curettage in 79.2% of the cases, and it is more efficient in 17.5% and less informative in 3.2% of the cases.

### Correlations between hysteroscopy and the histological diagnosis

| Authors | Correlations |
| --- | --- |
| Mencaglia [10] | 92% |
| Dargent [11] | 100% |
| Lasala [12] | 67.4 |

The endoscopical treatment can be offered when the progestative treatment (a sequence from the 5th to the 25th day of the cycle) has failed. The procedure is a traditional endometrectomy or a Yag laser treatment. The presurgery treatment with two injections of LH-RH antagonists or more simply a curettage to reduce the thickness of the mucosa makes the procedure simpler. A complete histological study is necessary and resection is the best technique to obtain it. If debris of resection show atypias, then hysterectomy is unavoidable.

In a personal series, the average age of the patients treated for a proliferative endometrial pathology was $46.4 \pm 1$ years. The results are satisfying in 76.6% of the cases with an average follow-up period of 23 months and with better stability than in the treatment of adenomyosis. The latter technique is relevant if the medical treatment fails. It is necessary to monitor these patients for a long time for an early diagnosis in case of some severe endometrial pathologies.

The observations to be found in the literature about the endometrium cancer after a hysteroscopical treatment (Decherney, Dequesnes) were about high risk patients (hyperplasia with atypias). The reported observations were not cases of endometrial resection but cases of destruction by Nd-Yag laser.

### The substitutive hormonal treatment of menopause

Endometrectomy is most often complete and results in amenorrhea or extreme oligomenorrhea. Thus, a substitutive hormonal treatment of menopause should always be undertaken with a strong antiestrogenic component. If abnormal bleeding appears in those patients under a substitutive treatment, investigations should be thorough and quick, particularly endoscopical investigations as not enough information is available to assess the long term endometrial risk in those patients.

### References

1.  Chamlian DL, Taylor HB (1970) Endometrial hyperplasia in young women. Obstet Gynecol 36:659-666
2.  Hendrickson MR, Kempson R (1980) Endometrial hyperplasia in surgical pathology of the uterine corpus. WB Saunders, Philadelphia, pp 285-318
3.  Kurman RJ, Norris HJ (1982) Evaluation of criteria for distinguishing atypical endometrial hyperplasia from well differentiated carcinoma. Cancer 49:2547-2559
4.  Archer DF et al (1991) Endometrial morphology in asymptomatic post menopausal women. Am J Obst Gynecol 165:317-322
5.  Osmers R et al (1992) Evaluation de l'endomètre dans la post ménopause par sonographie vaginale. Rev Rf Gynecol Obstet 87(6):309-315
6.  Grandberg D (1982) Clinical use of progestin in the menopausal patient. J Reprod Med 27:531-538
7.  Bourne TH et al (1990) Detection of endometrial cancer in post menopausal women by transvaginal ultrasonography and colour flow imaging. Br Med J 301-369
8.  Ferenczy A (1984) Out-patient endometrial sampling with endocyte comparative study of effectiveness with endometrial biopsy. Obstet Gynecol 63:295-302
9.  Gimpelson RJ, Rappolo HO (1988) A comparative study between panoramic hysteroscopy with directed biopsies and dilatation and curettage. Am J Obstet Gynecol 158:489-492
10. Mencaglia L, Perino A, Hamou J (1984) Hysteroscopic evaluation of endometrial cancer. J Reprod Med 29:701-704
11. Dargent D (1986) The value of the hysteroscopy curettage sequence under local anesthesia in the diagnosis of cancer of the endometrium in endometrial cancers. 5th Cancer Research Workshop, Grenoble, 1985, Karger Basel, pp 67-74

# Endometrectomy

B. Blanc, R. de Montgolfier

## Definition

Endometrectomy is the removal or destruction of the endometrium (functional and basal layers) by coagulation or photovaporization. The ablation reaches the internal level of the myometrium. Endometrectomy is indicated for treatment of hemorrhagic troubles of the cycle. Endometrectomy allows conservative treatment of benign disorders of the endometrium, when medical treatment has failed or is inappropriate. Thus, hysterectomy for benign lesions and functional uterine disorders can be avoided. Endometrectomy relies on correct assessment of the endometrium since carcinoma or associated pathologies could be contraindications. It is technically possible to resect or destroy a pathological mucosa but treatment will not heal the whole of the endometrium.

## Indications

Indications include bleeding disorders of the menstrual cycle such as menorrhagia, menometrorrhagia, and metrorrhagia caused by benign abnormalities of the endometrium (either functional or organic) such as hyperplasia of the endometrium, endometrial proliferation, subatrophic endometrium, benign pathologies of the myometrium, small-sized interstitial fibroids and adenomyosis. The surgical procedure is performed after careful local and regional preoperative assessment to ascertain that there are no intracavitary or intramyometrial abnormalities which can account for the bleeding troubles. The surgical procedure is not indicated for only one abnormality in the cycle though it could be considered after several medical treatments have failed.

Endometrectomy should not be offered to young women even if there is no desire for pregnancy. It should be reserved for patients over 40. After menopause, endometrectomy is still an indication in metrorrhagia either spontaneous or linked to substitutive hormonal treatment after diagnostic hysteroscopy and directed endometrial biopsies have proved there are no neoplasic endouterine lesions. Endometrectomy can be performed as a complement of an endouterine resection to improve functional results, which seem to be correlated to uterine volume and to the existence of associated adenomyosis. Endometrectomy is to be contraindicated for a large hysterometry (over 11 cm), polyfibromatous uterus and in case of deep diverticular adenomyosis visible in hysterography.

## Preoperative assessment

It is necessary to realize a rigorous preoperative evaluation to be sure there are no endometrium carcinoma or associated disorders which might be contraindications to conservative surgery (voluminous uterine myoma, deep diverticular adenomyosis or adnexial pathology).

The assessment should include:
- a careful review of the patient's history and a pelvic examination;
- smear tests if they have not been done before;
- pelvian and endovaginal ultrasonographies to evaluate the objective characteristics of the genital organs (uterus, adnexa);
- an office diagnostic hysteroscopy with endometrial tests (if the patient has not already been treated by hemostatic curettage).

If there is any suspicion of adenomyosis, hysterosalpingography may be necessary for diagnostic purposes as it is more informative than hysteroscopy and endovaginal ultrasonography. A hysterosalpingography is useful to evaluate the volume and depth of diverticular images. When all the examinations have been performed, endometrectomy may be indicated or not.

If there is no neoplasic pathology, vaginal hysterectomy may as well be an indication as endometrectomy. Endometrectomy is a simple, short (10 to 20 minutes) procedure involving a brief hospital stay, and preservation of the genital organs. Drawbacks are linked to risks of recurrences. The decision has to be taken with the patient who should be correctly informed.

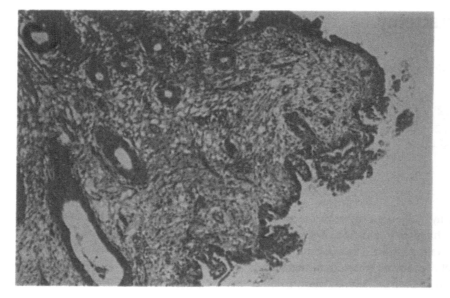

**Fig. 1.** Endometrectomy: histological exam

A recent randomized study including 200 patients was published by Dwyer, who compared endometrectomy by electroresection with abdominal hysterectomy. All his patients were examined 4 months after the surgery. After the hysterectomy, symptoms as menorrhagia, dysmenorrhea or premenstrual syndrome were improved. As for the length of the procedure, pre and postoperative morbidity, length of hospitalisation and return to regular sexual activity, endometrial ablation showed better results than hysterectomy.

## Preparation of the endometrium

Administration of preoperative medication should be discussed in view of its price and iatrogenous effects. The aim of the surgery is total or partial endometrium ablation or the destruction of the endometrium down to its basal layer. A treatment to thin down the endometrium so that the deeper regenerating layers may be more accessible should facilitate the procedure, particularly if coagulation of the endometrium is part of the indication.

Several methods are available:
- progestatives to thin the endometrium;
- GnRH agonists and danatrol (danazol) are potentially more efficient but limited by several factors,
  • side effects, hot flushes, metrorrhagia
  • rigidity of the cervical canal which might prevent the insertion of the resectoscope

• price of the medication

When preoperative medication, if any, is administered it can be followed by postoperative medication to prolong the resection effects. Brooks [1] reported the following results about a series of 172 patients treated from February 87 to October 92 with a follow-up time of more than 12 months:

Four groups were formed:
- Group 1   51 patients   no preoperative treatment
- Group 2   11 patients   progestative preoperative treatment
- Group 3   26 patients   Danatrol pre-operative treatment
- Group 4   84 patients   LH-RH agonist (leucoprolide) preoperative treatment

This study, however, was not prospective nor randomised and with very irregular number of people in the groups. It showed, however, favorable results obtained when the endometrium was prepared by LH-RH agonists.

## Operative techniques

### Ablation of the endometrium

It is better to use the 27CH resectoscope to obtain thick and big-sized debris. If it is impossible to introduce the equipment, then use the 26 or 21CH resectoscope. Distension fluids are glycine or mannitol. A

**Table 1.** Results (%) on the bleeding disorders [1]

| Group | Amenorrhea % | Hypomenorrhea % | Normal menstruation | Persistent menorrhagia |
|---|---|---|---|---|
| 1 | 24 – 47 | 21 – 41 | 2 – 4 | 4 – 8 |
| 2 | 6 – 55 | 2 – 18 | 1 – 9 | 2 – 18 |
| 3 | 12 – 46 | 11 – 42 | 2 – 8 | 1 – 4 |
| 4 | 57 – 68 | 20 – 24 | 5 – 6 | 2 – 2 |

high frequency electrical current is advisable. The cutting power has to be strong enough (45 w) to avoid carbonization which will leave a rough surface.

After exploring the uterine cavity, the first furrow is cut into the posterior wall by beginning near the left ostia. With the first furrow it is usually possible to find out the ideal depth. The other furrows are traced in the adjacent region according to the following sequence: 1) posterior face; 2) left border; 3) anterior face; 4) right border and 5) posterior face, from fundus toward isthmus (back to front) by pulling in the loop towards the hysteroscope in the cutting mode.

The resection procedure should avoid the cornua regions for the muscular wall is thin there, and with fluid distension making the uterine wall even thinner, there are risks of perforation. Besides, this procedure should keep away from both the isthmic portion of the uterus, because large vessels are very near, and the endocervical portion to avoid the appearance of synechia blocking the uterine cavity, thus preventing any ulterior follow-up. Hemostasis will be achieved at will by elective coagulation of the vessels. Myometrium should be reached at the level of the medium layer which can be recognized by its dense fasciculated structure. This depth is reached after one or two passages of the cutting loop. There is no glandular recess in the middle layer.

To maintain satisfactory control of the resection depth, two resected furrows should be separated by a mucous protusion so the surgeon knows where the initial level of the uterine cavity was. The protusions or bridges are resected afterwards in a second phase to level out the surfaces of the cavity. The course of the loop is 27 mm so that it is impossible to achieve resection of an average uterus (hysterometry 9-10 cm) in one movement. It is necessary to cut the furrow down to the bottom until the desired level is reached.

The surface of the resection is function of the desire to keep some degree of menstrual function. In case of partial endometrial resection, ablation should avoid the first supraisthmic centimeter. The ulterior

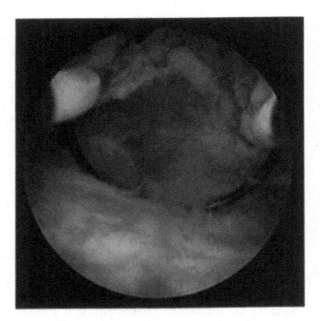

**Fig. 2.** Ablation of the endometrium beginning in the posterior wall

exploration of the uterine cavity is then theoretically possible but risks of recurrences are higher since the endometrium left in situ can colonize the uterine cavity.

In case of complete endometrectomy the endometrium should be removed down to the isthmic region. The risk of creating a low uterine synechia is high, and it may prevent any ulterior follow-up. Access to the fundus is difficult because of its curving shape as well as access to the pericornua regions. Therefore, it is often necessary to complete the ablation with a Rollerball electrode. The procedure starts around the cornua in the postostial region. The electrode is placed in contact with the endometrium, and the current of monopolar electrocoagulation is delivered till the tissues turn white. Then the electrode is moved from front to the back or transversally to coagulate the whole fundus and the periostial region.

During an endometrectomy procedure, the endometrial ablation is, however, never complete for there are still unresected parts of endometrium in the ostial and isthmic regions. They cause frequent failures of the procedure whatever the importance of the endometrial ablation.

During the procedure, debris obscure operative vision. The removal of resected tissues is always a difficult phase for inexperienced surgeons and their repeated removal lengthen the operative time. After shutting off the irrigation circuit, debris can be removed with the loop by pulling out the handle from the sheath or with a blunt curette. Debris extractors are available but their efficiency has to be objectively evaluated. Once the technique has been mastered, it is possible to avoid a drawback by pushing the debris towards the bottom of the uterine cavity and removing them once or twice during the procedure. In special cases of uterine hypoplasia, it is sometimes useful to get rid of the resected tissue after each resection for their accumulation prevents the procedure.

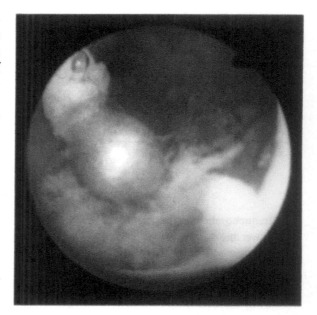

Fig. 3. Coagulation of the posterior wall

## Techniques of endometrial destruction

### Coagulation

The equipment is the same as the one described for the ablation of the endometrium. A 27CH resectoscope is particularly recommended. It has a specific electrode for coagulation (Rollerball). It is a sphere turning around an axis and coagulation is more homogeneous while reducing the risks of accidental effraction. The average power is between 35 to 45 watts.

The first phase of the coagulation procedure usually concerns the periostial and fundal areas.

Indeed, photocoagulation often results in uterine contractions which reduce the volume of the uterine cavity and prevent easy access to the area to be coagulated. The coagulation electrode is applied homogeneously and smoothly on the whole surface by pulling the electrode backwards towards the optical system. The coagulated zone turns white. The uterine fundus, the walls and the borders are then coagulated in succession. To keep menstrual cycles, a thin isthmic area is preserved.

The procedure is short (< 15 min). It is essential to let the electrode ride smoothly on the surface to be coagulated without staying too long in one area. Coagulation produces intense heat and bubbles. So irrigation should be started previous to the procedure and coagulation interrupted from time to time to remove the bubbles.

Because the per- and susostial areas are particularly thin, it is advisable to lower the coagulation power (20 watts). If necessary, the vessels can be selectively coagulated in case of vascular effraction. At the end of the procedure the uterine cavity should look smooth and white.

### Laser Nd Yag photocoagulation

The equipment is either a rigid hysteroscope or a fibrohysteroscope.

The rigid hysteroscope is a traditional operative hysteroscope with an operative channel (OD 2 mm) or a surgical hysteroscope with a double channel, one for the delivery of distending media and one for operative instruments. This equipment is unfortunately rigid and the laser fiber cannot be moved inside the whole uterine cavity. With the double circulation system, visualization of the uterine cavity and of the lesions is perfect.

The surgical fibrohysteroscope, however, should be preferred. No cervical dilation is called for and it allows easy exploration of uterine cavity and easy access to all its areas, being always perpendicular to the selected site. The same irrigation media are used as with resectoscopy (glycine, mannitol or hyskon used by American authors). The outside sheath has an OD of 5.2 mm and an operative channel (OD 2 mm) which allows laser penetration. Its tip should be protected by a teflon sheath to avoid lesions at the time of penetration. The protective sheath will be removed as soon as the laser is past the operative channel.

The most commonly used laser is the Nd Yag laser of high power (100 watts) with adequate coagulating effects and great penetrating power. It uses a quartz fiber of 400 to 600 microns. Uterine drainage is not automatic as there is no dual channel on the hysterofibroscope. This is not a real drawback as glycine leaks around the cervix.

Two types of techniques are available:

- the blanching (non-touch) technique allows deeper coagulation and is thus particularly adapted to total destruction of the endometrium. It is however time-consuming;
- the dragging (touch) technique creates parallel furrows on all the faces and uterus fundus.

The uterus fundus is most often treated with the non-touch technique and the lateral sides by the touch technique so as to reduce the procedural time for a power of 80 watts. Laser operates down to a depth of 5 mm for a pressure of 100 watts. It can operate down to a depth of 6 to 7 mm in the endometrium. The same safety measures must be applied to the treatment of the fundus and cornual areas.

### Combined techniques

They allow complete treatment with limited risks. It is possible to realize photovaporization or electrocoagulation of the fundal and cornual areas and resection of the wall and the lower part of the lateral wall.

### Postoperative period

There are usually no complications. In case of anesthesia, the return to consciousness should be quick. Hospitalisation is short, from 12 to 48 hours, and recovery takes 3 to 7 days. A serosanguineous discharge is usually present for 15 to 20 days and sometimes more severe metrorrhagia (bleeding) around the 10th day when the coagulated endometrium is eliminated. No postoperative medication is necessary apart from usual desinfection of the vulva. Patients should avoid any vaginal irrigation and sexual intercourse as long as the discharges continue.

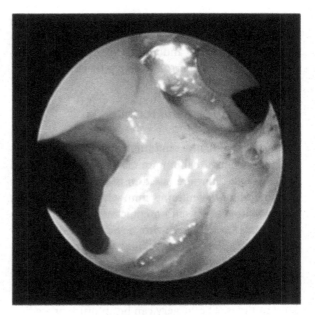

**Fig. 4.** Hysteroscopy six months after endometrectomy. Note the synechiae

### Intraoperative complications: incidents, accidents

Though surgical accidents are rare. Two of them may occur: bleeding and perforation. They can be avoided by meeting a certain number of requirements.

- progression of the hysteroscope under continuous visual control;
- application of the electrical current during the return movement of the loop;
- electroresection or coagulation under visual control;
- respect of the cornual areas (perforation risks because they are thinner);
- hemostasis on demand.

Generally the most dangerous accident for vital prognosis is vascular passage of glycine.

Side effects may be: 1) hypervolemia, because of important fluid resorption causing pulmonary edema; 2) hemodilution with hyponatremia causing cerebral edema; 3) acute renal insufficiency by interstitial nephropathy if glycine is metabolized to serine and glyoxylic acid; 4) encephalopathy.

It is essential to achieve early diagnosis of complications at the start of hemodynamic perturbations. An electrolytogram and hematocrit tests have to be performed when the procedure exceeds 50 minutes or in case of multiple vascular effraction or uterine perforation. Pauciparity and multiparity seem to be favorable elements as a personal study proved.

## Alternatives to endometrectomy

New systems such as endometrium thermocoagulation with a small balloon are currently being offered and assessed. They are based on the principle of heat destruction of the endometrium without using a high energy source as in endometrectomy. The system is made up of a catheter with a balloon linked to a control unit. The balloon is filled with a sterile liquid (5% dextrose) and is activated for a 0.5 cm deep destruction of the endometrium thanks to a thermal resistance. Temperature rises to 85° C and is maintained for 8 minutes. The surgery can be an office procedure with local paracervical block. There are no risks of glycine absorption and no dangers from high temperature sources. In case of balloon rupture there is fluid passage through the vascular network but no risks of vascular or electrolytic complications because of the small quantity of fluid used for the procedure (20 cc) and its immediate cooling. RS. Neuwirth reported the preliminary results on a series of 18 patients with 83% favorable results. (3 failures including two hysterectomies).

## Results

They are to be found on the following Table 2, which represents a compilation of the main results published in the literature.

Immediate complications are few in numbers. In the literature only 2% of complications can be found (uterine perforations, metabolic complications, menorrhagia or endometritis). These results are over-optimistic and do not do justice to clinical facts.

Our series of 121 endometrectomies started in January 1989 to January 1993. It included:
- 103 electroloop resection associated with a Rollerball electrode in the fundal and cornual areas;
- 9 electrocoagulations exclusively carried out with a Rollerball electrode;
- 9 cases of Laser Nd Yag photocoagulation (a limited number because of unavailability of the equipment).

Five patients dropped out. A patient died during the year following the endometrectomy by a rupture of an arterial aneurysm. For the 115 remaining patients the average follow-up period was 25 months (between 12 to 60 months). There were 77 good results (66.9%) (amenorrhea, oligomenorrhea or normal menstruation). The results seemed to deteriorate as time passed, from 90% good results after 6 months to 75% after 12 months. The results published in the literature are on average more favourable than ours, and the closest to ours are Dequesne [3] results: he obtained 78% of good results from a series of 71 endometrectomies after 24 months and 71% after 60 months.

## Comments

The notion of good results is a matter of interpretation. Amenorrhea cannot be considered as a good result if the objective was the restoration of a normal menstrual cycle. The risks of pregnancy are low but not entirely null. Hill recorded a pregnancy – with favourable evolution – three months after an endometrectomy and van Caille [5] one observation of a pregnancy after a Rollerball endometrectomy. Risks are higher with partial endometrial ablation; thus, made a contraceptive treatment has to be prescribed or even endoscopical sterilisation.

Risks of endometrium carcinoma have yet be assessed correctly. They are theoretically null with a complete endometrectomy but it is difficult to be certain. Two observations were published in the literature. It is impossible to realize a complete treatment of the fundal and cornual areas. Cancer could develop from those residual islets and would be really difficult to diagnose. With partial ablation of the endometrium, hysteroscopical screening is theoretically possible.

A hormone substitutive treatment of menopause is to be considered in the therapeutic indication. It may appear inconsistent to realise a conservative treatment which may be a contraindication to a substitutive hormonotherapy.

## Conclusion

Endoscopic treatment of benign lesions of the endometrium is an alternative to hysterectomy, if the evaluation of the mucosa is correct. Several points have to be taken into consideration for a therapeutic plan, particularly a substitutive hormonal treatment of menopause and ulterior risks of carcinoma of the endometrium.

**Table 2.** Endometrectomy main results published in literature

| Authors | Year | Type of procedure | No | Good (N) | Good (%) |
|---|---|---|---|---|---|
| Goldrath [6] | 1986 | Laser | 216 | 206 | 95 |
| Lomano [7] | 1986 | Laser | 89 | 49 | 89 |
| Loffer [8] | 1987 | Laser | 109 | 101 | 93 |
| Bagggish [9] | 1988 | Laser | 14 | 13 | 92 |
| Davis [10] | 1989 | Laser | 25 | 13 | 52 |
| Gimpelson [11] | 1988 | Laser | 70 | 68 | 97 |
| Hamou [12] | 1988 | Resect | 96 | 85 | 88 |
| Bertran [13] | 1989 | Laser | 22 | 21 | 95 |
| Brooks [14] | 1989 | Resect | 19 | 17 | 89 |
| Daniel | 1989 | Laser | 18 | 14 | 78 |
| Mac Lucas [15] | 1989 | Laser | 10 | 10 | 100 |
| Nezhat [16] | 1989 | Laser-resect | 18 | 11 | 60 |
| Vancaille [17] | 1989 | Resect | 171 | 151 | 88 |
| Shirk | 1989 | Laser | 48 | 46 | 96 |
| Dallay [18] | 1992 | Laser | 44 | 42 | 93 |
| Donnez [19] | 1991 | Laser | 50 | 49 | 98 |
| Serden [20] | 1991 | Resect | 91 | 82 | 93 |
| Magos [21] | 1991 | Resect | 234 | 210 | 90 |
| Rankin [22] | 1992 | Resect | 400 | 336 | 85 |
| Van Damme | 1992 | Laser | 200 | 194 | 97 |
| Kiswani [23] | 1993 | Resect-coag | 90 | 88 | 97 |
| Dequesne [3] | 1993 | Resect-laser | 71 | 50 | 71 |
| Brooks [1] | 1994 | Resect | 172 | 163 | 90 |
| Dallay [24] | 1994 | Laser | 107 | 99 | 90 |
| Garry [25] | 1994 | Laser | 600 | 500 | 83.4 |
| Vancaille [5] | 1994 | Coagulation | 90 | 74 | 84 |
| Blanc [26] | 1990 | Resect | 115 | 77 | 67 |

# References

1. Brooks PHG (1994) Resectoscopic endometrial ablation. Réf Gynécol Obst 02:Spécial Hystérectomies et Alternatives 202-205
2. Neuwirth RS, Dura AS, Singer† A et al (1994) The endometrial ablator: a new instrument. Obst Gynecol 8(3):792-796
3. Dequesne J, Lachat R, Sistek J et al (1993) Endometrectomy laparoscopic assisted vaginal hysterectomy vaginal or endometrial hysterectomy: reasoned indications. Gynaecological Endoscopy 2:93-95
4. Hill DJ, Maher DJ (1990) Pregnancy following endometrial ablation. AAGL 19th Annual Meeting, Orlando, Résumé des communications, p 12
5. van Caille TH (1994) Rollerball endometrial ablation. Réf Gynécol Obst Spécial Hystérectomies et alternatives 2:207-211
6. Goldrath MH (1986) Hysteroscopic laser obliteration of the endometrium. In: Sharp F, Jordan MA (eds) Gynecologic laser Surgery. Ithaca Perinatology Press Publ, p 357

7. Lomano JM (1986) Photocoagulation of the endometrium with the ND YAG laser for the treatment of menorrhagia. J Reprod Med 31:148
8. Loffer FD (1987) Hysteroscopic endometrial ablation with ND Yag laser using a non contact technique. Obstet Gynecol 69:679
9. Baggish MS (1988) New laser hysteroscope for neodymium yag endometrial ablation. Laser Surg Med 8:99-103
10. Davis J (1989)Hysteroscopic endometrial ablation with the neodymium yag laser. Br J Obstet Gynecol 96:928-932
11. Gimpelson RJ (1988) Hysteroscopic Nd Yag laser ablation of the endometrium. J Reprod Med 38:372
12. Hamou J, Mencaglia L, Perino A, Gilardi G (1988) L'électrocoagulation en hystéroscopie et microcolposcopie opératoire. In: Cittadini E, Scarselli G, Meucaglia L, Perino A (eds) Isteroscopia operativa e Laser chirurgia in ginecologia. CIC, Roma p 31
13. Bertrand JD (1989) AAGL 18th Meeting, Washington, Livre des communications
14. Brooks PHG (1989) AAGL 18th Meeting, Washington, Livre des communications

15. Mac Lucas B (1989) AAGL 18th Meeting, Washington, Livre des communications

16. Nezhat C (1989) AAGL 18th Meeting, Washington, Livre des communications

17. van Caille TH (1989) AAGL 18th Meeting, Washington, Livre des communications

18. Dalley D, Tissot H, Portal F (1992) Endométrectomie par hystérofibroscopie et laser Yag. J Gynecol Biol Reprod 21:431-435

19. Donnez J, Nisolle M (1991) Nd yag laser et hystéroscopie opératoire. Contrac Fertil Sex 19:299-305

20. Serden JP, Brooks PG (1991) Treatment of abnormal uterine bleeding with the gynecologic rectoscope. J Reprod Med 36(10):697

21. Magos A, Baumann R, Lockwood GM, Turnbull AC (1991) Expérience sur les 250 premières résections d'endomètre pour métrorragies. Lancet (FR) 41-46

22. Rankin L, Steinberg LH (1992) Transcervical resection of the endometrium: a review of 400 consecutive patients. Br J Obstet Gynecol 99:911-914

23. Kiswani L, van Herendael B (1993) Endometrial ablation: resectoscope or laser. A comparison of results. The hysteroscope (ESH), p 7

24. Brie M, Cambon D, Dallay D et al (1994) Endométrectomies par hystérofibroscopie et laser Yag. Réf Gynécol Obst Spécial Hystérectomies et Alternatives 2:197-200

25. Garry R (1994) Endometrial laser ablation. Réf Gynécol Obst Spécial Hystérectomies et alternatives 2:188-195

26. Boubli L, Blanc B, Bautrant E et al (1990) Le risque métabolique de la chirurgie hystéroscopique. J Gynecol Obstet Biol Reprod 19:217-222

27. Singer A, Almanza R, Guttierez A, Neuwirth RS et al (1994) Preliminary clinical experience with a thermal ballon endometrial ablation method to treat menorrhagia. Obstet Gynecol 83:732-4

# Endometrial ablation: a review

L. Mencaglia, D. Tonellotto

Endometrial ablation was first introduced at the beginning of the 1980's as a surgical intervention used to destroy the endometrium in patients diagnosed with "abnormal uterine bleeding". The purpose of this intervention was to reduce or irradicate completely the bleeding. Despite of some other "historic" precedents used against abnormal uterine bleeding, such as chemical substances or radioactive intracavital applications, the first successful case was described using a Neodymium YAG laser under uteroscopic control and attributed to Goldrath [1] in 1981. In 1983, De Cherney and Polan [2] reported an endosopic resector to do unipolar electrocoagulation and obtain identical final results.

Irregular bleeding, particularly in women older than 40, represents a well-known problem by gynecologists, not easily resolved from the medical point of view. In fact, hormone therapy usually causes a transitional effect and could not be applied for extended periods of time. The discovery and utilization of hysteroscopy on a large scale has solved a large portion of these cases, identifying the precise organic pathology responsible for the symptomatology and allowing the successive selective removal (i.e. polyps, submucous fibromyomas). There still remains a consistent number of patients in whom direct vision of the cavity and endometrial biopsy show no significant alterations. In a recent multicentric study by the European Society of Hysteroscopy [3] on 1075 patients with abnormal uterine bleeding, all of them undergoing diagnostic hysteroscopy and successive endometrial biopsy (Table 1), the histological data have demonstrated the presence of an endometrium layer functioning normally or paraphysiological (dysfunctional) in approximately 59% of the cases. This data is slightly lower (47%) if the women selected were in post-menopause (Table 2). The medical hormone treatment usually causes a difficult response in these patients because after an initial positive situation, in some cases after the suspension of the therapy, we observe a relapse in the symtomatology. Besides, all the medical therapies (i.e. progesterone and gestagen, danazol, similar LH-RH, etc.) have caused a number of side effects and are not well tolerated within time. Dilatation and curetage which has been frequently used for many years as the diagnostic and therapeutic method, has been shown to be totally inefficient. An in depth study by Lerner [4] in 1984 demonstrated, just like in reality, that this technique does not change the menometrorrhagia symptomatology, neither in the short nor in the long term.

Table 1. Histological and hysteroscopic results of 1075 patients with abnormal uterine bleeding [3]

|  | NO | % |
| --- | --- | --- |
| Functioning endometrium | 292 | 27.2 |
| Atrophic endometrium | 226 | 21.0 |
| Dysfunctional endometrium | 119 | 11.1 |
| Endometrial polyps | 99 | 9.2 |
| Hyperplasia | 217 | 20.2 |
| Endometrial carcinoma | 68 | 6.3 |
| Endometriosis | 34 | 3.2 |
| Leiomyoma | 7 | 0.6 |
| Other | 13 | 1.2 |

Table 2. Histological and hysteroscopic results of 447 patients in post-menopause

|  | NO | % |
| --- | --- | --- |
| Atrophic endometrium | 181 | 40.4 |
| Dysfunctional endometrium | 34 | 7.5 |
| Endometrial polyps | 55 | 12.3 |
| Endometrial hyperplasia | 105 | 23.4 |
| Endometrial carcinoma | 62 | 13.8 |
| Endocervical carcinoma | 2 | 0.4 |
| Other | 10 | 2.2 |

Hysterectomy is obviously efficient in these cases. Various interventions appear particularly utilized in these unusual bleeding cases. McDonald [5] reported that 50.000 woman every year get total hysterectomy in the UK, of whom ca. 18.500 have menorrhagia or correlated pathologies which could place them as possible candidates for endometrial ablation. Brooks [6] in 1991 refers to the fact that in the US there are about 650.000 hysterectomies per year, of which 200.000 for non oncological reasons. Even though there is no doubt about the efficiency of the intervention, it is disproportionately used in most of the cases. The reasons are its high risk, operation mobidity and most importantly, a high cost for the operation. These types of needs (cost, benefit report, hospital stay length) which are felt more in the US, and in this country as well, resulted in the development and the acceptance of endometrial ablation.

## Indications

As we have seen, the main indications for endometrial ablations are abnormal bleeding, resistance to pharmacological therapies [7] and the absence of cancerous or precancerous lesions of the endometrium. Recently, some authors [8] have proposed endometrial ablation even in cases of endometrial hyperplasia recurrence, even without cytological atypias. The inclusion of these indication forms seems logical from the theoretical point of view for the low oncological potential and for the elevated number of relapses after drug treatment.

Actually, it can be confirmed that endometrial ablation should be performed in patients presenting with an elevated hysterectomy surgical risk and in those who, for various reasons, don't want or just can't undergo traditional surgical interventions. Even the side effects due to the general anesthesia or in the presence of coagulopathies are indications for endometrial ablation, which can also be performed with a local anesthesia [9]. Recently, Lefler [10] proposed the use of endometrial ablation with success in pre-menstrual **dysmenorrhea** syndrome trying to reduce the same menstrual flux and the presence of intracavity clots.

Lastly, particularly in the US, there is a significant request by women to undergo the intervention as a solution to avoid the bother and the inconvenience of menstruating (athletes, managers). Ablation has also the advantage of influencing the negative acceptance of this type of procedure and because of this it has gained such a large success. It is defined, in certain social circles of the American population, as "cosmetic"

surgery. Certainly the knowledge of medicine, which is characteristic of the woman of this nation, has contributed to make endometrial ablation popular thanks to its execution simplicity and favorable results [11].

## Pre-surgery preparation

Absolute conditions to perform endometrial ablation are the certainty of neoplastic lesions, endometrium pre-neoplastic or of the uterine cavity lesions. It is necessary to perform a diagnostic hysteroscopy and an endometrium biopsy before going ahead with the surgical intervention. It is advisable to identify easy the benign pathologies such as endometrial polyps or submucous fibromyomas, which can be removed immediately before performing the ablation. Hysteroscopy associated with endometrial biopsy is normally capable of identifying the neoplastic lesion even in a early phase. In all, it remains to be defined exactly if some focal or early lesion, can escape the initial diagnosis and then be removed using hysteroscopic ablation. Mencaglia [12] reports the identification of two cases of endometrial adenocarcinoma well differentiated in the material sent to the histologist after ablation using resectoscope, the first in the context of a polyp and the other a submucous fibroma identified as benign from the initial hysteroscopic/histologic diagnosis. For now we recommend to use always resectoscope instead of simple destructive techniques which do not permit the histological analyses after the material is removed. The operation of a pure adenocarcinoma, in the initial phase of coagulation or with thermal "destruction" could have a direct effect such as hiding the lesion for a long time from clinical diagnosis [13].

The pre-surgery pharmacological treatment of the patients who undergo endometrial ablation is one of the basic steps for positive intervention results. It is in fact known that the thickness of the endometrium is variable in the different cycle phases and in the pathologic situations (dysfunctional endometrium-hyperplasia). It becomes necessary then to obtain a constant and possibly thin endometrium to be able to proceed with a homogeneous destruction of the mucosa. With Danazol therapy [14] and with the administration of GnRH analogous for approximately 2 months is sufficient to obtain a correct endometrial preparation [15]. Endometrial suppression is of particular importance in the cases where the Nd Yag laser is used because an unprepared endometrium bleeds a great deal and the energy of the Nd Yag laser is absorbed by the dark or red colours, causing superficial thermal destruction and homogeneity of the area. Resectoscope is without doubt the more adaptable technique in those cases which cannot undergo pre-surgery pharmacological therapy, for example in cases where there is massive bleeding or for progressive anemia of the patient. The resection of the endometrium allows in fact the visual identification of the myometrium in the majority of cases, and therefore to adjust the resection thickness to that of the endometrium. Some authors [12] recommend a curettage or an aspiration of the endometrium before the intervention just in case it is not possible to give the patient an adequate pharmacological therapy.

Goldrath [16] suggests a suppression treatment of the endometrium even after post-surgery. Brook et al [6] and Mecaglia et al [8] utilized a preventive antibiotic treatment for two days after surgery.

## Endometrial ablation technique

From the very first attempt up today, there have been many diverse methods more or less efficient in the effort to completely destroy the endometrium. Whatever technique used, some fundamental points have to be followed:

1) it is necessary to destroy the endometrium and all its extensions completely otherwise small islands of endometrium can be areas of epithelium recolonization;

2) it is necessary to destroy the thickness of the endometrium which can be variable depending on the cycle phase (proliferous, secretive) or due to the pathologic situation (atrofia, hyperplasia).The extension should not be too deep in the myometrium to prevent immediate complications and to avoid activation of the scarring process in the area causing complete adhesion syndrome;

3) normally we tend to save epithelium in the isthmus to prevent a possible Ascherman syndrome.

4) it would be ideal to maintain the uterine cavity penetrable in a way that allows for follow ups of this patient;

5) the techniques under uteroscopy control seem preferable to the blind methods because hysteroscopic method is more efficient showing intrauterine lesions of all types.

## Radioactive-chemical substances

Used at the end of the 60's, the substances were blindly injected transcervically so as to create a complete adhesion of the wall of the cavity. The agents which were experimented were mainly the corrosive chemicals such as quinacrine, formaldehyde, oxalic acid or adhesive substances such as **methylcyanoacrilate** or silicon. This type of procedure was abandoned for the potential damage due to the passage of these substances in the peritoneum and for the poor results obtained which required multiple applications. The intracavity applications of radioactive chemicals have been efficiently demonstrated, but were abandoned for the high risk of using radioactive substances.

## Cryosurgery

Proposed in 1987 by Droegemuller [17], it has never been popular for the numerous technical difficulties.

## Destruction of the endometrium using high frequency radio waves

It is a method recently proposed [18, 19], it has to still be considered in the experimental phase [20].

## Resectoscope

It is an instrument which has an urologic derivation, in that it is made up of an optical part and two external sleeves which allow for infusion and contemporary aspiration of the liquid medi for distension of the cavity. To extend the uterine cavity a continual flux pumping system is used, with a sorbitol/mannitol solution that maintains the constant clear vision. Using the resectoscope, two diverse techniques are possible, resection and coagulation. The first consists in shaving endometrial slices 3-5 mm thickness using a resectoscope attached to a electrosurgical source and under direct endoscopic control. This technique is more used in Europe, with the advantage that it permits istopathological analysis of the materials removed. It requires a discrete surgical ability for the removal of all the endometrium without penetrating too deep in the myometrium. The monopolar electrosurgical source must be capable of reaching 50-100 Watts and can be connected to an endoscopic system. On the terminal part of the resector there **is a handle** (U-shaped) which allows the resectioning process to be under endoscopic control.

## Rollerball coagulation

It is a variation of the method stated earlier [21]. In the same way a resector endoscope is used, but at its terminal end it is substituted with a Rollerball, consisting in a metallic, ball attached to a monopolar electrosurgical source which is then used to perform a systematic coagulation of the entire endometrium. This method is technically more simple than resection in that the endometrium is coagulated and there is no risk of penetrating too deep into the myometrium [22]. As a whole, it has the disadvantage of not allowing post-surgical histopathological analysis. Most authors [6, 8] therefore recommend the initial resection using resectoscope and then using the Rollerball to coagulate the vascular bed area reaching the tubal cornua.

## Neodymium Yag laser coagulation

Basically it can be compared to electrosurgical coagulation though the coagulation here is accomplished using a laser [23]. The neodymium Yag laser has a noted coagulative/destructive ability and can be transported using fiber very fine (600 microns). The fiber is introduced into the operation canal of the hysteroscope and under visual control we proceed with the point to point coagulation of the endometrium. The fiber provokes thermal damage to the endometrium with a penetration depth of 5mm from the contact surface. If the fiber is forced into the myometrium we obtain obviously a deeper penetration. Even for laser ablation there are two distinct techniques. The first defined by Goldrath [24] as "dragging" or "touching" consists of forcing the fiber into the endometrial lining till the myometrium is reached, in a way which creates a complete destruction of the epithelium. The second method is described by Loffer [25] as "blanching" or "non touching" which consists of bringing the fiber very close to the endometrial surface, withose cortag. Even in this case most Authors [26] suggest a combination of the two laser techniques to obtain the best results. For Nd Yag ablation it is necessary to have a range from 50 to 70 Watts of power. One of the critical points of this procedure is the uterine cavity width in which the laser does not appear particularly adapted to cavities greater then 8 cm wide. The diameter of the fiber in fact is quite thin (600 microns), therefore requiring a noted amount of time (variable from 40 to 100 minutes) to cover the entire endometrial surface. Some Authors [27] have proposed a method to reduce the time required for the intervention by increasing the power of the laser; it has been demonstrated an existing risk if the intervention is not correctly followed [28]. The cost of the equipment and the impossibility of ever having removed material to be examined histologically represent the two evident limits of this procedure. Other types of lasers such as $CO_2$,

Argon and the KTP 532 revealed to be not usable or are not particularly adapted to this technique.

## Results

The ideal aim of this intervention is to obtain a state of amenorrhea, even if a reduction of the symptomatology big enough to prevent ulterior surgical interventions, including a successive endometrial ablation, has to be considered a positive result. The percentage of amenorrhea is variable, from 7% stated by Baggish [29] to 19% Loffer [25]. It depends in fact on the technique and the variations used and from the selection and the preparation of the patient. Some Authors [8] have also considered the normalization of the menstrual flux a better result than that of amenorrhea and tend to be less aggressive in the surgical procedure. The results which appear to be constant in all cases excluding the experience of Daniell [30] and Davis [31], is that the percentage of failures varies from 3% to 11%. It is necessary to underline that no author has considered in his case histories the percentage of successes which were obtained in these patients that persisted in the hemorrhage symptomatology. In fact, Garry [32], Goldrath [1], Loffer [25], Davis [31] and Mencaglia [8] have demonstrated how it is possible to obtain an amenorrhea, thanks to a second endometrial ablation intervention in approximately 93% of the cases.

Even in terms of comparison, the resectoscope and the laser seem equal in the ability to supply optimum results (amenorrhea-hypomenorrhea): 83% and 86%, respectively.

Lefler [33] reported favorable results even in the treatment of dysmenorrhea, with a 70% improvement of the symptomatology in 99 patients. No author except Mencaglia [8] reported precise results of the incidence of intrauterine synechias in the follow-up exams of these patients. The presence of a total synechia is verified in fact in 8% of the cases. Goldrath [24] refers that after the ablation (dragging) with the Nd Yag laser the cavity is reduced a great deal and in a tube form. This data is also confirmed by Brooks [6].

## Complications

Complications due to endometrial ablations are few. An intraoperation or a postoperation hemorrhage is an occurrence due the techniques which destroy and remove the endometrium [34]. Goldrath [1] reported 13 cases of postoperation bleeding in a total of 335 cases. Mencaglia [8] considered 2 cases which required hospitalization of the post-surgery patients both treated with pharmacological therapy (oxytocin). Many Authors [35] refer the possibility to an intravascular passage of the distension medium. Even if this is possible in all the surgical hysteroscopic procedures, it is necessary to remember that this situation could be very serious with an irreversible encephalitis in case of a massive overloading. The passage of the distension medium is tied to the experience of the operator and the execution time, as well as the liquid pumping pressure. The technique which removes and destroys the endometrium (resection-coagulation) favors the naked placing of the vascularization myometrial and therefore the passage of the distension medium.

Uterine perforation is an event which is quite rare [36], even if Loffer [35] refers to some serious cases of intra-abdominal lesions, which caused the death of the patient in both the Nd Yag laser and resectoscopy techniques.

## Conclusion

Endometrial ablation is not just a simple experimental procedure but a reality in the field of gynecological surgery [37]. The results demonstrate clearly that it is possible to prevent a large percentage, near 50%, of hysterectomies in patients with abnormal bleeding who are resistant to pharmacological therapies. The advantages of hysteroscopic surgery are evidently tied to the short hospitalization period of the patient (day surgery), the low morbidity and to the optimum results obtained. Some weak points must still be cleared, for example, the risk of destroying the neoplastic lesions which are not identified, the chance of hiding them, or the long term follow up of these patients. It is probable that this intervention will become even more simple in the future. Actually the resectoscope seems to be the more popular technique due to how easy it is to learn and to its low exercise cost.

In terms of cost-benefit, imagine that in approximately 200,000 hysterectomies which are done in the US per year, roughly 90,000 could be prevented due to endometrial ablation with a calculated savings of 180 million dollars.

As it is, the medical organization in our country is quite different, but the above data is indicative even in our own reality.

## References

1. Goldrath MH, Fuller TA, Segal S (1981) Laser photovaporization of endometrium for the treatment of menorrhagia. Am J Obstet Gynecol 140:14

2. De Cherney A, Polan ML (1983) Hysteroscopic management of intrauterine lesions and intractable uterine bleeding. Obstet & Gynecol 61:392

3. Mencaglia L, Colafranceschi M (1990) Hysteroscopy in abnormal uterine bleeding: a multicentric study. Abstract IVth European Congress of Hysteroscopy and Endoscopic Surgery, Losanna, Svizzera pp 13-15, 18

4. Lerner HM (1984) Lack of efficacy of prehysterectomy curettage as a diagnostic procedure. Am J Obstet Gynecol 15:1055

5. Mac Donald R (1990) Modern treatment of menorrhagia. Br J Obstet Gynecol 97:3

6. Brooks P (1991) Unpublished data

7. Wren BG (1998) Dysfunctional uterine bleeding. Aust Fam Physician 27(5):371-377

8. Mencaglia L, Taticchi F, Mommi R, Gilardi G (1990) Ablazione endometriale per via isteroscopia. In Atti del LXVI Congresso della Societa' Italiana di Ginecologia ed Ostetricia, Roma, CIC Ed, p 889

9. Magos AL, Baumann R, Cheung K, Turnbull AC (1989) Intrauterine surgery under intravenous sedation as an alternative to hysterectomy. Lancet 925

10. Lefler HT (1989) Premenstrual syndrome improvement after laser ablation of the endometrium for menorrhagia. J Reprod Med 34:905

11. Nagele F, Rubinger T, Magos A (1998) Why do women choose endometrial ablation rather than hysterectomy? Fert Steril 69(6):1063-1066

12. Mencaglia L (1991) Hysteroscopic resection of submucous fibroids and endometrial polyps. Gynecol End (in press)

13. Margolis MT, Thoen LD, Boike GM, Mercer LJ, Keith LG (1995) Asymptomatic endometrial carcinoma after endometrial ablation. Int J Gynaecol Obstet 51(3):255-258

14. Fraser IS, Healy DL, Torode H, Song JY, Mamers P, Wilde F (1996) Depot goserelin and danazol pre-treatment before rollerball endometrial ablation for menorrhagia. Obstet Gynaecol 87(4):544-550

15. Romer T (1998) Benefit of GnRH analogue pretreatment for hysteroscopic surgery in patients with bleeding disorders. Gynaecol Obstet Invest 45 [Suppl 1]:12-20; discussion 21, 35

16. Goldrath MH (1990) Use of danazol in hysteroscopic surgery for menorrhagia. J Reprod Med 35:91

17. Droegemuller W, Greer BE, Davis JR (1978) Cryocoagulation of the endometrium at the uterine cornua. Am J Obstet Gynaecol 131:1

18. Philips JH, Lewis BV, Roberts T, Prior MV, Hand JW, Edler M, Field SB (1990) Treatment of functional menorrhagia by a radio frequency induced thermal endometrial ablation. Lancet 335:374

19. Lewis BV (1995) Radiofrequency induced endometrial ablation. Baillieres Clin Obstet Gynaecol 9(2):347-355

20. Thijssen RF (1997) Radiofrequency induced endometrial ablation: up date. Br J Gynaecol 104(5):608-613

21. Valle RF (1995) Rollerball endometrial ablation. Bailliers Clin Obstet Gynaecol 9(2):299-316

22. Paskowitz RA (1995) "Rollerball" ablation of the endo-metrium. L Reprod Med 40(5):333-336

23. Osei E, Tharmaratnam S, Opemuyi I, Cochrane G (1995) Laser endometrial ablation with the neodynium: yttrium-aluminium garnet (Nd-Yag) laser: a review of ninety consecutive patients. Acta Obstet Gynaecol Scand 74(8):619-623

24. Goldrath MH (1990) Intrauterine laser surgery. In: Keye WR (ed) Laser Surgery in Gynecology and Obstetrics. GK Hall Mass Publisher, Boston, p 93

25. Loffer FD (1987) Hysteroscopic endometrial ablation with the ND: Yag laser using a non-touch technique. Obstet & Gynecol 69:679

26. Loffer FD (1988) Laser ablation of the endometrium. In: De Cherney AH (ed) Hysteroscopy. Obstetricial and Gynecological Clinics of North America, WB Saunders Philadelphia, p 77

27. Indmna PD (1991) Highpower Nd: Yag laser ablation of the endometrium. J. Reprod Med 36:501

28. Perry CP, Daniell LF, Gimpelson RJ (1990) Bowel injury from Nd: Yag endometrial ablation. J Gynecol Surg 6:199

29. Baggish MS, Baltoyannis P (1988) New techniques for laser ablation of the endometrium in high risk patients. Am J Obstet Gynaecol 159:287

30. Daniell LF, Tosh R, Meisels S (1986) Photodynamic ablation of the endometrium with the Nd: Yag laser hys-teroscopically as a treatment of menorrhagia. Colpos-copy & Gynecologic Laser Surgery 2:43

31. Davis JA (1989) Hysteroscopic endometrial ablation with the neodymium-Yag laser. Brit J Obstet Gynecol 96:928

32. Garry R, Erian J, Grochmel SA (1991) A multi-centre collaborative study into the treatment of menorrhagia by Nd: Yag laser ablation of the endometrium. Brit J Obstet Gynecol 98:357

33. Lefler HT, Sullivan GH, Hulka JF (1991) Modified endo-metrial ablation: electrocoagulation with vaso-pression and suction curettage preparation. Obstet Gynecol 77

34. Loffer FD (1995) Endometrial ablation and resection. Curr Opin Obstet Gynaecol 7(4):290-294

35. Loffer FD (1992) Complications related to uterine dis-tending media. In: Corfman RS, Diamond MP, De Cherney AH (eds) Complications of endoscopic proce-dures: intra-abdominal and intra-uterine. Blackwell Scientific Publ, Cambridge,

36. Hulka JF, Peterson HA, Phillips JM, Surrey MW (1997) Operative hysteroscopy: American Association of Gynecologic Laparoscopists' 1993 membership survey. J Am Assoc Gynaecol Laparosc 2(2):131-132

37. Hart R, Magos A (1997) Endometrial ablation. Curr Opin Obstet Gynaecol 9(4):226-232

# Endometrial ablation in an office setting

F.D. LOFFER

## Historical background

Endometrial ablation was probably first described in 1937 using an electrical method [1]. No further work was done until 1971 when endometrial destruction was attempted by cryotherapy. The results obtained with the equipment available at that time were inadequate [2]. Finally, in 1981 excellent results were achieved using the Nd:Yag laser [3]. The author was the second person to employ laser energy for endometrial ablation and using a slightly different technique confirmed excellent clinical results [4]. It is a historical anomaly that high technology laser energy was used for endometrial ablation before electrical energy since the latter had long been used in operative surgery. Removal of the endometrium using a modified urological resectoscope with a loop electrode was not accomplished until 1983 [5]. The first description of the use of a bail ended electrode was in 1988 [6]. However, this report was in a Japanese journal and it was not until the following year that clinical results were available [7].

## Traditional results

Excellent results have been achieved using both the Nd:Yag laser and the resectoscope method and they provide a gold standard for the newer technology being developed [8]. The largest published Nd:Yag laser series reports on 524 patients followed between 6 and 42 months. Twenty seven percent were amenorrheic; 66% had continuing menses and 7% required a hysterectomy [9]. To achieve these results there were 75 patients who had a repeat procedure. Similar results were found in a smaller series of 100 patients followed 6 to 130 months [10]. In this group amenorrhea occurred in 23% and hypomenorrhea in 60% of patients. Seven percent of patients returned to eumenorrhea and the procedure failed to control menorrhagia in 10%.

Long term follow-up with electrical methods have also produced excellent results. In a follow-up of 130 patients between 6 and 84 months amenorrhea was achieved in 26% of patients, hypomenorrhea in 51% and eumenorrhea in 16%. There was a 7% failure rate [10]. Slightly poorer results were obtained in this series with a resection technique as compared to a rouer ablation technique. In 128 patients who underwent roller ball ablation and were followed 12 to 52 months, amenorrhea was achieved in 25%; hypomenorrhea in 57% and normal menses in 4%. Failure to control bleeding occurred in 14% [11].

Using the life-table analysis of 525 patients treated by endometrial resection 80% of women had no further surgery and 91% had not had a hysterectomy [12].

Although the Nd:Yag laser and the resectoscope ablation procedures are very efficacious in experienced hands and appear to the casual observer to be quite simple to accomplish, they are very skill dependent. The first cases in an operator's hands yield much poorer results than after experience has been achieved [13].

While laser and electrical endometrial ablation procedures have been done in an office setting they are usually done in an outpatient or hospital operating facility. The reasons for this are several fold. The equipment, especially the Nd:Yag laser, are very expensive and cannot be economically justified unless they are used by several specialties. There is discomfort not only with cervical dilatations but more importantly with the necessary manipulation within the uterine cavity. Finally, the risk involved in these procedures, primarily excessive fluid intravasation, are more easily monitored in a true operating room setting.

## Benefits of the new technology for endometrial ablation

Minimally invasive surgical procedures have resulted not only in longer cost and quicker patient recovery when done in traditional operating room settings but also have encouraged the movement of many procedures into an office setting. It was logical that endometrial ablation, a procedure needed by many thousands of women and accomplishable without any incisions, should move towards being done in an office.

The newer technologies will have obvious appeal especially if they are easier to do in a non-hospital setting. However, they need to be of equal or greater effectiveness; be less costly to accomplish; be more readily done under local anesthesia and require less skill in achieving more uniform results.

Virtually all of the new technologies are blind procedures. Many are not suitable for use in patients whose uterine cavity is distorted by a septum, large fibroids or polyps. Therefore, in addition to knowing about the endometrial histology, the size and shape of the cavity must frequently be determined by either ultrasound or hysteroscopy.

Although many of the newer endometrial ablation techniques appear to be more suitable for office use and have been accomplished in office settings, many are still done in an outpatient or hospital operating room setting. In part this is because of the anesthetic and pain management requirements of all endometrial ablation procedures. Intraoperative and postoperative cramping can be a significant problem frequently requiring the use of conscious sedation in addition to non-steroidals and a paracervical block. Before endometrial ablation can become widely adapted for office use, gyneçologists will have to become more familiar and comfortable with providing higher levels of pain relief than are now generally used.

## Indications for endometrial ablation

In spite of the less skills required in implementing these new technologies, it is extremely important that rigid standards of work up and surgical indications should be adhered to. Endometrial ablation is primarily designed for ovulatory women with menorrhagia or menometrorrhagia whose uterine cavity is normal or can be made essentially normal in size and configuration by removing polyps or submucous myomas. Since no ablation procedures can be sure that all endometrium is destroyed, no patient with a malignant or premalignant condition, nor a patient who is predisposed to an endometrial malignancy should be considered for this procedure. It should not be used in patients who want to become pregnant. Although the procedure is not a sterilization technique, it severely limits a patient's ability to become pregnant and to sa-

fely carry a pregnancy. Finally, both patients and their physicians must recognize that amenorrhea cannot be guaranteed by any technique.

## Methods of tissue destruction

All technologies except cryotherapy depend on tissue destruction by thermal energy. The means of creation of that energy and its delivery to the uterine cavity varies according to the technology. In the following section, a description will be given to the power source, the method of delivery, the tissue effects, the results and complications if known. The type of technologies will be divided into laser, electrical, heated fluids, microwave, cryotherapy and photodynamic therapy. Only a few of the newer technologies have been studied in detail and their clinical effectiveness proven.

### Laser energy

The Nd:Yag laser develops a wave length of 1,064 nm. This is ideally suited for use with an operative hysteroscope. It can be transmitted into the uterine cavity through a flexible 600 or 800 micron fiber and the energy is not absorbed by fluids. This allows distension of the uterine cavity with a physiological saline solution thus avoiding the risks of hyponatremia but not hypervolemia. The laser energy can be applied to the surface by a dragging technique in which the fiber is drug along the surface vaporizing the endometrium and penetrating into the uterine musculature to further complete the destructive process [3]. A nontouch technique in which the laser fiber is brought as close and perpendicular as possible to the uterine surface was developed in order to decrease intraoperative fluid intravasation and postoperative bleeding [4]. Technically it is ceasier to use a non-touch technique in the fundal area and a dragging technique in the longer uterine segment and many physicians use this combined approach. A side fire fiber which allows the lateral uterine walls to be approached in a non-contact technique has provided very good results [14].

A new fiberoptic delivery system similar to an IUD has also been developed which is inserted collapsed into the uterus and opens to conform to the configuration of the uterine cavity [15]. No uterine distension is required in 5 patients studied using the Nd:Yag laser with an output of 30 watts in a continuous mode for 5 minutes; the maximum serosal temperature was 41 degrees centigrade. The first 2 patients of the 10 who underwent this therapy had an immediate hysterectomy to study tissue effects. Seven of the remaining patients who were followed from 6-17 months were amenorrheic and 1 patient had a hysterectomy for pain.

The GyneLase™ or Elitt™ (ESC Medical Systems Ltd., Israel) uses a similar intrauterine device and a continuous wave GaALAs diode laser with a wavelength of 830 nm and a variable power up to 21 watts with an automated programmed exposure time. This system is currently being investigated. Clinical results have not yet been published.

## Electrical energy

The gynecologic resectoscope using a roller ball or bar electrode requires similar electrosurgical generating equipment as is used for transurethral prostatectomies. There is no uniformity of opinion among clinicians as to the type of wave form that is best used. Some authors believe a continuous wave form (cutting current) at about 100 watts provides the best in depth destruction. The author has had good results using a modulated (coagulating) current at 75 watts. There seems to be good evidence to support this power [16]. The tissue effect is to vaporize the softer endometrium and coagulate the endometrium to a sufficient depth to destroy the deep encroachment of endometrial glands into the myometrium and the vascular supply that might help regenerate residual endometrium. When a loop electrode is used, a power setting of 100-110 watts of a continuous (cutting) wave form allows the endometrium and myometrium to be resected. Some operators prefer to then roll over the irregular surface with a roller in order to enhance the effectiveness of this technique [17].

The resectoscope is a unipolar instrument and necessitate the use of non-electrolyte distending media for adequate tissue effects to be obtained. Because of this, there is a greater risk with the resection technique of excessive fluid intravasation resulting in hyponatremia. In order to avoid this, a sheath has been developed (ERA Sleeve Conceptus Inc, San Carlos, CA) which fits over the resectoscope converting it to, in essence, a unipolar piece of equipment which can use saline as a distending media. Higher power settings are used than with the conventional resectoscope.

The OPERA Star system (FemRx Inc, Sunnyvale, CA) is a modified disposable resectoscope which uses physiological fluid as a distending media. This is accomplished by both electrical poles being incorporated in the resectoscope. The loop end is designed to cut and coagulate the endomyometrial surface and a built-in morcellator removes the tissue. Over 200 resection-ablations have been done without complications of fluid overload [18]. Detailed clinical results are not available.

Another electrical instrument which allows the use of saline is the Versapoint™ (Gynecare, Ethicon, Menlo Park, CA). This system uses a dedicated power source and a disposable probe. The probe can be used through a standard 5 French operating hysteroscope channel. The technology has also been developed into a modified resectoscope. It functions as a bipolar instrumentation because the electrical current traverses from the tissue being treated through the saline back to the return electrode further up the probe. Although designed for vaporization and transaction of myomas, polyps, septums and adhesions, it has been used for endometrial ablation. No clinical trials have been published to support its efficacy or safety.

The Vesta block™ system (Vesta Medical, Valley Lab, Boulder, CO) uses a modified electrosurgical generator and a disposable inflatable device containing 12 electrodes. Each electrode is controlled by a separate thermistor which after a warm up interval lasting between 90 and 150 seconds automatically keeps the electrode at 75 degrees C for 4 minutes. A continuous (cutting) current of 45 watts is used in this unipolar system.

Results in a randomized study comparing the Vesta block™ system against endometrial resection followed by roller ball ablation shows statistically similar results were achieved in diminishing blood loss and obtaining amenorrhea [17]. General or epidural anesthesia was used in 16.7% of the Vesta™ procedures and 80% of the roller ball procedures. The remainder of the procedures were done using paracervical block and intravenous sedation. More adverse events occurred in the roller ball ablation than in the Vesta™ arm of the study. A problem unique to this system is muscle fasciculation which required discontinuing the procedure in 1 of 18 cases.

A true bipolar system being currently clinically evaluated is the Novasure™ (Novacept, Palo Alto, CA). This system uses a dedicated bipolar high frequency electrosurgical generator and a disposable ablation device. The intrauterine portion of the probe consists of a 24 carat gold plated disposable mesh with non-conducting portions on the anterior and posterior midline surface as well as along each side. The effect of this configuration is a bipolar system in which current flows through endometrial tissue from one portion of the mesh electrode to the other. Once the device is opened in the uterine cavity, a negative pressure is applied thus pulling the endometrial and uterine surface against the electrode. The device was used in 22 pre-hysterectomy cases. The power delivered to perform the procedure range between 54 and 145 watts. Treatment time is generally between 1 and 2 minutes. Only in 1 case was any endometrium identifiable when evaluated by diaphorase stain. The 21 patients treated in the feasibility study were pretreated with a GNRH agonist. All had iv. conscious sedation without paracervical block or NSAID's. Of 18 patients evaluable at 12 months, amenorrhea was achieved in 16 patients. The other 2 patients were hypomenorrheic. In 14 patients without pre-treatment, followed up to 6 months, 2 patients were hypomenorrheic and 12 were amenorrheic. No significant complications were identified in either group [19].

## Heated fluid systems

The ThermaChoice™ System (Gynecare Products Division, Ethicon Inc., Menlo Park, CA) uses a dedicated generator which monitors pressure, temperature and treatment time. A disposable 5 mm probe with a latex balloon at one end containing a thermistor and heating element is inserted into the uterine cavity. After demonstrating the integrity of the catheter by filling with sterile 5% dextrose and water and then creating a negative pressure, the balloon is inserted into the uterus. The catheter is refilled with 5% dextrose and water until a pressure of 170-180 mmHg is achieved. At this pressure the balloon will conform to the shape of the uterine cavity. A treatment time of 87 degrees for 8 minutes is monitored by the generator.

In a randomized study comparing the ThermaChoice™ system to the standard roller ball ablation, statistically similar decreases in days of menstrual flow and decrease in diary scores was shown [20].

Amenorrhea rates at one year were statistically different with the roller ball at 27.2% and the ThermaChoice™ system at 15.2%. However, by 24 months the difference had narrowed with the amenorrheic rate in the rouer bail at 21.7% and ThermaChoice at 13.3%. In this study, 84.1% of patients in the roller ball group had general anesthesia but only 53.7% in the ThermaChoice™ group. At one study site, 12 of the 13 ThermaChoice™ patients were done in an office setting. No intraoperative adverse events were recorded with the Therma-ChoiceTM system and no significant postoperative problems developed.

A new ThermaChoice™ catheter is being developed which has the ability to mix the heated fluid within the intrauterine silicone balloon. *In vitro* and *in ex-vivo* extrapated uteri studies, there appears to be an increased thermal effect on the posterior uterine surface which would appear to increase the depth of destruction by 1 mm. It would be anticipated that this would increase effectiveness without altering safety.

The Cavaterm™ system (Wallsten Medical, Morges, Switzerland) uses a battery operated generator and disposable catheter with a silicone balloon. At the distal end of this 8 mm catheter is a heating element, thermistor and mixing unit. Treatment temperature is 75 (+-5) C for 30 minutes. Glycine is used as the distending media. The balloon is pressured to 170-180 mmHg.

At 18-28 months of follow-up, 29 of 32 suitable candidates for the procedure (91%) reported significant reduction in bleeding. Three patients continued to bleed heavily but less than before the treatment. No significant complications have been reported [21]. In another study using the Cavaterm system, 50 patients were followed between 6 and 24 months (mean 15 months)[22]. Thirty-four (68%) had complete amenorrhea; 12 (24%) spotted, and 2 (4%) had normal menses. There were 2 treatment failures and no significant complications.

The Hydro ThermAblator™ (BEI Medical Systems, Hockensack, NJ) circulates heated saline into the uterine cavity [23]. The procedure is monitored hysteroscopically and the fluid is circulated through a disposable hysteroscope sheath. A pressure of 75-80 mmHg is used which prevents outflow through the tubes. The safety of the device relies on direct visualization of the uterine cavity during treatment and an automatic shut down of the system should a deficit of 10cc occur. Preliminary results are excellent. Amenorrhea and hypomenorrhea rates are of 41% each and eumenorrhea of 6% at 1 year [24]. No significant complications have occurred. This system is currently being compared in a randomized study to the roller ball ablation.

The EnAbl™ system (US Surgical Corp, Norwalk, CT) also circulates a heated saline for 15 minutes at a temperature of 70-85° C [25, 26]. Results of clinical studies are not available.

## Microwave endometrial ablation

The MEA system (Microsulis, Waterlooville, Hampshire, UK) is a microwave system composed of a computerized control unit, a coaxial microwave cable and reusable uterine probes. The shaft diameter is 8.5 mm which delivers a 9.2 GHz microwave to the uterine cavity. A power of 30 watts is used with a mean treatment time of 147 seconds. In 180 women followed up to 2 years amenorrhea rates were approximately 35% [27]. Approximately 89% of patients received no further re-treatment after the first microwave endometrial ablation. No intraoperative complications have been reported.

## Radiofrequency electromagnetic energy ablation

The Menostat™ system (Rocket Medical, Watford, UK) uses a conductive intrauterine probe. The patient wears an external electrode around her waist. In an international study of 1.280 cases, 944 patients were followed between 6 and 54 months [28]. Amenorrhea resulted in 184 patients (19%) with hypomenorrhea in 557 patients (59%). Poorer results occurred in 199 patients (21%). Serious complications developed with this device and further safety enhancements were felt to be necessary before wide spread use could be considered.

## Cryotherapy

Cryotherapy for uterine ablation appears to have promise [29]. It is being evaluated (Cryogen Inc, San Diego, CA). The system uses a control unit and reusable intrauterine probe which measures 5.5 mm in diameter. Three to 5 cc of saline are instilled into the uterine cavity and the intrauterine probe is placed in one horn where 4 minute freezing cycle is followed by a 2-3 minute thawing cycle. The probe is then placed in the opposite horn for an additional 4 minute maximum freezing [30].

The Gynecare Soprano Cryotherapy System (Gynecare Products Division, Ethicon, Inc, Menlo Park, CA) is an uniquely small cryoablation system about the size of a personal computer. It is a closed loop system. The re-useable probe is 5 mm in diameter and has a rounded atraumatic tip. The active freezing zone is 4 cm in length.

Long term results are not yet available and a pivotal trial are being conducted on both systems.

## Photodynamic ablation therapy

An interesting concept for endometrial ablation is the photosensitization of endometrium and the subsequent treatment with light. A variety of photosensiti-

zers are available including 10 ethyl etiopurprin (SnET2) and Benzyoporphyrin [32, 31]. The interaction between light and the sensitized endometrium induces an oxidation reaction. Singlet oxygen which is produced by such a reaction is toxic to the endometrium. Specific wavelengths of light are necessary to optimize the reaction depending on the sensitizing agent used. An intrauterine light probe has been designed to provide adequate light coverage of the uterine cavity [33]. This is still an experimental technique and no clinical trials are available to evaluate.

## The future

All endometrial ablation techniques currently available and probably all of those technologies being developed can be done in an office setting. The limiting factors in moving endometrial ablation into the office would appear to be the cost of the equipment involved and the need to provide pain management beyond simply a paracervical block and non-steroidal. The newer technologies appear to be less skill dependent than the Nd:Yag or resectoscope procedures and therefore provide more uniform results. This coupled with their generally shorter treatment times makes them ideally suited for office use.

## References

1. Bardenheuer FH (1937) Elektrokoagulation der uterusschleimhaut zur Behandlerung klimakterischer Blutengen. Zentralblatt Gynaekologic 59:209-216
2. Droegemueller W, Makowski E, Macealka R (1971) Destruction of the endometrium by cryosurgery. Am J Obstet Gynecol 110:467-469
3. Goldrath MH, Fuller TA, Segal S (1981) Laser photovaporization of endometrium for the treatment of menorrhagia. Am J Obstet Gynecol 140:14-19
4. Loffer F (1987) Hysteroscopic endometrial ablation with the ND: Yag laser using a nontouch technique. Obstet Gynecol 69:679-682
5. DeCherney AH, Polan ML (1983) Hysteroscopic management of intrauterine lestons and intractable uterine bleeding. Obstet Gynecol 61:392-397
6. Lin BL, Miyamoto N, Tomomatu M et al The development of a new hysteroscopic resectoscope and its clinical applications on transcervical resection (TCR) and endometrial ablation (EA). Jap J Obstet Gynecol Endosc 4:56-61
7. Vancaillie TG (1989) Electrocoagulation of the endometrium with ball-end electrode. Obstet Gynecol 74:425-427

208     F.D. Loffer

8. Loffer FD (1992) Endometrial ablation-where do we stand? Gynaecol Endosc 1:175-179

9. Garry R, Shelley-Jones D, Mooney P et al (1995) Six hundred endometrial laser ablations. Obstet Gynecol 85:24-29

10. Loffer FD (1995) Endometrial ablation and resection. Curr Op Obstet Gynecol 7:290-294

11. Chullapram T, Song J, Fraser I (1996) Medium-term follow up of women with menorrhagia treated by rollerball endometrial ablation. Obstet Gynecol 88:71-76

12. O'Connor H, Magos A (1996) Endometrial resection for the treatment of menorrhagia. New Eng J Med 335: 151-156

13. Unger JB Meeks GR (1996) Hysterectomy after endometrial ablation. Am J Obstet Gynecol 175:1432

14. Everett, RB (1999) Five year review of endometrial ablation with the SideFire laser fiber. J Am Assoc Gynecol Laparosc 6: 65-70

15. Donnez J, Polet R, Mathieu P et al (1996) Endometrial laser interstitial hyperthermy: a potential modality for endometrial ablation. Obstet Gynecol 87:459-464

16. Farnsworth A, Itzkowic D, Catt M et al (1994) Rollerball endometrial ablation: a histological study in danazol pretreated patients. Aust NZ J Obstet Gynaecol 34:200-207

17. Corson SL, Brill AI, Brooks PG et al (1999) Interim results of the American Vesta trial of endometrial ablation. J Am Assoc Gynecol Laparosc 6:45-49

18. Isaacson KB, Olive DL (1999) Operative hysteroscopy in physiologic distension media. J Am Assoc Gynecol Laparosc 6: 113-118

19. Seth Stabinsky (1999) Novacept, Palo Alto, California (Personal communication)

20. Meyer WR, Walsh BW, Grainger DA et al (1998) Thermal balloon and rollerball ablation to treat menorrhagia: a multicenter comparison. Obstet Gynecol 92: 98-103

21. Friberg R, Persson BRR, Willen R et al (1998) Endometrial destruction by thermal coagulation: evaluation of a new form of treatment for menorrhagia. Gynaecol Endosc 7:73-78

22. Hawe JA, Phillips G, Erian J et al (1998) Endometrial ablation with the Cavaterm endometrial balloon (Abst) 5:Sl9

23. Goldrath MH, Barrionuevo M, Husain M (1997) Endometrial ablation by hysteroscopic instillation of trot saline solution. J Am Assoc Gynecol Laparosc 4: 235-240

24. Weisberg M (1998) BEI Medical Systems, Hockensock, NY (Personal communication)

25. Baggish M, Paraiso M, Breznock EM et al (1995) A computer-controlled continuously circulating, trot irrigating system for endometrial ablation. Am J Obstet Gynecol 173:1842-1848

26. Bustos-Lopez HH, Ibarra-Chavarria A, Vadillo-Ortega F et al (1996) Endometrial ablation with the EnAbl System. J Am Assoc Gynecol Laparosc 3 [Suppl]: S5

27. Sharp NC, Feldberg IB, Hodgeon DA et al (1998) Microwave endometrial ablation. In: Sutton C, Diamond MP (eds) Endoscopic surgery for gynecologists. 2nd ed WB Saunders, London, pp 630-637

28. Thijesen RFA (1997) Radiofrequency induced endometrial ablation: an update. Br J Obstet Gynecol 104:608-613

29. Rutherford TJ (1996) Cryosurgery is a simple modality for endometrial ablation. J Am Assoc Gynecol Laparosc 3 [Suppl]:S44

30. Williams J, Townsend D, Dobak J et al (1998) In vivo uterine endometrial cryoablation with ultrasound visualization. Presented at 27th annuel meeting of the American Association of Gynecologic Laparoscopists. Atlanta, Georgia, November 10-15

31. Rocklin GB, Kelly HG, Steve AA et al (1996) Photodynamic therapy of rat endometrium sensitized with tin ethyl etropurpurin. J Am Assoc Gynecol Laparosc 3: 561-570

32. Horung R, Fehr MK, Tromberg BJ et al (1998) Uptake of the photo sensitizer benzoprophryin deriverative in human endometrium after topical application in vivo. J Am Assoc Gynecol Laparosc 5:367-374

33. Tadir Y, Horung R, Pham T et al (1999) Intrauterine light probe for photodynamic ablation therapy. Obstet Gynecol 93:299-303

# Thermoablation of the endometrium

B. Blanc

A survey by the WHO on heavy uterine bleeding reported a stable prevalence of menorrhagia in 19% of the 5322 women interviewed in 14 different countries. Menorrhagia can be invalidating and its limitations on active, social and family life for the concerned women are severe. It is a common cause for anemia by iron loss in women.

Heavy uterine bleeding is the most frequent cause for consultation in women in the perimenopausal period. It is managed by progestative treatments but when they fail they are followed by surgical procedures, particularly hysterectomy. With the development of endoscopic techniques, surgical conservatory alternatives such as endometrectomy are now available. These new techniques require highly specialised training.

Thermocoagulation of the endometrium is a new technique using an intrauterine balloon (UBT gynecare catheter). It is an interesting alternative which can be carried out without technical difficulty in the treatment of refractory bleeding.

International studies were first published by Surger et al. in Northern America in 1988 followed by Haber in Canada in 1993. In France, a preliminary multicentre study was launched in 1994 (Hurriet's Law). The four centres chosen for this study were Prof. Fernandez' Department in Clamart, Prof. Dallay's centre in Bordeaux, Prof. Body's department in Tours, and Prof. Blanc's department in Marseille.

In the short term, the preliminary results of this therapy are comparable to the results reported by Anglo-Saxon authors with an 89% success rate [1-3].

The feasibility and short-term efficacy (3 to 6 months) having been demonstrated, we now report long-term evaluation of the technique (ranging between 10 to 24 months) through the study of 66 cases in the four French centers.

## Our study

Thermocoagulation of the endometrium was evaluated in 66 patients presenting with dysfunctional menometrorrhagia. The patients were treated between November 1994 and February 1996. Evaluation was carried out in December 1996 with a follow-up period ranging from 10 to 24 months according to the patients. Theses were questioned about reduction of blood flow or continuous menorrhagia before and after treatment. Success was defined as a clear reduction of menses to eumenorrhea or even amenorrhea.

## Technique

### Description

The uterine balloon therapy system (UBT Gynecare catheter) is specific for treatment of dysfunctional menorrhagia by thermal ablation of the endometrium. It consists of a latex balloon fixed at the end of a catheter (OD 5 mm) which is inserted into the uterus and then filled with 2 to 30 ml of a 5% dextrose solution to distend all the folds. The heating unit is housed in the distal tip of the catheter inside the balloon and keeps an 87° C temperature during 8 minutes. The heating produces thermocoagulation of the endometrial tissues. The catheter is linked to a controller unit which monitors the temperature and duration of the treatment cycle and pre-set intraballoon pressure. The balloon is filled with fluids till a mean pressure of about 170 mmHg is achieved.

For safety, the device automatically deactivates when the pressure falls below 45 mmHg or reaches 210 mmHg and above. Moreover, if the temperature inside the balloon exceeds 95° C, the heating unit shuts itself off and the heating cycle is stopped. At the end of the cycle, the balloon is emptied and the catheter is delicately removed from the uterus.

### Selection criteria for the patients (Table 1)

Eligible candidates were premenopausal women, with no desire for preservation of fertility, no antecedents of malignancy, and presenting with functional menometrorrhagia. They were otherwise in good health.

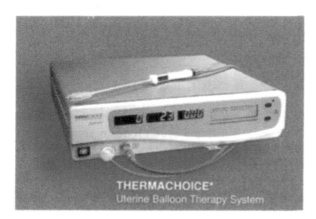

**Fig. 1.** The uterine balloon therapy system

**Table 1.** Selection criteria

---

Dysfunctional menometrorrhagia
 • Premenopausal women with no desire for further fertility
 • No history of malignant or pre-malignant lesions
 • Normal uterine cavity
 • Uterine cavity depth from 6 to 12 cm
 • General good health

---

## Contraindications (Table 2)

Contraindications to the therapy include:
- allergy to latex, for the balloon is made of the material;
- intrauterine fibroids or polyps which distort the uterine cavity and may impede the uniform application of the heating balloon against the uterine mucosa;
- abnormalities of the uterine cavity which prevents the balloon from adapting to the endometrium;

**Table 2.** Contraindications to thermo-coagulation

---

 • Latex allergy
 • Intrauterine fibroids or polyps
 • Pathologies distorting the uterine cavity
 • Genital tract infections
 • Uterine cavity depth < 6 cm or > 12 cm

---

- uterine infection as for any intrauterine maneuver;
- hysterometry inferior to 6 cm for the balloon cannot be correctly expanded inside the uterine cavity but hysterometry over 12 cm is no good as it is bigger than the balloon.

## Preoperative preparation

Before any thermocoagulation are requested:
- negative cervical smears within a year;
- hysteroscopy with normal endometrial biopsies (no malignancy or suspicious lesions).

## Population

Twenty-five patients were treated in Clamart, 27 in Marseilles, 6 in Tours, and 8 in Bordeaux. The description of the population is schown in Table 3.

The mean age of the patients was 45-56 years old. The majority of the patients was multiparous (71.21%) and 68.18% had a previous progestative treatment or even a treatment of LHRH analogs.

Twenty-seven patients (40%) were followed-up from 10 to 18 months and 39 (59%) were followed-up from 19 to 24 months. The uterine data are to be found in Table 4.

Even though thermocoagulation is an outpatient procedure, with local anesthesia, the majority of our

**Table 3.** Description of the population

---

 Mean age: from 45 to 56 years
  • Min. 34 years
  • Max. 54 years
 Mean parity: 2.16
  • Min. 0
  • Max. 9
  • Nulliparous: 2 (3%)
  • Primiparous: 17 (25.75%)
  • Multiparous: 47 (71.21%)

---

**Table 4.** Uterine characteristics (58 patients)

---

| | | | |
|---|---|---|---|
| • | Anteverted | 24 (41.37%) | |
| • | Mid-position | 25 (43.10%) | |
| • | Retroverted | 9 (15.51%) | |
| • Depth (cm) | Mean: 8.86cc | Min. 6 | Max. 12 |
| • Volume (cm) | Mean: 12.62cc | Min. 4 | Max. 52 |

---

patients were hospitalised due to a problem of administrative organisation in our services at the beginning of study (Table 5).

**Table 5.** Types of anesthesia

| | |
|---|---|
| General: | 50 (75.75%) |
| Local: | 15 (22.72%) |
| Regional: | 1 (1.51%) |

## Results

A durable clinical improvement was observed in 61 patients, thus in 91% of the cases. We compared blood loss before and after thermocoagulation as objectively as possible (Table 6). The difference is statistically significant.

Five patients, 9%, experienced no improvement and had to undergo a hysterectomy. The debris of hysterectomies all showed anatomopathological anomalies which could explain why thermocoagulation failed. Some uteri were polyfibromatous and others presented with deep adenomyosis. The presence of several fibroids whatever their location may explain the failure of the thermocoagulation treatment which only cures the endometrium.

As for adenomyosis, failure is also understandable as adenomyosis lesions occur in the uterine muscle but coagulation performed with the UBT catheter only reaches the endometrium with a maximal coagulation depth of 4 mm.

No per-operative complication occurred. Three cases of endometritis 72 hours after the treatment were reported, but an appropriate antibiotic therapy cured them. One case of cervical stenosis was also described.

## Discussion

Conventional treatments of menorrhagia are either medical or surgical (curettage, endometrectomy, hysterectomy).

Medical therapy traditionally comes first for both the gynecologist and the patient, who prefers a non invasive cure. However, medical treatments with progestatives or oral contraceptives combined with LHRH analogs are long term cures which are not always successful and need proper compliance. Side effects include weight gains, peripheric edemas, depression with progestatives and weight gains, severe metrorrhagia with combined contraceptives. Prices for drugs and visits to the doctor may be expensive for these long term treatments.

Amongst surgical cures, curettage is still the most common treatment to manage dysfunctional menometrorrhagia but the improvement such as reduction in blood flow or disappearance of the bleeding may be temporary and the treatment has to be repeated. Though complications are rare, uterine perforations, severe bleeding and infections have been reported.

Hysterectomy is another cure of dysfunctional bleeding but its morbidity rate is important for a functional disease (3%) and with its long hospitalization and recovery period [4, 5], it is an expensive method.

Given the poor results of curettage and the morbidity rate of hysterectomies, a new surgical approach has been developed, endometrectomy. Its success rates vary according to the teams from 75 to 100%. Specialised training is necessary to master the new hysteroscopic material and techniques, which explains the great variability amongst the results according to the experience of the surgeons [6-8]. Complications due to endometrectomy are few (8.6/1000) but may be severe, even fatal and generally due to the inexperience of the surgeon [9].

**Table 6.** Pre- and postoperative bleeding patterns

| Menstrual pattern | Before | | | After | | |
|---|---|---|---|---|---|---|
| Min/Max | N | Mean Pads/day | | Min/Max | N | Mean Pads/day |
| 0 – 12 | 51 | 7.68 | | 2 – 12 | 47 | 3 |
| Days/Cycles 0 – 9 | 51 | 9.41 | | 5 – 28 | 47 | 3.79 |
| Pads/Cycles 0 – 72 | 50 | 74.07 | | 25 – 224 | 47 | 14.66 |

So therapeutic alternatives in the treatment of menorrhagia have their own advantages and drawbacks. Thermocoagulation is a valuable alternative in the management of menorrhagia. Its efficacy is less than in the case of hysterectomy (91 vs. 100%) but it does not have the same morbidity rate since only three cases of infections and a cervical stenosis were attributed to the thermoablation of the endometrium. These are minor complications as opposed to the intra-abdominal infections and the hemorrhage risks linked to a hysterectomy.

With endometrectomy, the challenge is different. Results in terms of efficacy are comparable (75 to 100% according to the teams for endometrectomy as against 89 to 91% for thermocoagulation) [6, 10]. However, endometrectomy needs an experienced surgeon to avoid complications which may be severe such as absorption of the distending liquid with adverse side effects, perforations, and lesions of neighbouring organs or hemorrhages. An inexperienced surgeon can get away with thermocoagulation as the technique is easy, simple and does not need any special training.

Indications for endometrectomy are wider than for thermocoagulation and intracavitary lesions are no contraindications; on the contrary, they can be treated at the same time. Finally, comparison with a medical treatment is not relevant as thermocoagulation is an easy, efficient and definitive treatment, while the medical therapy is not.

Cost comparisons would be interesting if they were possible. Progestative treatments are widely used in the treatment of functional menometrorrhagia (when the uterus is healthy, without any fibroids). In France, they account for an annual cost of 800 MF for 6 million women. Yet it is difficult to assess the exact number of patients specifically treated for functional menometrorrhagia, and thus the exact cost of progestative treatments. The monthly cost of a progestative treatment is about 75 FF per day, that is 900 FF per year, plus office visits and blood tests.

In France the direction of the Economic and Financial Services of the Clamart Hospital made a comparative study of the costs of traditional hysterectomy, endometrectomy and thermocoagulation by UBT of Gynecare in March 1995. Economies were realised on the length of the procedure, the costs in staff, anesthesia, hospitalisation and small equipment. Thermocoagulation related 50% less expensive than abdominal hysterectomy and 30% less expensive than the cost of vaginal hysterectomy, with or without laparoscopy. Thermocoagulation costs less than surgical hysteroscopy, (6000 FF for an endometrectomy as against 4411 for a thermocoagulation procedure).

Therefore, thermocoagulation appears as an interesting alternative in the treatment of dysfunctional menometrorrhagia with good long term results (5 failures and 61 satisfied patients) and its cost seems competitive.

The patients need to be carefully screened, the indications are specific and success depends on strict respect of the criteria. In our studies the five patients who ultimately needed a hysterectomy had other pathologies which could account for the metrorrhagia but were not accessible to the thermal uterine balloon therapy system treatment.

## Conclusion

Endometrial thermocoagulation therapy by intra-uterine balloon is a reliable, efficient alternative in the management of menometrorrhagia. This technique is reproducible, easily performed without a long training period. It is the least expensive treatment for menometrorrhagia. If indications and contraindications are duly respected, thermoablation is a valuable conservative technique choice.

## References

1. Neuwirth RS, Duran AA et al (1994) The endometrial ablator: a new instrument. Obst And Gyn 83:792-796
2. Rudigoz RC, Marchal L et al (1994) Complication de l'hystéroscopie. J Gyn Obst Biol Repr 23(5):503-510
3. Singer A, Almanza R, Gutierez A et al (1994) Preliminary clinical experience with a thermal balloon endometrial ablation method to treat menorrhagia. Obst Gyn 83(5):1
4. Carlson J, Nichols D, Schiff I (1993) Indications for hysterectomy. N Engl J Med 328:856-860
5. Cosson M, Querleu D, Crepin G (1994) Voies d'abord des hystérectomies pour lésions bénignes. Réf Gynécol Obst
6. Cravello L, d'Ercole C, Rogé P, Boubli L, Blanc B (1996) Hysteroscopic management of menstrual disorder, a review of 395 patients. Eur J Obs Gyn Rep Biol 67(2):163-167
7. Cravello L (1994) Le traitement hystéroscopique des lésions endo-utérines bénignes. Thèse Marseille
8. Jourdain O, Joyeux O, Lajus C et al (1996) Endometrial Nd-Yag laser ablation by flexible hysteroscopy. Long term follow-up of 137 cases. Eur J Obs Gyn Rep Biol
9. Cravello L, d'Ercole C et al (1995) Complication of hysteroscopic resection. Cont Fert Sex 5: 335-340
10. Friberg B, Person BRR et al (1996) Endometrial destruction by hyperthermia. A possible treatment of menorrhagia. Acta Obst Gyn Scand 75:330-335

# Uterine fibroids

B. BLANC, R. de MONTGOLFIER

Fibroids are benign encapsulated tumors made up of uterine muscular tissues. They are to be found in one out of three women over 35 years old. Their localisation in the uterus accounts for the symptoms and their treatment.

The interstitial fibroid or myoma lies in the depth of the uterine muscle. It may be voluminous and remains outside the range of the endoscopical treatment.

The sub-serous fibroid cannot be treated by hysteroscopy. It does not cause bleeding.

The intracavitary and the submucous fibroids cause bleeding by mechanical irritation, which accounts for the failure of the medical hormonal treatment. The right treatment is endoscopical resection. The perilesional endometrium needs a medical treatment or an endoscopical treatment (endometrectomy) so as to avoid a functional failure of the treatment.

## Clinical and paraclinal data

### Circumstances of discovery

Menstrual troubles are frequent and varied: menorrhagia, metrorrhagia, menometrorrhagia with adverse consequences on the general state of health such as anemia. Fibroids are rarely involved in sterility and are only investigated for sterility if all the other investigations have led to nothing.

### Paraclinical tests

#### Endovaginal and pelvic ultrasonography

It is the first investigation to be performed. It discloses precise localisation of the fibroid in relation to the uterine cavity and the endometrium. The intracavitary fibroid is to be found between the two faces of the endometrium.

The submucous fibroid pushes the endometrium with more or less force according to its interstitial or submucous location. The vaginal ultrasonography should be performed around the tenth day of the cycle. The interstitial myoma is exclusively intramural and away from the endometrium. The ultrasonography detects the depth of the interstitial insertion and the location of the deepest interstitial part in relationship with the uterine serous membrane. Risks of uterine perforation during uterine resection are high when the serous membrane is less than 1 cm away from the deep intramural base of the myoma. Ultrasonography also discloses the number, biometry and structure of the myoma. The volume of the interstitial base is usually undervalued even in vaginal ultrasonography.

#### Hysterosalpingography

It is still the best investigation to assess myomas revealed by severe bleeding, but the efficacy of diagnostic hysteroscopy as an outpatient procedure is gaining ground.

In the case of an intracavitary and submucous myoma, hysterography reveals regular, round or oval images, particularly visible on the X-rays, taken when the cavity is filling with fluids or at the end when it is emptying.

In the case of an interstitial myoma, the uterine cavity is enlarged but distorted on the side of the lesion. The edge is lengthened and stretched out. The uterine tube is lifted if the myoma is near the fundus. When the myoma develops inside the uterine cavity, the submucous jutting dome is visible at the beginning and end of the operation under the shape of a regular opacity. The image pales and sometimes disappears when the uterine cavity is full. As the interstitial base cannot be evaluated with precision, it is most important to assess the size of the dome to be resected. Diagnostic hysteroscopy seems more interesting in this indication.

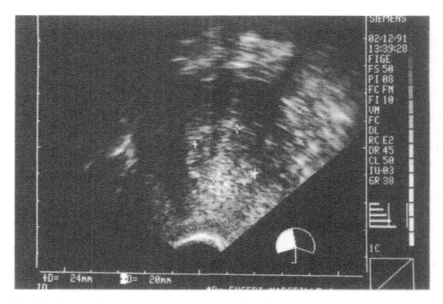

**Fig. 1.** Endovaginal ultrasonography: submucous fibroid

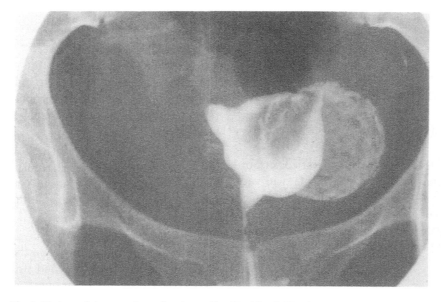

**Fig. 2.** Hysterosalpingography: voluminous fibroid with calcifications

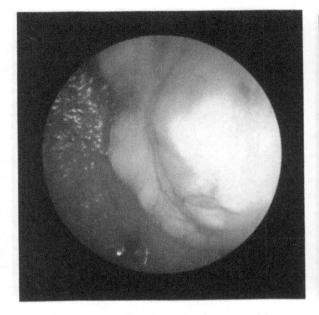

Fig. 3. Hysteroscopy: endocavitary fibroid (acute angle)

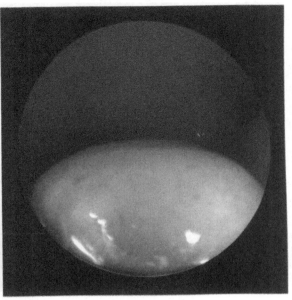

Fig. 4. Hysteroscopy submucous myoma (obtuse angle)

## Diagnostic hysteroscopy

It should be performed at the beginning of the cycle so as to evaluate the state of the endometrium around the myoma.

In the case of an intracavitary myoma, hysteroscopy discloses the endocavitary nature of the fibroid, its volume, location, type, pedicular or sessile nature, vascularisation and the angle formed by the lesion and the endometrium wall.

The myoma must be examined from all angles. If a voluminous lesion fills the uterus cavity, the hysterofibroscope is particularly useful because of its flexibility, as it can be pushed between the uterine wall and the myoma to explore the fundus and the ostial regions. The endocavitary myoma is an excellent indication for the endouterine resection under hysteroscopy as it is possible to resect the whole of the myoma without harming the myometrium. The presence of an acute angle formed by the myoma and the uterine wall is a precious indication for hysteroscopy.

In case of a submucous myoma, hysteroscopy allows the assessment of the jutting dome, its diameter, vascularisation but particularly the angle between the dome and the uterine wall. If the angle is 90°, the interstitial base is as voluminous as the jutting dome.

If the myoma is not too voluminous, resection can be performed with reasonable chances of success by an experienced surgeon. So evaluation by ultrasonography to measure the biometry of the myoma is important.

When the linking angle is obtuse, the base is predominant and the surgeon who decides to perform a uterine resection has to be very careful. A two-stage treatment can be envisaged according to the following therapeutic sequence:

- resection of the jutting dome and Laser ND Yag treatment of the interstitial insertion base so as to obtain devascularization and secondary lysis;
- resection of the submucous superficial part of the insertion base, control and secondary resection (2-3 months) of the interstitial base which has often moved towards the uterine cavity and is thus more accessible to resection. A preoperative LH-RH agonist treatment may be undertaken to reduce the volume of the myoma;
- in case of an interstitial myoma slightly distorting the uterine cavity, there is no reasonable indication for any uterine resection. It can, however, be performed if the myoma is small or when an endometrial resection has laid the myoma bare. Interstitial myomas can be treated with a Yag laser fibre introduced *in situ* through several points. The laser Yag produces a more or less complete devascularization of the myoma which develops a painful necrobiosis. Its volume is progressively reduced.

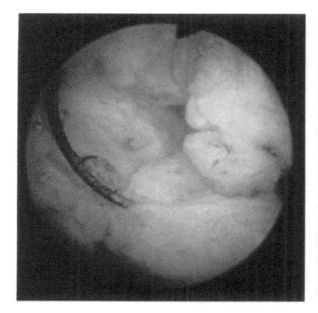

Fig. 5. Endocavitary fibroid: beginning of resection

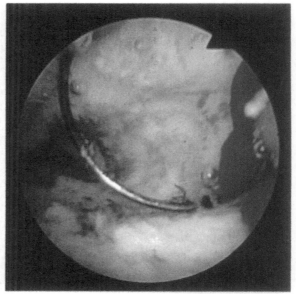

Fig. 6. Same patient: end of resection

## Hysteroscopic treatment of myomas

### Resection

It is the simplest procedure, derived from the urology techniques of prostatic lesion resection [3]. In case of an intracavitary fibroid, the myoma is easily resected for it is completely located in the uterine cavity and its bigger diameter is intrauterine when the linking angle of the myoma with the uterine wall is acute. After dilatation of the cervix, the resector is inserted under visual control to avoid a false passage and the irrigation system is started as soon as the equipment is introduced into the exterior orifice. The first stage is an exploration of the uterine cavity with identification of the tubal ostia and the associated lesions (polyps, hyperplasic endometrium, adenomyosis). The intervention begins by progressively moving the electrode to coagulate the bigger vessels of the myoma and its pedicle.

There are three ways of performing the resection:

- the resection of the base can be performed first, particularly if the lesion is pedunculated or sessile, with a narrow base, so that the uterine wall can be assessed immediately. It is only possible if the myoma is small;
- another possibility is to begin by resecting the free side of the myoma;

- finally, the myoma may be divided and resection be performed on each side of the myoma.

Whatever the technique, the common strategy is always to resect under visual control by moving the loop from back to front and never the reverse. During the intervention, the debris accumulate inside the uterine cavity. They can be extracted with a deep, blunt curette or by bringing them towards the cervix with the deactivated resecting electrode. Their extraction is time-consuming and significantly lengthens the time of the procedure. Hemorrhages are rarely severe and easy to treat by coagulating the bleeding vessel.

If the endocavitary fibroid has a pedicle, the limits of the resection are obvious but it may be more difficult to decide for a submuous sessile lesion. After resecting the endocavitary portion, the interstitial portion has to be resected and the limits of its location will be evaluated thanks to certain "effects". With the tip of a deactivated electrode, massage the limits of the resected zone, so the myometrium will contract and the interstitial portion of the myoma will be projected into the cavity. This can be obtained with a curettage to dispose of the debris or under a perfusion of ocytocine. The interstitial portion can thus be resected if the manoeuvre is repeated several times. When the myoma is deeply incased into the muscle, the risks of perforation have to be considered. A pre- and peroperative ultrasonographic control is necessary to evaluate the limits between the deep interstitial part of the myometrium and the serous membrane. A healthy myometrium has a more fasciculated structure, is pinker and bleeds more easily than the myometrium. The surgeon will have to be very careful in the treatment of subcornual lesions because of fluid distension. The wall is very thin (3 to 5 mm) so there are risks of perforation.

At the end of the resection, the debris are extracted and the operator should make sure there is no hemorrhage by exploring the uterine cavity after the irrigation is shut off. The barohemostasis phenomenon comes to an end and it is easier to see if there is bleeding and take care of it. When the indication is menometrorrhagia in a premenopausal woman, it may be necessary to perform an endometrectomy as the perilesional endometrium may be heterogeneous. For fertility troubles, a small resector (21CH) has to be used to limit cervix dilatation and avoid any lesion of the adjacent mucosa.

## The ND-Yag laser

The surgical hysteroscope (or hysterofibroscope) is introduced under visual control inside the uterus. The distending medium is glycine. It is more advisable to use the hysterofibroscope because of its size (OD 5 mm) and flexibility. After exploration the laser fiber is inserted inside the operating channel. It is advisable to associate the two laser techniques. The non-touch technique is used to devascularize the pedicle or the base of the myoma. The touch technique drills into the myoma to obtain an effect of delayed myolysis. The laser shots are aimed at all the surface of the myoma and the impacts are spaced out every 3 mm. A laser destruction of the endometrium can be associated. There are advantages in using the hysterofibroscope. The cervix trauma is small or absent and myomas embedded inside the uterine wall which are little accessible to resection can thus be treated. The adjacent mucosa is respected but the procedure is often long and results are measured after several weeks.

## Association of the two techniques

It can be considered for myomas distorting the uterine cavity but whose bigger diameter is located in the depths of the uterine muscle. It is thus possible to resect the jutting dome inside the uterine cavity and perform the laser Yag treatment of the intramyometrial lesion.

## Post-operative surveillance

No postoperative treatment is necessary. A control hysteroscopy will be performed two to three months after the resection if a pregnancy is wished for.

## The results

Table 1. Main results in the literature

| Authors | Number of UR | Good results (%) |
|---|---|---|
| Neuwirth [4] | 28 | 61 |
| Dargent [5] | 25 | 84 |
| Hallez [6] | 61 | 83 |
| Hamou [7] | 111 | 83 |
| Mergui [8] | 111 | 79.3 |
| Blanc [19] | 239 | 81 |

## Results of personal series [9]

Two hundred and thyrty-nine patients presenting with intra-cavitary fibroids were enrolled in our study between October 1987 and December 1992.

## The patients

Mean age was 45 years and one month. The youngest was 25 and the oldest 67.

## Indications

**Menstrual disorders.** One hundred and ninety-six patients suffered from bleeding symptoms, either menorrhagia, metrorrhagia or menometrorrhagia. In 21 cases, bleeding had induced anaemia under 10 gHb, including two cases of severe anemia under 4 gHb.

**Sterility.** Siwteen patients suffered from primary or secondary sterility.

**Post-menopausal metrorrhagia.** Twenty-seven patients under a hormonal substitutive treatment were concerned.

## Nature of the lesions

**Number.** There were 290 myomas for 239 patients, 23 having two and 13 having three.

**Size.** The mean diameter of the lesions was 2.23 cm. In 5 cases, the myoma was over 5 cm.

**Localisation.** The localisation of the myomas inside the uterine cavity is represented by the following diagram.

## Preoperative treatment

**Progestatives.** Fifty-nine patients were under progestatives before the endo-uterine resection. Progestatives from the 19-norprogesterone group (promegestone, nomegestrol) were chosen rather than progestatives from the 19-nortestosterone group (lynestrenol, norethisterone).

**Danazol.** We never used it because of the androgenic properties of the molecule. Baggish [10] uses it systematically eight weeks before the endouterine ND laser Yag treatment of the myomas. Corson [11] uses it for voluminous myomas (diameter over 4 cm).

**LH-RH agonists.** Thirty-nine patients received a preoperative treatment of LH-RH agonists. The maximum effect was obtained in three months and was not improved by continuation of the treatment. Advantages include reduction of the myoma volume (30%) and thus length of the resection procedure, reduction of the bleeding and better timing for the surgery. Drawbacks are estrogen deficiency, endocervical stenosis, relative vaginal atresia and the cost of the treatment (three injections). Findings by Pace [12] confirm our observations. He reports a smaller volume of the myomas, a shortened operative time and reduction of the bleeding.

The efficacy of analogies is proved. Yet the systematic prescription of a preoperative expensive treatment has no justification except in some situations:

- an intra cavity voluminous myoma with a diameter over 4 cm;

- troubles of the menstrual patterns with anaemia for which chemically induced amenorrhea associated with iron intakes restores blood count and thus the possibility of the intervention.

## The procedure

Two hundred and thirty-nine patients, two hundred and seventy-nine uterine resections:
- 93.5% with general anesthesia
- length of the procedure: 41.5 minutes
- glycine: 4.04 litres
- length of hospitalisation: one day and a half
- complications
  - infectious      0/279    0%
  - hemorrhagic    2/279    0.7% (Table 2)
  - perforations   7/279    2.5% (Table 3)

## Repeat resections

Thirty-nine patients are concerned. There were two indications for a repeat resection:
- the initial resection was not complete in 23 cases;
- the resection was interrupted, mean length of the procedure: 59 minutes.

A two-time operative strategy had been adopted either because of the volume of the myoma (3.36 cm for the diameter) or because of the number of myomas (2 to three in 28% of the cases) or because of the localisation of the myomas (submucous myomas in 35% of the cases). The Bleeding resumed in 16 cases.

In 15 cases, bleeding resumed after the cycles had become normal. The repeat resection was performed after a mean delay of 17 months (from 6 to 52 months).

**Long term results.** For the 39 patients, poor long-term results correspond to 10.2%; success for all the other cases was 89.8%. Thus, a first incomplete resection or the need for a repeat resection does not mean that the method should be given up. It is better to of-

Table 2. Hemorrhagic complications after endouterine resection

| Authors | Number of Cases | Treatment |
|---|---|---|
| De Cherney [16] | 1 | Foley catheter |
| Loffer [17] | 3 | Foley catheter |
| Corson [11] | 1 | Foley catheter |
| Serden [13] | 4 | Foley catheter |
| Istre [15] | 1 | Hysterectomy at day 1 |
| Hill [18] | 5 | Foley catheter |
| | 1 | Progestatives |
| | 1 | Hysterectomy at day 21 |
| Blanc [19] | 2 | Foley catheter |

**Table 3.** Uterine perforations during resection of myomas

| Authors | HSS | Perforations | Therapeutic complications | Consequences |
|---|---|---|---|---|
| Hamou [7] | EUR | 2/96 (2%) | intestine burn | endometrectomy |
| Dargent [5] | EUR | 2/25 (8%) | 0 | 2 laparoscopies |
| Hallez [6] | EUR for myoma | 1/92 (1%) | hemoperitoine | hysterorrhaphy laparotomy |
| Blanc [19] | EUR | 7/279 (2.5%) | | laparotomy |
| Cravello [9] | for myoma | | | laparoscopy with myomectomy |
| Corson [11] | EUR | 3/92 (3.3%) | | |
| Serden [13] | EUR | 1/216 (0.5%) | | |
| Hucke [14] | EUR | 1/39 (2.6%) | | |
| Mergui [8] | EUR | 1/111 (0.9%) | | |
| Istre [15] | EUR | 2/20 (10%) | | |

fer a repeat hysteroscopic resection than a vaginal hysterectomy.

**Associated endometrectomy.** The endouterine resection of myomas was associated to an endometrectomy in 31 patients. In 19 cases, the endometrectomy was decided on the spot. In 12 cases, the endometrectomy was performed during a repeat resection because of recurrent bleeding.

## Control hysteroscopy

An outpatient control hysteroscopy at the beginning of the second cycle after the resection was performed in two cases: a young woman of child-bearing age, an incomplete resection.

The control hysteroscopy may reveal iatrogenous synechiae (10% in our series). They were mucous synechiae easily collapsed with the bevelled tip of the hysteroscope.

## Results

Two hundred and thirty-nine patients underwent surgical hysteroscopy for endocavitary myomas between October 1987 and December 1992. Two hundred and twenty-one were followed-up and 17 lost to the follow-up. The mean follow-up period is 2 years and 5 months with extremes going from 6 months to 5 years and a half.

So the bleeding symptoms disappeared in 81.1% of the cases. The results after a follow-up period of 2 years and 6 months can be considered as durable. The rate of favorable results is stable and the delay is now long enough to ascertain the efficacy of the transcervical resection of endocavitary myomas which is in our opinion the only reference treatment of intracavitary myomas.

**Table 4.** Fertility results after endoscopical surgery

| Authors | Year | Number | Pregnancies (%) | Viability (%) of cases |
|---|---|---|---|---|
| Valla | 1990 | 16 | 10 | 8 |
| Loffer | 1990 | 12 | 7 | 7 |
| Corson | 1991 | 13 | 11 | 9 |
| Derman | 1991 | Not given | 21 | 18 |
| Hucke | 1992 | 14 | 4 | 2 |

**Table 5.** Myoma resection for bleeding symptoms

| Authors | Number of cases | Good results |
|---|---|---|
| Hallez [6] | 61 | 83% |
| Hamou [7] | 111 | 83% |
| Cornier [20] | 28 | 64% (laser Nd Yag) |
| Pace [12] | 59 | 100% |
| Serden [13] | 90 | 92% |
| Loffer [17] | 53 | 75% |
| Corson [11] | 80 | 81% |
| Derman [21] | 94 | 76% |
| Hucke [14] | 29 | 100% |
| Blanc [9] | 239 | 78.2% |

**Failures.** Twenty-two cases. Analysis of the data of those 22 cases points at a number of common features:

- the size of the resected myomas was slightly superior to the mean size of the series 2.46 as against 2.32;
- multiple intracavitary localisations are frequent (1.42 myomas per patient);
- 9 patients presented with polymyomatosis;
- adenomyosis was discovered in 4 out of the 12 surgical pieces. Indications for surgical hysteroscopy rest more on the associated lesions than on the volume of the myomas. Hysterectomy, preferably vaginal hysterectomy, is more adapted for a big uterus with polymyomatosis or adenomyosis.

## References

1. Blanc B, Boubli L (1991) Manuel d'Hystéroscopie opératoire. Vigot, Paris, p 39
2. Blanc B (1983) Atlas d'hystérosalpingographie comparée. Sandoz, Rueil Malmaison, p 78
3. Neuwirth RS, Amin HK (1976) Excision of submucous fibroids with hysteroscopic control. Am J Obst Gynecol 126:95-99
4. Neuwirth RS (1983) Hysteroscopic management of symptomatic submucous fibroids. Obstet Gynecol, 62 (4):509-511
5. Dargent D, Mellier G, Jacquot F (1988) Electro-résection endoutérine: une série préliminaire de 25 cas. J Gyn Obst Bio Rep 17(7):940
6. Hallez JP (1987) Résection endoutérine trans-cervicale J Gyne Obst Bio Rep 16:781-785
7. Hamou JE, Salat-Baroux J (1988) Hystéroscopie et microhystéroscopie. Mise à jour en gynécologie-obstétrique. Collège National des Gynécologues-Obstétriciens, Paris, pp 111-197
8. Mergui JL, Renolleau C, Salat-Baroux J (1994) Traitement des fibromes utérins par hystéroscopie opératoire. Gynecol Internat 4(1):12-22
9. Cravello L (1994) Le traitement hystéroscopique des lésions endo-utérines bénignes. Thèse de Médecine, Marseille
10. Baggish M, Szehm Morgan G (1989) Hysteroscopic treatment of symptomatic submucous uterine myomas with the ND Yag Laser. J Gynecol Surg 5: pp 27-3
11. Corson SL, Brooks PG (1991) Resectoscopic myomectomy. Fertil Steril 55(6):1041-1044
12. Pace S, Labi FL, Lotti G et al (1992) LHRH analogues in the preparation of hysteroscopic resection of uterine fibromyoma. Minerva Ginecol 44(5):245-250
13. Serden SP, Brooks PG (1991) Treatment of abnormal uterine bleeding with the gynecologic resectoscope J Reprod Med 36(10):697-699
14. Hucke J, Campo RL, Debruyne F et al (1992) Hysteroscopic resection of submucous myoma. Geburtshilfe Frauenheilkd 52(4):214-218
15. Istre O, Schiotz H, Sadik L et al (1991) Transcervical resection of endometrium and fibroids: initial complications. Acta Obstet Gynecol Scand 70(4-5):363-366
16. De Cherney AH, Diamond MP, Lavy G et al (1987) Endometrial ablation for intractable uterine bleeding: hysteroscopic resection. Obstet Gynecol 70(4):668-670
17. Loffer FD (1990) Removal of large symptomatic intrauterine growths by the hysteroscopic resectoscope. Obstet Gynecol 76:836
18. Hill D, Maher P, Wood C et al (1992) Complications of operative hysteroscopy. Gynecol endosc 1:185-189
19. Cravello L, D'Ercole C, Boubli L, Blanc B (1995) Les complications des résections hystéroscopiques. Contracep Fertil Sexual (in press)
20. Corniere E (1990) Traitement des métrorragies par hystéroscopies opératoires et Laser ND Yag. Contracept Fertil Sex 18(12):1111-1117
21. Derman SG, Rehnstrom J, Neuwirth RS (1991) The long-term effectiveness of hysteroscopic treatment of menorrhagia and leiomyomas. Obstet Gynecol, 77(4): 591-594
22. Valle RF (1990) Hysteroscopic removal of submucous leiomyomas. J Gynecol Surg 6:89-96

# Intrauterine synechiae

B. Blanc, R. de Montgolfier

Uterine synechiae are intrauterine adhesions. They result from the coalescence of the uterine walls whatever their location and are caused by the destruction of the endometrium:
- most often by abrasion of the endometrium during obstetrical manoeuvers;
- by infectious diseases such as tuberculosis or parasitosis (bilharziosis);
- by its disappearance through trophic alterations after menopause.

Our series is concerned with traumatic synechiae, whose numbers are as high as before elective abortion was legalised "Karman has not displaced Asherman" [1, 2]. Therapy involves endoscopic techniques and diagnostic hysteroscopy has become the indispensable exploration for diagnosis, treatment and postoperative surveillance.

## Etiology

Synechiae may appear after any endouterine mechanical trauma by destruction of the basal layer of the endometrium. Pregnancy is the cause in 85% of the cases [3-5] and the risk is higher in a prolonged pregnancy, in case of a miscarriage or in the postpartum phase.

Synechiae may appear outside pregnancy (15%), after DC, myomectomies and cervix surgery. They may also be a consequence of endouterine resection (8.5%) in our series. In that case, they are often difficult to manage as they are widespread, complex and muscular particularly after resection of interstitial myomas and coagulation of a bleeding endometrium with a rollerball.

## Physiopathology

The initial causes are uterine trauma but risks are increased by some circumstances such as a soft uterus (advanced pregnancy, or retention of a dead foetus or a post-partum uterus), surgical conditions such as the surgeon's experience, the technique chosen to empty the uterus. A curette causes more trauma than aspiration. Manual uterine revision is little traumatic.

## Endometritis

The destruction of the basal layer and the trauma reaching down to the underlying myometrium gives rise to granulous tissues. When there are identical lesions on both sides of the uterus, a mucosal bridge develops between the abraded surfaces in contact. The process of scarring turns into fibrosis. Successful cure of synechiae is function of the neighbouring endometrium. If it is healthy, a cure may be obtained. If not, there will be recurrences.

## Anatomic pathology

A synechia may be total (5%), corporeal (5%), isthmo-corporeal (21%) or cervico-isthmic (18%). The endometrium surface is reduced by the presence of synechiae.

### Histology: evolution of synechiae

When sinechiae first appear are just soft, thin mucous bridges which a radiological examination or diagnostic hysteroscopy will break apart. During a second phase, fibrous and strong conjunctive tissues develop between the two faces of the uterine cavity. About a year later, muscular fibers have developed from side to side filling in all the gaps.

Hamou [6] described 3 types of histological lesions (X 20 magnification):
- mucous or endometrial synechiae. They have the same aspect as the adjacent endometrium, are very thin and easily collapsed by the hysteroscope. They bleed easily;
- fibro-conjunctive synechiae. They are translucent, not very thick, nor covered with the endometrium and poorly vascularized. When synechiae are divided, they bleed a little and the stumps retract after lysis;
- muscular synechiae are covered with a thin pale endometrium, showing several glandular orifices (X 20 magnification). They are richly vascularized

and cannot be easily divided. When they are dissected, the cleavage is never complete and leaves irregular stumps with muscular structures.

## Adjacent endometrium

Its role is essential. If it is healthy, it will allow the colonization of the treated zones. When the synechiae are small, the endometrium is generally healthy. When the lesions are large, it may be deeply modified. Glandular epithelium is flat and non functional as a result of local trauma or disturbed receptivity to normal hormonal secretions. Islets of endometrium in the middle of scarry bridges may turn into adenomyosis so dysmenorrhea is frequent.

Foix [7] reported:
- secretory epithelium (80%);
- proliferative endometrium (12%);
- atrophic epithelium (5%);
- hyperplastic endometrium (3%).

## Underlying myometrium

The amount of fibrous tissue in a uterus with recurrent synechiae is three to four times more important than in a uterus without synechiae. Yaffe [8] suggested that synechiae could be part of a pathological process progressively turning the myometrial tissue into fibrosis.

## Symptoms

### Reproduction disorders

#### Sterility

Synechiae are the most frequent symptoms (43% according to Schenker [5]). Synechiae indeed cause sterility in a certain number of cases (cervico-isthmic, corporeal or total synechiae). Amar [9] also insisted on cases of false sterility which were in reality disorders of the nidification process leading to an early termination of pregnancy.

#### Repeated abortions and premature delivery

Repeated abortions can be caused by a distorted uterine cavity or by a traumatic incompetent cervix.

#### Placenta insertion

Placenta praevia and placenta accreta may lead to the discovery of synechiae.

### Disorders of the cycle

#### Amenorrhea

It is a frequent occurrence and a revealing symptom. Schenker [5] found it in 37% of the cases. It is normohormonal and hormonoresistant.

#### Hypomenorrhea

Schenker [5] found it in 31% of the cases, when the surface of the active endometrium is reduced and sometimes when there are changes in the mucosa around scarry bridges.

#### Dysmenorrhea

It is rarely the only symptom but when it is associated with hypomenorrhea, it can be a symptom of adenomyosis developing on the endometrium around the synechiae.

### Asymptomatic synechiae

Intrauterine synechiae are often discovered by chance as they cause no functional disorders. (1.5% of hysterographies are performed for other reasons than unfecondity).

## Diagnosis

Complementary examinations are necessary to establish a diagnosis of uterine synechiae. They involve hysterosalpingography and hysteroscopy [10].

### Hysterosalpingography

With hysterography, it is possible to evaluate the number, location and development of the synechiae and the associated lesions. The images were perfectly described by Asherman [2]. There is a characteristic image, a clear-cut lacuna showing the junction of the

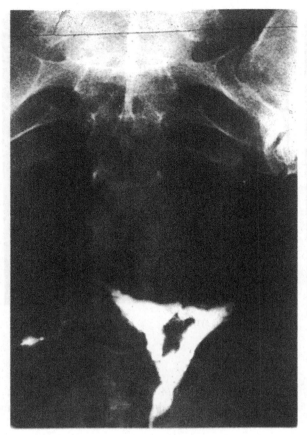

**Fig. 1.** Hysterography: central synechiae

### Isthmic synechiae

They are either a glove finger-like image or a candle flame

Toaff, Krochik and Ballas [11] described four grades of synechiae according to their sizes:

- grade 1 = lacuna images occupying less then 1/10 of the cavitary surface;
- grade 2 = lacuna images occupying 1/5 of the cavitary surface;
- grade 3 = lacunar images occupying 1/3 of a cavity and with edges distorted by marginal lesions;
- grade 4 = lacunar images in the middle of a seriously distorted cavity.

### Diagnostic hysteroscopy

Asherman recommended it as early as 1950 [2]. It reveals the existence of the coalescence. With hysteroscopy, it is possible to know whether the tissues are mucous, muscular or conjunctive and to assess the surrounding endometrium and establish a prognosis. Associated lesions such as polyps of the endometrium or submucous myomas which are not correctly seen in hysterography can also be evaluated. Hysteroscopy provides a more objective approach of the operative possibilities according to the aspect of the endometrium, the number of synechiae, their location either central or marginal, their thickness, their degree of vascularisation and the ability to see one or two tubal ostia.

Several aspects are listed:

- central synechiae are like bridges linking the posterior and the anterior walls of the uterus far from the edges. The uterine cavity may be explored on either side of the synechiae;
- marginal synechiae appear like thickened edges hiding part of the cavity and sometimes the tubal ostia;
- mucous synechiae are thin, lamellar, well vascularised and their color is very much like the color of the surrounding endometrium. They can easily be torn and prognosis of uterine restoration is excellent as the endometrium of the lesion or perilesional has not been harmed;
- muscular synechiae are far thicker, covered with atrophic endometrium. They tear less easily and rarely completely. The prognosis of restoration is not so good as the endometrium on the synechiae and around it is often altered and dystrophic;
- fibrous synechiae are not covered by the endometrium and are poorly vasculariz ed. They have

two walls of a uterus. The junction is distorted and irregular, either linear or angular with distinct and clear-cut edges.

### Total synechiae

The uterus is a full organ. Only the cervico-isthmic region is darkened with a glove finger-like image.

### Centro-corporeal synechiae

They are often multiple with irregular images.

### Fundic marginal synechiae or images in the cornua

They are images of lacunae which emulate a uterine malformation (synechiae of the uterine fundus).

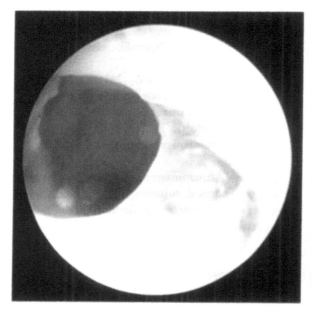

Fig. 2. Hysteroscopy: mucous marginal synechiae

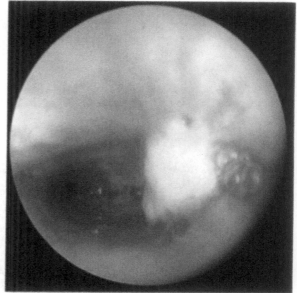

Fig. 3. Old fibrous synechia

been compared to dead tree trunks. Their destruction rarely draws blood. The perilesional endometrium is altered and sometimes absent. Prognosis of restoration is not poor.

The two exploratory techniques are complementary and have to be carried out at the same time, though the radiological exam has to come first.

Hysterography is used to assess the location of the lesions and the state of the uterine tubes, whether they are obstructed or not.

Hysteroscopy allows the surgeon to evaluate the nature of the synechiae (mucous, muscular or fibrous) which cannot be seen on the X-rays. In case of total synechiae, radiography allows the surgeon to distinguish them from isolated isthmic synechiae.

Confrontation between the results of the two procedures shows a good correlation in 90% of the cases in our experience.

When the assessment is complete, the synechiae can be graded with the classification used by the American Society of Fertility. This classification does not evaluate the central or marginal location of synechiae nor their correlation with the tubal ostia. March [13] established a classification in three degrees for corporeal synechiae (having excluded cervico-isthmic synechiae):

- Severe: more than the 3/4 of the uterine cavity are concerned; 2 walls have been merged into a fibro-muscular block; ostia and the higher portion of the cavity are not visible;

- Mild: from 1/4 to 3/4 of the cavity are concerned; simple fibrous synechiae of the two walls; ostia and uterine fundus are partly visible
- Minor: less than 1/4 of the cavity is concerned; mucous synechiae; ostia and uterine fundus are totally visible.

## Treatment

### Operative protocol

Apart from recent mucous synechiae of small volume which can be collapsed in the office during a diagnostic hysteroscopy or salpingography, the treatment of synechiae must be performed with ultrasonic control to reduce the risks of uterine perforation or false passages. The distending media are always liquids. We generally use a 21CH resector, a cutting electrode and glycine as distending medium for it affords an excellent intrauterine visibility. Hysteroscopic treatment of small-sized central synechiae may be very easy. Treatment of complex marginal synechiae hiding one or two tubal ostia may be very difficult.

### The date of the surgery

If the patient is amenorrheic, the procedure can take place at any time. For a menstruating woman, it has to take place between the seventh and the twelfth days to avoid a proliferative endometrium. A preoperative treatment can be used with progestatives such as 19 Nor progesterone, preferably, or Donatrol (2 pills to start on the fifth day of the cycle to be continued for 20 days afterwards). We think that the treatment by LHRH analogs is dangerous in this indication because of its atrophic effects on the cervical canal and the uterine walls and increases the risks of false passages and uterine perforation.

## Endoscopic technique

Synechiae have to be released or cut down while respecting the neighbouring endometrium.

1-It is possible to release them without anesthesia or just local anesthesia. The bevelled tip of the endoscope with its forobliquity can be used in a to and fro movement starting at the weakest level of the coalescence and collapses the recent, mucous and small-sized synechiae. This adhesiolysis is usually successful and draws little bleeding for it concerns mucous lesions. The technique only applies to central mucous synechiae as the endoscope needs to be plied around a central coalesced partition, so indications for this surgical technique are limited.

2-With the help of small flexible scissors introduced into the side channel of a surgical hysteroscope. Indications are limited to small-sized synechiae whatever their structure. Section sometimes causes bleeding.

3-Electroresection with an electrode equipped with a central bar or at the tip of a resector is the usual technique. The cutting electrode is 5 mm long and its angle with the sheath may be 45 or 90 degrees. It is better to use the 21CH resector or the 24 CH intermediate resector as patients usually have sterility problems and the uterine cavity may be reduced by synechiae. Section should be controlled with the tip of the instrument to evaluate the texture of the synechiae before treating them. Ultrasonographic control is necessary particularly when the synechiae are marginal to avoid harming the myometrium as much as possible. Risks of perforation are particularly important with synechiae in the fundus or on the edges.

## ND laser Yag destruction

The tip of a Yag laser fiber can be inserted through the side channel of a surgical hysteroscope. The absence of a dual fluid circulation and the rigid nature of the hysteroscope are obstacles for the end of the laser fiber cannot be in contact with lateral synechiae. So it is preferable to use a flexible surgical hysteroscope (OD 5.5 mm) with a side operative channel (OD 2.2 m) which can accommodate an ND Yag laser fiber. The synechiae, whatever their location, can be reached thanks to its distal rotating tip.

Marginal synechiae should be treated with the "touch" technique since the limit of the coalescence with the myometrium is not easily visualized. With central synechiae, the two techniques of touch and no touch can be used, the synechiae being destroyed after de-vascularisation. ND Yag laser vaporisation is particularly effective for it allows an elective destruction of the coalescence while preserving the surrounding endometrium and myometrium. It is particularly useful in the hypoplastic cavities exposed to DES.

## Follow-up

### Ultrasonographic control

It is absolutely necessary to cut the synechiae as close as possible to the myometrium with abdominal ultrasonographic control. Sometimes it is possible to have an endorectoral ultrasonographic control.

### Laparoscopic control

It is of no interest in comparison with hysterographic control.

### Hysterographic control

If possible, the section of the synechiae should be controlled by a hysterosalpingography performed in the operating theatre. It can be particularly useful in case of complex synechiae to check the section and carry out corrective surgery if necessary.

### Surgical procedures

Complex synechiae (stage III of the AFS classification) which could not be treated endoscopically or because of peroperative complications (repeated perforations) have to be managed surgically.

**Musset's procedure** [9]. Laparotomy and blind treatment of synechiae with a metallic bougie in the uterine cavity and control with the other hand holding the uterus to prevent any false passages. Hysterotomy with dissection of the synechiae under visual control. The two surgical procedures are exceptional and their morbidity is higher than endoscopical treatments.

## Adjuvant treatments

They should avoid recurrences and prevent infectious complications.

### Prevention of recurrences

Estrogenotherapy seems useful. Good results are measured by the state if the surrounding endometrium which should colonize the surgical wound. We prescribe a sequential pill or a continuous estroprogestative treatment associating a natural estrogene given by itself for 14 days and an estroprogestative for the 12 following days. It is preferable to use a progestative with luteomimetic action to obtain maturation and desquamation of the endometrium (Retro Progesterone, 19 Nor Pregnane). The sequential treatment should be observed for three cycles.

### Endocavitary devices

Several equipments such as flexible drains, Folley's catheter, vaseline compresses, a silastic blade, Massouras IUD have been tried. Ambulatory hysteroscopical controls can be started during the following cycle.

### Prevention of infectious complications

An associated antibiotic treatment is necessary. We practise a peroperative antibiotic flash and an antibiotic treatment for the ten following days.

## Therapeutic indications

There are three main situations with different therapeutic solutions.

### Isolated, central or partially central synechiae

They may be recent mucous synechiae or older muscular or fibrous synechiae. Treatment is easy for the synechiae visible on both faces:
-   release of mucus synechiae;

-   electroresection of fibrous or muscular synechiae.

Peroperative ultrasonographic control is necessary to treat the synechiae as near as possible of the myometrium when the section is near the uterine fundus. Prognosis depends on the age of the synechiae, their vascularization and the quality of the perilesional endometrium. Prognosis is excellent with mucous synechiae, and less so with muscular and particularly fibrous synechiae. A follow-up hysteroscopy during the following cycle is necessary.

### Isolated but marginal synechiae

Treatment is less easy because only one side of the coalescence is visible. Ultrasonographic control is necessary to avoid uterine perforations. A small resector is used for electroresection with a cutting electrode. Prognosis depends on the structure and the quality of the surrounding endometrium.

### Complex synechiae

Synechiae may be complex because of their number (isthmic and corporeal or corporeal in tiers) or they may be complex because of the distorted uterine cavity.

There may be several possibilities:
-   uterine cavity with several tiers in annular synechiae;
-   amputation of a cornua;
-   synechiae in tiers with visible ostia;
-   disappearance of the two tubal ostia.

Treatment involves electroresection with strict ultrasonographic control. If there is one visible ostium, it is easier to direct the cutting electrode inside the intrauterine cavity. If the two ostia have disappeared, the uterine cavity appears cylindrical and very hypoplastic. The surgical procedure starts with the bevelended tip of the hysteroscope cautiously exploring the endometrium trying to localise one ostium or the uterine fundus. Dissection of the synechiae can then begin under strict ultrasonographic control. When the endoscopic treatment fails, Musset's [9] procedure has to be considered. Functional results are not guaranteed.

### Synechiae and uterine septa

The endoscopical treatment of the two disorders should be performed at the same time by electroresection. Small, centro-partial or marginal synechiae near the uterine septum are involved. Peroperative ultrasonographic control is necessary.

### Synechiae and DES syndrome

Synechiae reduce the size of an already hypoplastic uterine cavity. It is preferable to use a small diameter flexible hysteroscope adapted to this kind of uterus. Section of the synechiae will be obtained with the laser ND Yag fiber.

## Surgical cure

Indications for traditional surgery are exceptional and should only be considered after several failures of the hysteroscopical treatment. The procedure described by Musset [9] should be chosen first as it avoids the hysterotomy of the uterus. After laparotomy, synechiae are released with a bougie inserted into the uterine cavity. The surgeon holds the uterus with his other hand to avoid perforation. Sometimes hysterotomy is necessary to destroy the synechiae under visual control.

## Results

### Anatomic results

They vary from 63.8 to 97.4% of perfect anatomic results (Table 1). The table shows the increase of good

results by comparison with the surgical treatment. The reasons are visual control of the endoscopical procedure so the surrounding endometrium and the endocervical canal are protected (no postoperative incompetent cervix and peroperative ultrasonographic control), so there are fewer risks of uterine perforation.

### Functional results

They are excellent from 77.7 to 100% with cure of amenorrhea and oligomenorrhea.

### Obstetrical results

They are less successful (Table 2) and cannot be easily compared as the different authors do not differentiate between isolated and complex synechiae and do not take the number, type, age, volume, of synechiae nor the associated lesions into account. After a cure of the intrauterine adhesive disease, one woman out of two will become pregnant and one out of four will have a living child.

### Our results

Working on our series of patients hysteroscopically treated for the adhesive disease we have established a decisional algorithm to calculate the probabilities of success while always considering that an incomplete result is a failure. The rate of a perfect result after a

Table 1. Anatomic and functional results after endoscopical and surgical cure of the adhesive disease

| Author | Year | Number of cases | Technique | Anatomic results | Functional results |
|---|---|---|---|---|---|
| Amar [9] | 1974 | 436 | Surgery | 83.3% | |
| Sugimoto [15] | 1978 | 192 | Endoscopy | 77.6% | 45% |
| Parent [16] | 1980 | 116 | Endoscopy | 89.6% | 94% |
| March [12] | 1981 | 38 | Endoscopy | 97.4% | 100% |
| Schenker [5] | 1982 | 1250 | Surgery | 84% | |
| | (review of the literature) | | | | |
| Hamou [17] | 1983 | 39 | Endoscopy | 63.8% | 85.58% |
| Lancet [18] | 1986 | 137 | Endoscopy | 97.3% | 100% |
| Friedman [19] | 1986 | 30 | Endoscopy | 90% | |
| Siegler [20] | 1988 | 775 | Endoscopy | 87.2% | |
| | (review of the literature) | | | | |
| Valle [21] | 1988 | 187 | Endoscopy | 97.14% | 89.3% |
| Personal series [24] | 1986 | 103 | Endoscopy | 72.1% | 69.9% |

**Table 2.** Fertility results after endoscopical surgery and classical surgery

| Author | Year | Number of cases | Pregnancies (%) | Viability (%) |
|---|---|---|---|---|
| Musser [9] | 1974 | 436 | 41 | 22 |
| Parent [16] | 1977 | 55 | 32 | 27 |
| Sugimoto [15] | 1977 | 192 | 41 | 23 |
| March [12] | 1981 | 38 | - | 79.1 |
| Hamou [17] | 1983 | 39 | 53.1 | 38.4 |
| Israel | 1987 | 38 | 75 | 63 |
| Valle [21] | 1988 | 187 | 76.4 | 60.9 |
| Friedman [19] | 1986 | 30 | 80 | 76.6 |
| Personal series [24] | 1996 | 37 | 51.3 | 32 |

first cure can be 70%, some extra 20% can be obtained with a repeat procedure. There is no further progression after a third treatment.

# References

1.  Asherman JG (1948) Amenorrhea traumatica J Obstet Gynecol Br Emp 55:23

2.  Asherman JG (1950) Traumatic intra uterine adhesions J Obstet Gynecol Br Emp 57:892

3.  Butram UC, Turati G Uterine synechie: variation inn severity and some conditions wich may be conductive to severe adhesions Int J Fertif 22:98-103

4.  Polishuk WZ, Siew FP, Gordon R (1977) Vascular changes in traumatic amenorrhea and hypomenorrhea. Int J Fertil 22:189

5.  Schenker JG, Margalioth EJ (1982) Intra uterine adhesions: an updated appraisal. Fertil Steril 37:593-610

6.  Hamou JE, Cittadini E, Perino A (1983) Diagnostic of intra uterine adhesions by microhysteroscopy. Act Europ Fertil 14:117

7.  Foix A, Bruno RO (1966) The pathology of post curetage intra uterine adhesion. Am J Obst Gyn 96(7):1027-33

8.  Yaffe H, Ron M, Polishuk WZ (1978) Amenorrhea, hypoamenorrhea and uterine fibrosis. Am J Obst Gyn 1305:599-600

9.  Ammar A (1974) A propos de 346 cas de synéchies utérines. Thèse de médecine Montpellier

10. Blanc B (1983) Atlas d'hystérosalpingographie comparée. Sandoz Rueil Malmaison p 240-271

11. Toaff R (1966) Quelques observations sur les adhérences utérines post-traumatiques. Rev Franc Gynec Obstet 61(7-8):550-552

12. American Fertility Society (1988) The american fertility society classification of adnexal adhesions, distal tubal occlusion, tubal occlusion secondary to tubal ligation, tubal pregnancies, mullerian anomalies and intra uterine adhesion. Fertil Steril 49:944

13. March CM, Israel R (1981) Gestational outcome following hysteroscopic lysis of adhesions. Fertil Steril 36:455-459

15. Sugimoto O Diagnostic and therapeutic hysteroscopy for tramatic intrauterine adhesions Am J Obst Gym 1978;131(5); 539-47

16. Parent B, Barbot J, Dubuisson JB (1981) Synéchies utérines EMC Paris Gynécologie 140 A 10, Supplément 1988

17. Hamou J, Salat Baroux J, Siegler AM (1983) Diagnosis and treatment of intra uterine adhesions by microhysteroscopy Fertil steril 3 : 39

18. Lancet M, Kessler I (1986) Traitement du syndrome d'Asherman par l'hystéroscopie J gynecol Obstet Biol Reprod. 15 : 464

19. Friedman A, Defazio J, de Cherney AM (1986) Severe obstetric complication following hysteroscopic lysis of adhesions. Obstet Gynecol 67 : 864

20. Siegler AM, Valle RF (1988) Therapeutic hysteroscopic procedures Fertil Steril 50 : 685-701

21. Valle RF, Sciarra JJ (1988) Intra uterine adhesions : hysteroscopic diagnosis classification treatment and reproductive outcome Am J Obstet Gynecol 158 :1459

22. Frenz Z, Huang Y, Sunj F and al (1989) Diagnostic and therapeutic hysteroscopy for traumatic intrauterine adhesion. Clin Med J JUL 102 (7) 553-33

# Intrauterine adhesions (Asherman's syndrome)

R.F. VALLE

Many eponymic terms have been used to describe intrauterine adhesions or scars resulting from trauma to the endometrial lining in the early postpartum or postabortal period. Nonetheless, it is the term Asherman's syndrome that has been uniformly accepted as the best way to term this condition. While Asherman described amenorrhea following endometrial trauma in the early postpartum that he termed amenorrhea traumatica atretica, two years after his first description he added to the syndrome the partial occlusion of the uterine cavity secondary to adhesions [1, 2]. At present, the term Asherman's syndrome includes both pathologic entities.

While in the past this condition, particularly when hypomenorrhea or eumenorrhea was present, was not diagnosed consistently due perhaps to the lack of a reliable method that could determine its presence, with increased awareness of this condition, particularly after the introduction of better methods to evaluate the uterine cavity, such as hysteroscopy and ultrasound, the condition was diagnosed more frequently and the treatment established earlier than before. Furthermore, because the condition may result in infertility, menstrual abnormalities (particularly amenorrhea or hypomenorrhea), pregnancy complications such as habitual abortions, missed abortions, premature deliveries, and placental insertion abnormalities (such as placenta previa and placenta accreta), it is of most importance to arrive at early diagnosis and establish treatment when the adhesions can be removed easier and more completely [3].

## Etiology

Intrauterine adhesions are scars that result from trauma to a recently pregnant uterus. Over 90% of the cases are caused by curettage [4-6]. Usually the trauma has occurred because of excessive bleeding requiring curettage 1 to 4 weeks after a delivery of a term or preterm pregnancy or after an abortion. During this vulnerable phase of the endometrium any trauma may denude or remove the basalis layer causing the uterine walls to coapt each other and form a permanent bridge, distorting the symmetry of the uterine cavity. In rare occasions, non puerperal conditions such as abdominal metroplasties or myomectomies may cause intrauterine adhesions, but these adhesions are usually due to misplaced sutures rather than the true coaptation of denuded areas of myometrium that occurs following postpartum or postabortal curettage [3].

The type and consistency of the adhesions vary; some are focal, some extensive, some mild and filmy, and some thickened and dense, with extensive fibromuscular or connective tissue components. The extent and type of adhesion causing uterine cavity occlusion correlate well with the extent of endometrial trauma during the vulnerable phase of the endometrium following a recent pregnancy. Some adhesions are focal, others completely occlude the uterine cavity, consistency of adhesions usually follows the longevity and duration of these adhesions, the older ones being thickened and dense, and formed by connective tissue [7-9].

## Symptomatology

Intrauterine adhesions frequently result in menstrual abnormalities, such as hypomenorrhea or even amenorrhea, depending upon the location and extent of uterine cavity occlusion. Patients with long standing intrauterine adhesions may also develop dysmenorrhea (25%). Over 75% of women with moderate or severe adhesions will have either amenorrhea or hypomenorrhea. Patients with significant uterine cavity occlusion secondary to intrauterine adhesions experience menstrual abnormalities particularly amenorrhea (37%) and hypomenorrhea (31%). Patients with minimal or focal intrauterine adhesions may not demonstrate obvious menstrual abnormalities and may continue to have normal menses [3, 6].

Some patients may also exhibit problems in reproduction, particularly pregnancy wastage, should the adhesions only partially occlude the uterine cavity. When total amenorrhea and total uterine cavity occlusion exist, the patient will generally be infertile. Other problems associated with intrauterine adhesions are premature labor, fetal demise and ectopic pregnancy. When pregnancy is carried to term, placental insertion abnormalities such as placenta accreta, percreta or increta may occur. Schenker and Margalioth [6] evaluated 292 patients who did not receive treatment for intrauterine adhesions. Of these, 133 women conceived (45.5%) and of these, only 50 (30%) achieved a term pregnancy; 38 (23%) had preterm labor, and 66 patients had a spontaneous abortion (40%). In 21 patients (13%) placenta previa, ectopic pregnancy and abnormal placental insertions, such as placenta accreta, were diagnosed.

## Diagnosis

The most important clue to the diagnosis of intrauterine adhesions is a history of trauma to the endometrial cavity, particularly curettage following a delivery or an abortion. Secondary to that is a history of amenorrhea or hypomenorrhea. Because intrauterine adhesions are not related to hormonal events, an intact hypothalamic-pituitary-ovarian-axis should result in a biphasic basal body temperature chart supporting ovulation; failure to withdraw from a progesterone challenge test in a patient who is amenorrheic will strengthen the diagnosis. Uterine sounding has been used to ascertain obstruction of the internal cervical os, but this test should be abandoned, because of an increased danger of uterine perforation as well as inaccuracy of diagnosis. The most useful screening test for intrauterine adhesions is a hysterosalpingogram. It provides evaluation of the internal cervical os and uterine cavity; delineation of the adhesions, and information about the condition of the rest of the uterine cavity, if adhesions do not completely occlude this area. About 1.5% of hysterosalpingograms performed for infertility evaluation demonstrate intrauterine adhesions [10]. When hysterosalpingograms are performed for repeated abortions, about 5% will show intrauterine adhesions. A history compatible with intrauterine adhesions will increase the yield of hysterosalpingography for intrauterine adhesions in about 39% of patients [3, 6]. These adhesions will appear as star-like, stellate irregular shape filling defects, with ragged contours and variable locations through the uterine cavity. They are most commonly found in

the central corporeal uterine cavity and less frequently at the uterotubal cones and lower uterine segment.

Despite the usefulness of hysterosalpingography as a screening method for patients suspected of having intrauterine adhesions, the final diagnosis is determined only by direct visualization with hysteroscopy, because about 30% of abnormal hysterosalpingograms may not be confirmed by hysteroscopy [11]. The diagnosis can be confirmed by visualization, and the appropriate treatment can be provided once the adhesions are observed endoscopically.

Hysterosalpingography is useful in determining the extent of uterine cavity occlusion, but it cannot provide an appraisal of the consistency and type of intrauterine adhesions. For this reason, hysteroscopy becomes a useful adjunct to hysterosalpingography by confirming the extent and type of intrauterine adhesions.

Other techniques, such as ultrasonography and magnetic resonance imaging (MRI), have been used to make this diagnosis, but their accuracy is not well established and not enough experience exists with these techniques to supplant the hysterosalpingogram and hysteroscopy [12]. Furthermore, the cost may be prohibitive.

## Methods of treatment

Treatment of intrauterine adhesions is surgical, consisting of removing those adhesions by selective endoscopic division. In the past, blind methods of division were used with curettes, probes or dilators, or hysterotomy assisted division of these adhesions under direct vision, but these techniques have failed to produce acceptable results and have been largely abandoned. Introduction of modern hysteroscopy has permitted transcervical division of adhesions under visual guidance; hysteroscopic methods have used mechanical means, such as hysteroscopic scissors, thin electrodes, and fiberoptic lasers (Figs. 1-4).

## Treatment of intrauterine adhesions with hysteroscopic scissors

Because intrauterine adhesions in general are avascular and are divided, not removed, the treatment has been similar to that used for division of a uterine septum. The adhesions are divided centrally, allowing the uterine cavity to expand upon division of the adhesions. This is performed utilizing flexible, semirigid and occasionally rigid or optical scissors. The

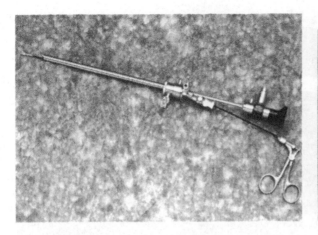

**Fig. 1.** Operative rigid hysteroscope, 7 mm in outer diameter with hysteroscopic scissors in place

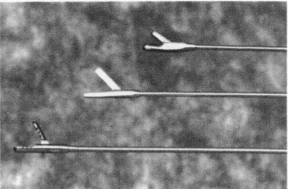

**Fig. 2.** Semirigid hysteroscopic instruments. *Top to bottom:* biopsy forceps, scissors, grasping forceps

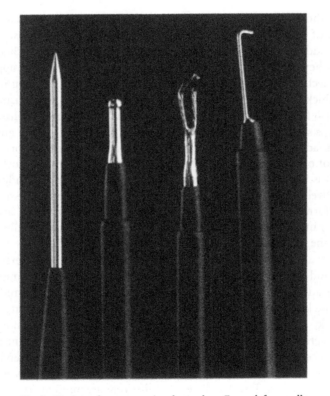

**Fig. 3.** Various hysteroscopic electrodes. *From left:* needle shape, blunt, spoon type, hook-shape

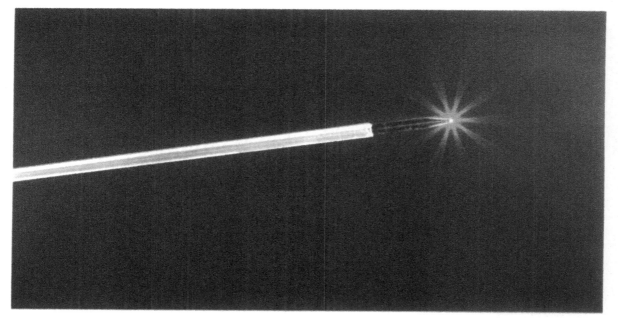

**Fig. 4.** Sculpted sharp fiber laser

most commonly used method is the semi-rigid hyste-roscopic scissors because of the increased facility ma-nipulating the scissors and by selectively dividing these adhesions when they retract upon cutting. Occasionally, thick connective tissue adhesions are present that form very thick stumps and benefit not only from division but also from removal. To achieve this effect, a biopsy forceps sometimes becomes most useful when lateral thick adhesions are present and the technique involves not only division of the adhe-sions but also removal. It is important to use a sharp biopsy forceps to selectively sculpture the uterine cavity to achieve a uniform symmetry. This tech-nique is also useful at the uterotubal cones, particu-larly at the junction of the tubal openings and the uterine cavity.

While the semi-rigid and flexible scissors are most useful for the division of adhesions by hysteroscopy, the rigid optical scissors are less helpful in this endea-vor. Because of the thick, sturdy configuration of these scissors, when the uterine wall is thin and scle-rotic, there is greater chance of uterine perforation, particularly because a panoramic view is somewhat impaired by the distally fixed scissors. Targeted dissec-tion, which is easily obtained with the flexible and semi-rigid scissors, is hampered and difficult with op-tical scissors.

Fluids with electrolytes should be used when divi-ding these adhesions, because of increased chances of intravasation and because the adhesions are cut close to the myometrial tissue and the extensive area of de-nudation may predispose to fluid intravasation. Normal saline, Dextrose 5% in half normal saline and Ringer's lactate are most appropriate. Care must be taken to measure the amount of fluid infused and the amount recovered when using the hysteroscope, par-ticularly if the instrument has inflow and outflow per-mitting an estimate of the amount of fluid non-reco-vered and potentially absorbed by the patient. In the absence of a continuous flow system, care must be ta-ken to measure the total inflow of fluids and ascertain that the intrauterine pressure does not exceed the mean arterial pressure of about 100 mm Hg. These procedures must be expedited to avoid excessive in-travasation of fluid.

Depending upon the extent of uterine cavity oc-clusion, division is done under visual control by cut-ting the adhesions in the middle to avoid uterine da-mage at the level of the uterine wall. When there is total uterine cavity occlusion, selective dissection of adhesions begins at the internal cervical os until a neocavity is created and then the dissection progresses until the uterotubal cones are free. When extensive adhesions are present, the hysteroscopist should be alert to perforation. Upon completion of the proce-dure, indigo carmine is injected transcervically to test for tubal patency (Figs. 5-10).

New thin electrodes have been designed that can be used through the hysteroscopic channel of a conti-nuous flow hysteroscope. The shape of these elec-

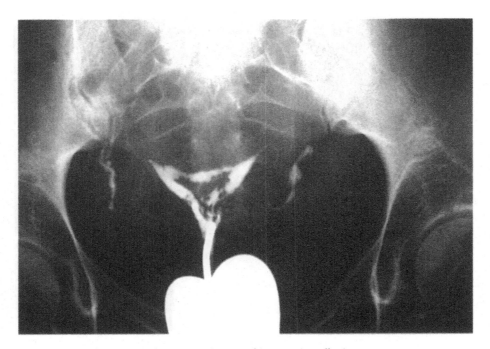

**Fig. 5.** Hysterosalpingogram shows extensive central intrauterine adhesions

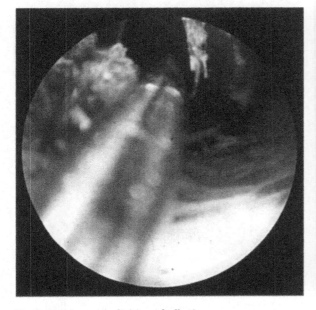

**Fig. 6.** Hysteroscopic division of adhesions

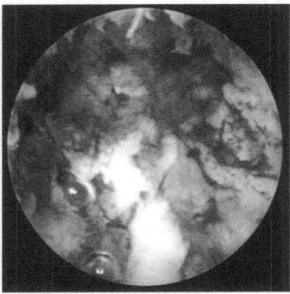

**Fig. 7.** Rugged aspect of uterine cavity following division of adhesions

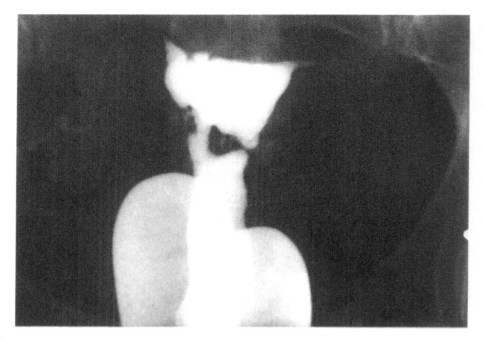

**Fig. 8.** Hysterosalpingogram shows focal intrauterine adhesions

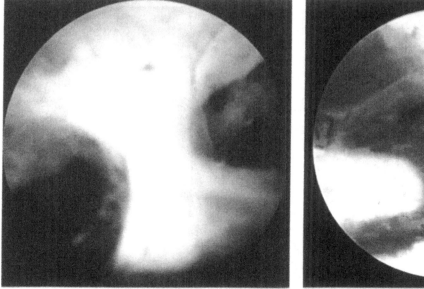

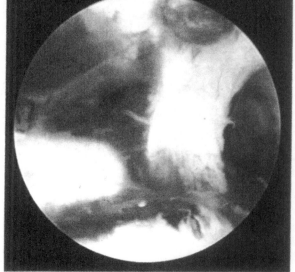

**Fig. 9.** At hysteroscopy a central adhesion is seen connecting the uterine walls

**Fig. 10.** Extensive connective tissue adhesions occluding the entire cavity. Small portion of uterine cavity free of adhesions is seen on right

trodes varies from sharp points to hooktype electrodes. By decreasing the distal end of these electrodes, electrical scattering may be decreased permitting selective division of the adhesions. Nonetheless, because of their sharp configuration, care must be taken to avoid uterine wall damage and/or perforation. Additionally, because they coagulate as they cut, the visual appraisal of juxtaposed myometrial layer, may not be as clear as when mechanical scissors are used. Only fluids devoid of electrolytes can be used when electrosurgery is performed.

The procedure is performed by systematically dividing the adhesions and cutting as much as feasible, particularly when there is total uterine cavity occlusion [8, 9, 13-18].

The advantages of using hysteroscopic scissors for the division of intrauterine adhesions are those of mechanical methods. Mechanical tools provide excellent landmarks when dividing these adhesions, particularly when approaching the juxtaposed myometrium. Bleeding may be observed at the myometrium and this warns the hysteroscopist to stop the dissection so as to avoid perforation. No scattering of energies is produced to damage the small areas of healthy endometrium which are the reservoir for future reepithelialization. This is an important consideration, because no extensive healthy endometrium can be found when extensive intrauterine adhesions are present. The disadvantages are that it may sometimes be difficult to manipulate semi-rigid instrumentation, particularly to the lateral walls of the uterine cavity. Scissors do not provide the sharpness or mechanism to cut these adhesions, as the scissors do not close well distally and need to be readjusted and sharpened frequently (Figs. 11-15).

## Treatment of intrauterine adhesions utilizing the resectoscope and hysteroscopic electrodes

As an alternative to mechanical tools, the resectoscope can be used to divide intrauterine adhesions either with a resecting loop, a loop bent forward or with specifically designed electrodes that can be directly applied to the adhesions dividing them easily. These are in the form of knives or wires that must be specifically and selectively directed to the adhesions, particularly those in the lateral portion of the uterus or to the uterotubal cones. When utilizing the resectoscope, fluids without electrolytes must be used, e.g., Dextrose 5% in water, glycine 1.5%, Sorbitol 3.5% or Mannitol 5%, that provide excellent visualization and are useful distending media. When dividing these adhesions, the resectoscope loop may not be the appro-

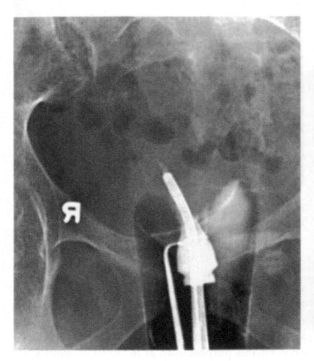

Fig. 11. Hysterosalpingogram fails to show any uterine cavity

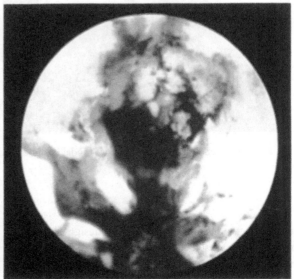

Fig. 12. Following lysis of adhesions a small uterine cavity is created. Note stumps of remaining adhesions

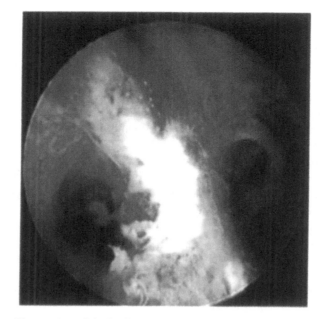

**Fig. 13.** Central thick adhesion connecting uterine walls

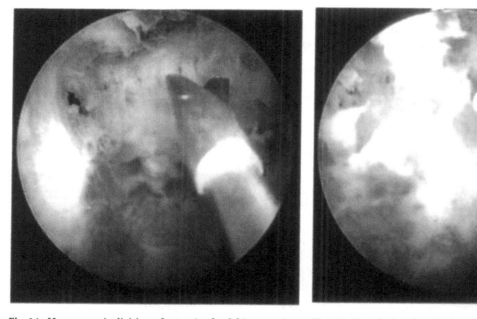

**Fig. 14.** Hysteroscopic division of extensive fundal intrauterine adhesions

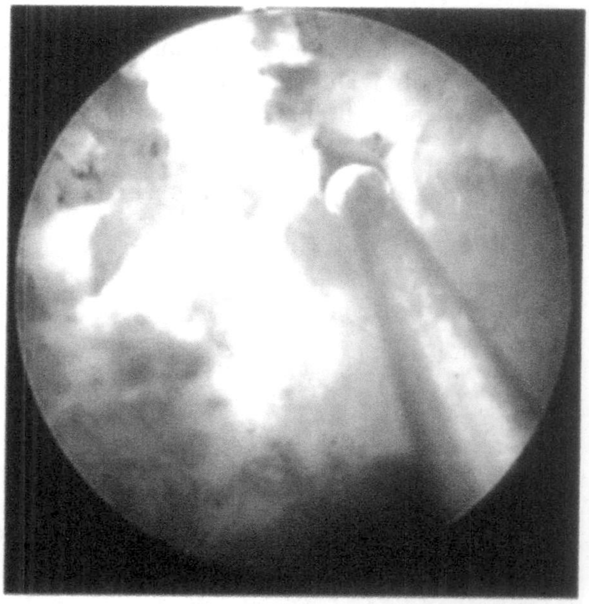

**Fig. 15.** Completing the division of fundal intrauterine adhesions

priate electrode to use, because it is designed to resect rather than to selectively divide centrally the adhesions. When the resectoscopic loop has been used, several complications have occurred, particularly due to future sacculations of the uterus, dehiscences and perforations. Ascertaining where the adhesions finish and

when the normal myometrium begins is difficult, and the resections may be so deep that a portion of the myometrium may be shaved during division of the adhesions [19]. Electrodes have been specifically designed for this purpose such as the knife or wire-types that can selectively be directed to the adhesions and divide them systematically. Nonetheless, concern remains about scattering the energy and damaging the peripheral healthy endometrium. With the use of specific electrodes, this effect may be somewhat decreased. It is important to monitor the operation with concomitant sonography or laparoscopy, because the landmarks of junction between adhesions and myometrium may be lost, and the coagulating effect this energy may produce in the myometrium may obscure a view of small vessels that, when bleed, warns the hysteroscopist to stop further dissection.

Attempts to guide the hysteroscopist by using concomitant fluoroscopy have been made with the use of radio-opaque material injected directly through the hysteroscopic channel or by injection transcervically or transfundally via small needles. However, the procedures add to the complexity of hysteroscopic division and remain of little help in the operation itself that should rely upon distinction and recognition of tissues while the operation is taking place. Additionally, the use of fluoroscopy adds to the cumulative radiation the patient is receiving in the pelvis [20-22].

Use of the resectoscope has several advantages: bleeding is decreased during dissection; the resectoscope allows estimation of the deficit of fluid, decreasing the chances of fluid overload. The disadvantage is that monopolar energy must be used, therefore the patient must be grounded and only fluids devoid of electrolytes can be used. This decreases the threshold for possible fluid overload if excessive amounts are absorbed. Additional disadvantages are electrosurgical damage of peripheral endometrium and the loss of landmarks while coagulating close to the myometrium, resulting in inadvertent perforation of this area [19].

## Treatment of intrauterine adhesions with fiberoptic lasers

Fiberoptic lasers, such as the Neodymium-Yag, Argon, KTP/532, can also be used to divide intrauterine adhesions, but their application has been somewhat limited. The Neodymium-Yag laser with sculpted or extruded fibers can be a useful tool to selectively divide intrauterine adhesions, particularly those that are lateral and fundal [23, 24]. Care must be taken to use these fibers by contact and selectively be aware of the overall symmetry of the uterine cavity, because the coagulating power of the laser may cause a similar effect than electrosurgery, that is coagulation and cutting, and the landmarks of the juxtaposed myome-

trium may be lost while performing division of the adhesions. Small arteries that cross the myometrium may not bleed, so dissection may proceed further than necessary. The manipulation of the fiberoptic lasers is very easy under hysteroscopy and can be facilitated greatly with the use of foreoblique vision. The Argon and KTP/532 utilize the sharpest fibers to cut rather than to coagulate.

Because lasers are not conductive, fluids with electrolytes should be used. Normal saline, Dextrose 5% in half normal saline, or Ringer's Lactate provide excellent visualization and have sodium on board that prevents hyponatremia, should excessive fluids be used. The utilization of these electrolyte-containing fluids will not prevent pulmonary edema but will increase the threshold; therefore, more fluid may be used than when using fluids without electrolytes. Ideally, a hysteroscope with a continuous flow system should be used, or one with true inflow and outflow, to collect the injected fluid and have a perfect account of the deficit or non-recovered fluid.

Use of the laser is attractive and has the benefit of easy manipulation, but requires more time than the use of mechanical tools such as hysteroscopic scissors. It is important, therefore, when utilizing this type of energy, to expedite the procedure as much as possible, to avoid excessive fluid from being intravasated.

New methodologies in the treatment of Asherman's syndrome have been suggested. From blind dissection with curved probes or dilators of the lateral aspects of the uterine cavity close to myometrium, in order to convers an occluded uterine cavity in a septate shape, myometrial scoring with an electrical knife performing 4 mm deep longitudinal sulci into the myometrium, to the renewal of hysterotomy for lysis of adhesions and placement of intrauterine and intratubal stents postoperatively [25-27]. All these procedures were attempted in few patients and remain to be validated as a true advance in the treatment of severe Asherman's syndrome.

## Other adjunctive therapy

The principal goal of therapy is to remove the adhesions surgically. Because most of these patients have a sclerotic or destroyed endometrium, they need other adjunctive therapy to promote reepithelialization and also a mechanical separation of the uterine walls to prevent the reformation of adhesions. These adjuncts are intrauterine splints, prophylactic antibiotics and estrogens and progesterone to promote reepithelialization.

Prophylactic antibiotics are used routinely in these patients in view of a traumatized endometrium and extensive manipulation these patients usually require. The antibiotics used are in the form of a cephalosporins, Kefzol 1 gram IV piggyback half an hour before the procedure, to be followed with Keflex 500 mg qid orally for a week, particularly when intrauterine splints are used. In those patients with extensive intrauterine adhesions an indwelling catheter is placed of the pediatric type number 8 with 3-3 1/2 ml of a sterile solution instilled and left in place for a week to prevent reformation of adhesions. Adjunctive hormonal therapy consists of natural estrogens in the form of Premarin 2.5 mg twice a day for 30 or 40 days, depending on the extent of uterine cavity occlusion and the type of adhesions found. The more extensive and old the adhesions are, the more prolonged the hormonal treatment needed. In the last 10 days of this artificial cycle, 10 milligrams of medroxiprogesterone acetate (Provera) a day are given orally. Upon completion of the hormonal treatment, and once withdrawal bleeding has ceased, a hysterosalpingogram is performed to assess the results of the operation and decide upon further therapy or initiation of attempts to conception. Those patients with filmy, focal adhesions may not require hysterosalpingography but an office hysteroscopy to assess uterine cavity symmetry [28].

## Results of therapy

The results of hysteroscopic treatment of intrauterine adhesions have correlated well with the extent of uterine cavity occlusion and the type of adhesions present. Normal menstruation is restored in over 90% of patients. The reproductive outcome correlates well with the type of adhesions and the extent of uterine cavity occlusion. Of 187 patients treated hysteroscopically by Valle and Sciarra [28], removal of mild, filmy adhesions in 43 cases gave the best result, with 35 (81%) term pregnancies; in 97 moderate cases of fibromuscular adhesions 64 (66%) term pregnancies occurred, and in 47 severe cases of connective tissue adhesions, 15 (32%) term pregnancies occurred. Overall restoration of menses occurred in 90% of the patients, and the term pregnancy rate was 79.7%. These results demonstrate a much better reproductive outcome than was previously obtained with blind methods of therapy (Table 1).

Results following treatment of intrauterine adhesions utilizing the resectoscope have been similar; nonetheless, the reported postoperative complications may be serious and should be kept in mind when utilizing this type of instrument. A few series report lysis of adhesions with fiberoptic lasers but when the lasers are used appropriately, results should not vary much from those reported with electrosurgery.

## Prognosis and classification

Reproductive outcome seems to correlate well with the type of adhesions and the extent of uterine cavity occlusion. It is useful to have a way of classifying these adhesions as filmy and composed of endometrial tissue, fibromuscular, or composed of connective tissue [37]. The degree of uterine cavity occlusion also is important. Attempts to classify intrauterine adhesions by hysterosalpingography give a good appraisal of the extent of uterine cavity occlusion, but it is impossible to determine by hysterosalpingography the type of adhesions that are present. When using hysteroscopy alone, it is difficult to assess the extent of uterine cavity occlusion by visualization, because the axis to the hysteroscopist is from the cervix to the fundus and not perpendicular to the uterine body, as hysterography is, outlining the uterine cavity from a different axis. For this reason, the combination of hysterosalpingography and hysteroscopy has been used most commonly to assess not only the extent of uterine cavity occlusion, but also the type of adhesions found by hysteroscopy at the time of treatment. Valle and Sciarra [28] utilized a three stage classification of the extent and severity of intrauterine adhesions (mild, moderate and severe), based on the degree of involvement shown on hysterosalpingography and the extent and type of adhesions found on hysteroscopy. Three stages of intrauterine adhesions are defined: *mild adhesions*, filmy adhesions composed of basalis endometrial tissue producing partial or complete uterine cavity occlusion; *moderate adhesions*, fibromuscular, characteristically thick, still covered with endometrium that may bleed upon division, which partially or totally occlude the uterine cavity; *severe adhesions*, composed of connective tissue only, lacking any endometrial lining and not likely to bleed upon division. These adhesions may partially or totally occlude the uterine cavity (Fig. 16).

Recently the American Fertility Society has proposed a classification of intrauterine adhesions based on the findings at hysterosalpingography and hysteroscopy, and their correlation with menstrual patterns [38]. Using a uniform classification for intrauterine adhesions greatly enhances our ability to report, evaluate and compare results of different treatments of intrauterine adhesions, particularly when utilizing these modalities by the hysteroscopic approach.

**Table 1.** Hysteroscopic lysis of intrauterine adhesions

| Author | No. patients | Medium | Technique | Menses nl. no. (%) | Reproductive outcome pregnancy no. (%) | Term no. (%) |
|---|---|---|---|---|---|---|
| Levine and Neuwirth [13] | 10 | Hyskon | Flexible scissors | 5 (50) | 2 (20) | |
| Edstrom [29] | 9 | Hyskon | Biopsy forceps | 2 (22) | 1 (11) | 1 (11) |
| Siegler and Kontopoulos [17] | 25 | $CO_2$ | Target abrasion/ scissors/curettage | 13 (52) | 11 (44) | 2 (44.4) |
| March and Israel [15] | 38 | Hyskon | Flexible scissors | 38 (100) | 38 (100) | 34 (79.1) |
| Neuwirth et al. [14] | 27 | Hyskon | Scissors alongside | 20 (74) | 14 (51.8) | 13 (48.1) |
| Sanfilippo et al. [30] | 26 | $CO_2$ | Curettage | 26 (100) | 6 (100) | 3 (50) |
| Hamou et al. [31] | 69 | $CO_2$ | Target abrasion | 59 (85.5) | 20 (51.3) | 15 (38.4) |
| Sugimoto et al. [32] | 258 | Hyskon/ normal saline | Target abrasion/ Kelly forceps | 180 (69.7) | 143 (76.4) | 114 (79.7) |
| Wamsteker '84 [33] | 36 | Hyskon | Scissors/biopsy forceps | 34 (94.4) | 17 (62.9) | 12 (44.4) |
| Friedman et al. [19] | 30 | Hyskon | Resectoscope/ scissors | 27 (90) | 24 (80) | 23 (76.6) |
| Zuanchong and Yulian [34] | 70 | Normal saline | Biopsy forceps/ flexible scissors | 64 (84.3) | 30 (85.7) | 17 (48.5) |
| Valle and Sciarra [28] | 187 | $D_5W$/Hyskon | Flexible/semirigid/ rigid scissors | 167 (89.3) | 143 (76.4) | 114 (79.7) |
| Lancet and Kessler [35] | 98 | Hyskon | Flexible scissors/ electrosurgery | 98 (100) | 86 (87.8) | 77 (89.5) |
| Pabuccu et al. [36] | 40 | Glycine | Murphy probe scissors | 33 (82.5) | 27 (67.5) | 23 (57.5) |
| Totals | 923 | | | 766 (83.0) | 562 (60.8) | 458 (81.5) |

(Modified from Siegler AM, Valle RF, Lindemann HJ, Mencaglia L (1990) Therapeutic Hysteroscopy. Indications and Techniques. CV Mosby Company, St Louis, Baltimore, Philadelphia, Toronto, Chapt 6, p 103)

## Summary and conclusions

Intrauterine adhesions are not an unusual entity and should be strongly suspected when there is trauma, usually in the form of a curettage, of the endometrial lining following a delivery or an abortion. The earlier the diagnosis is obtained, the better the prognosis and the reproductive outcome after treatment. The treatment of intrauterine adhesions can be accomplished by three different techniques: scissors, resectoscope, and fiberoptic lasers. All have advantages and disadvantages and must be used with knowledge of each

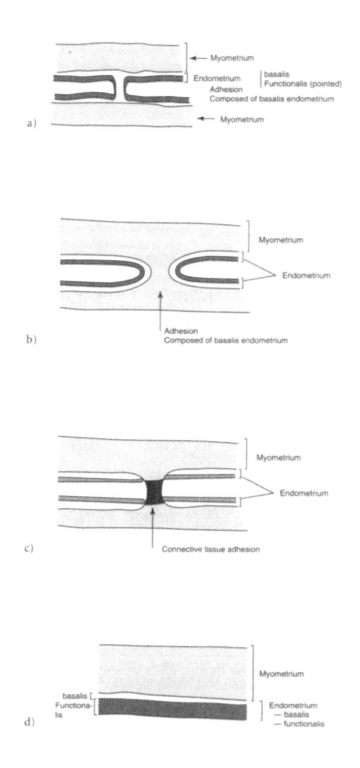

**Fig. 16.** Diagram of type of intrauterine adhesions: a) endometrial, filmy; b) fibromuscular, dense, and c) connective tissue adhesions, thick and lacking endometrium

particular technology and its drawbacks. Each method should be tailored not only to the anatomy, pathology and etiology of each process, but also to the experience of the operator. The gynecologist should select the appropriate method and technique for each patient. Results of therapy should be a successful viable pregnancy for those patients who desire reproduction, keeping in mind the safety of the patient with the least morbidity possible, the absence of complications and overall effectiveness and diminution of unnecessary costs. Versatility plays a significant role in the selection of therapeutic alternatives the surgeon has, to intelligently select the best method for each individual patient.

The hysteroscopic treatment of intrauterine adhesions should be considered the standard treatment for this condition and the selection of the specific method for hysteroscopic treatment must be done according to individual experience and the extent and type of intrauterine adhesions present.

# References

1. Asherman JG (1948) Amenorrhea traumatica (atretica). J Obstet Gynaecol Br Emp 55:23-30

2. Asherman JG (1950) Traumatic intrauterine adhesions. J Obstet Gynaecol Br Emp 57:892-896

3. Klein SM, Garcia CR (1973) Asherman's syndrome: a critique and current review. Fertil Steril 24:722-735

4. Forssman L (1965) Post-traumatic intrauterine synechiae and pregnancy. Obstet Gynecol 26:710-713

5. Foix A, Bruno RO, Davidson T, Lema B (1966) The pathology of post curettage intrauterine adhesions. Am J Obstet Gynecol 96:1027-1033

6. Schenker JG, Margalioth EJ (1982) Intrauterine adhesions; an updated appraisal. Fertil Steril 37:593-610

7. Sugimoto O (1978) Diagnostic and therapeutic hysteroscopy for traumatic intrauterine adhesions. Am J Obstet Gynecol 131:539-547

8. Valle RF, Sciarra JJ (1984) Hysteroscopic treatment of intrauterine adhesions. In: Siegler AM, Lindemann HJ (eds) Hysteroscopy. Principles and Practice. Lippincott, Philadelphia pp 193-197

9. Polishuk WZ, Siew FP, Gordon R, Lebenshoft P (1977) Vascular changes in traumatic amenorrhea and hypomenorrhea. Int J Fertil 22:189-192

10. Dmowski WP, Greenblatt RB (1969) Asherman's syndrome and risk of placenta accreta. Obstet Gynecol 34:288-299

11. Valle RF (1980) Hysteroscopy in the evaluation of female infertility. Am J Obstet Gynecol 137:425-431

12. Confino E, Friberg J, Giglia RV, Gleicher N (1985) Sonographic imaging of intrauterine adhesions. Obstet Gynecol 66:596-598

13. Levine RU, Neuwirth RS (1973) Simultaneous laparoscopy and hysteroscopy for intrauterine adhesions. Obstet Gynecol 42:441-445

14. Neuwirth RS, Hussein AR, Schiffman BM, Amin HK (1982) Hysteroscopic resection of intrauterine scars using a new technique. Obstet Gynecol 60:111-113

15. March CM, Israel R (1978) Gestational outcome following hysteroscopic lysis of adhesions. Am J Obstet Gynecol 130:653-657

16. March CM, Israel R, March AD (1978) Hysteroscopic management of intrauterine adhesions. Am J Obstet Gynecol 130:653-657

17. Siegler AM, Kontopoulos VG (1981) Lysis of intrauterine adhesions under hysteroscopic control: A report of 25 operations. J Reprod Med 26:372-374

18. Jewelewicz R, Khalaf S, Neuwirth RS, Vande Wiele RL (1976) Obstetric complications after treatment of intrauterine synechiae (Asherman's syndrome). Obstet Gynecol 47:701-705

19. Friedman A, Defazio J, DeCherney AH (1986) Severe obstetric complications following hysteroscopic lysis of adhesions. Obstet Gynecol 67:864-867

20. Lancet M, Mass N (1981) Concomitant hysterography and hysteroscopy in Asherman's syndrome. Int J Fertil 26:267-272

21. Ikeda T, Morita A, Imamura A, Mori I (1981) The separation procedure for intrauterine adhesion (Synechia uteri) under roentgenographic view. Fertil Steril 36:333-338

22. Sanders B, Machan LS, Gomel V (1998) Complex uterine surgery: a cooperative role for interventional radiology with hysteroscopic surgery. Fertil Steril 70:952-955

23. Newton JR, Mackenzie WE, Emens MJ, Jordan JA (1989) Division of uterine adhesions (Asherman's syndrome) with the Nd-YAG laser. Br J Obstet Gynaecol 96:102-104

24. Chapman R, Chapman K (1996) The value of two stage laser treatment for severe Asherman's syndrome. Br J Obstet Gynaecol 103:1256-1258

25. McComb PF, Wagner BL (1997) Simplified therapy for Asherman's syndrome. Fertil Steril 68:1047-1050

26. Protopapas A, Shusham A, Magos A (1998) Myometrial scoring: a new technique for management of severe Asherman's syndrome. Fertil Steril 69:860-864

27. Reddy S, Rock JA (1997) Surgical management of complete obliteration of the endometrial cavity. Fertil Steril 67:172-174

28. Valle RF, Sciarra JJ (1988) Intrauterine adhesions: Hysteroscopic diagnosis classification, treatment and reproductive outcome. Am J Obstet Gynecol 158:1459-1470

29. Edstrom K (1974) Intrauterine Surgical procedures during hysteroscopy. Endoscopy 6:175-181

30. Sanfilippo JS, Fitzgerald MR, Badaway SZ, Yussman MA (1982) Asherman's syndrome: a comparison of methods. J Reprod Med 27:328-330

242     R.F. Valle

31. Hamou J, Salat-Baroux J, Siegler AM (1983) Diagnosis and treatment of intrauterine adhesions by microhysteroscopy. Fertil Steril 39:321-326
32. Sugimoto O, Ushiroyma T, Fukuda Y (1984) Diagnostic and therapeutic hysteroscopy for traumatic intrauterine adhesions. In: Siegler AM, Lindemann HJ (eds) Hysteroscopy: Principles and Practice, Lippincott, Philadelphia, pp 186-192
33. Wamsteker K (1984) Hysteroscopy in Asherman's syndrome. In: Siegler AM, Lindemann HJ (eds), Hysteroscopy: Principles and Practice, Lippincott, Philadelphia, pp 198-203
34. Zuanchong F, Yulian H (1986) Hysteroscopic diagnosis and treatment of intrauterine adhesions. Clinical analysis of 70 cases. In Symposium on Hysteroscopy. Shanghai, Family Planning Association, p179

35. Lancet M, Kessler I (1988) A review of Asherman's syndrome, and results of modern treatment. Int J Fertil 33:14-24
36. Pabuccu R, Atay V, Orhon E, Urman B, Ergun A (1997) Hysteroscopic treatment of intrauterine adhesions is safe and effective in the restoration of normal menstruation and fertility. Fertil Steril 68:1141-1143
37. Sugimoto O (1978) Diagnostic and Therapeutic Hysteroscopy. Igaku-Shoin, Tokyo-New York, p 148
38. The American Fertility Society (1988) Classifications of adnexal adhesions, distal tubal occlusion, tubal occlusion secondary to tubal ligation, tubal pregnancies, Mullerian anomalies and intrauterine adhesions. Fertil Steril 49:944-955

# Falloposcopy in an office setting

E.S. SURREY

Several investigators have suggested that, in a population of infertile patients, 11 to 16% will be determined to have various tubal abnormalities. [1, 2] Significant prognostic factors include a history of pelvic infection, sexually transmitted diseases, tubal or ovarian surgery, endometriosis, or use of various intrauterine devices [3, 4]. Distal tubal disease most commonly stems from either prior infection or as a response to such inflammatory insults as prior pelvic surgery or endometriosis. Proximal tubal occlusion may result from inflammation or infection as well but may also stem from salpingitis isthmica nodosa, spasm amorphous casts, or extrinsic compression from adenomyosis, endometriosis or leiomyomata [5, 7]. These disorders may result in total tubal occlusion but may also result in more subtle dysfunction in the face of patent fallopian tubes.

The fallopian tube has a much greater role in the reproductive process than that of a passive conduct between ovary and uterus. The fallopian tube has a vital role in the reproductive process in humans. Its functions include sperm transport, ovum pick up, and embryo transport. The fallopian tube is the site for sperm capacitation, oocyte fertilization, as well as early embryo development and maintenance. Tubal transport depends upon the endocrine milieu, cilial function, muscular contractions and adrenergic innervation [8, 9].

The primary means of assessing the fallopian tube have traditionally included hysterosalpingography (HSG) and laparoscopy. The accuracy of findings at HSG in comparison with those obtained from laparoscopy have been debated. Investigators from a multicenter World Health Organization trial found that only 55% of 125 women undergoing both laparoscopy and HSG had similar findings [10]. Swart and colleagues [11] recently performed a meta-analysis of 20 previously published studies comparing the accuracy of diagnosis of tubal patency or peritubal adhesions by HSG in comparision to laparoscopy. Point estimates for tubal patency of 0.65 and 0.83 for sensitivity and specificity, respectively, were calculated. This means that although tubal disease is very likely in the presence of an abnormal HSG, tubal patency on HSG does not rule out pathology. Neither HSG nor laparoscopy allow the clinician to differentiate between true proximal occlusion and either spasm at the utercornual ostium or the presence of occlusive mucous plugs. Thus, a patent tube is not necessarily a normal tube.

Falloposcopy is a transcervical transvaginal approach for visualizing the follopian tubal lumen from the uterotubal junction to the fimbria. The first reports of the successful use of this microendoscopy technique were provided in 1990 by Kerin and coworkers [12, 13]. A variety of falloposcopes have been developed as modifications of fiberoptic angioscopes. These flexible instruments measure approximately 1.5 m in length and 0.45-0.5 mm in outer diameter (Conceptus, San Carlos, CA; Medical Dynamics, Englewood, CO; Intramed, San Diego, CA; Olympus, Lake Success, NY) (Fig. 1). Although the majority of the data regarding both diagnostic and therapeutic applications of falloposcopy have been derived from procedures performed under general anesthesia in a hospital setting, the potential for office based falloposcopy is great.

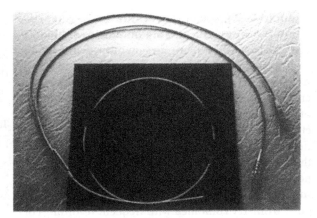

Fig. 1. Coaxial falloposcope with 0.45 mm OD and camera attachments (Conceptus, San Carlos, CA)

Prior to subjecting a patient to microsurgical anastomosis at laparotomy or tubal bypassemploying the assisted reproductive technologies, a thorough assessment of the tubal lumen may reveal such findings as spasm of the uterotubal ostium, intralumenal polyps or mucous plugs which may lend themselves to less invasive therapy. Similarly, the finding of an irreparably damaged tubal lumen may allow the patient to avoid laparoscopy altogether and be referred directly *in vitro* fertilization-embryo transfer.

The patient with hydrosalpinges diagnosed radiologically may also benefit from this outpatient procedure. Although falloposcopy provides no information regarding peritubal disease, should the endothelial lining prove to be badly damaged beyond repair, further surgical investigation would be unwarranted. In contrast, a patient with less severely damaged endothelial lining noted at falloposcopy could then be scheduled for a laparoscopic procedure to assess the extent of peritubal disease and potentially perform endoscopic tubal reconstruction.

A third indication is the patient with otherwise unexplained infertility after a standard evaluation. Patients with normal findings at hysterosalpingography and laparoscopy have been noted to have intralumenal adhesions and abnormal endothelial vascular patterns during tubal microendoscopy [7].

Contraindications to office based falloposcopy include active pelvic infection or uterine bleeding, and an intolerance to local anesthetic agents. Patients with such endometrial pathology as synechiae or submucous myoma which prevent visualization and access to the uterotubal ostium are poor candidates as well.

## Technique

Falloposcopy is most easily performed during the mid-follicular phase of the menstrual cycle after cessation of menses. Patients are administered antibiotics prophylactically. In their series on outpatient falloposcopy, Scudamore and co-workers [14] administered naproxen femazepam and uterosacral lignocaine as anesthesia to 14 patients after dissatisfaction with two other regimes in 7 other patients. In contrast, Venezia et al. [15] premedicated eight patients in an outpatient setting with atropine sulfate benzodiazepine without complication. Dunphy [16] employed intravenous fentanyl and a benzodiazepine with similar success. Intraoperative monitoring of patients with pulse oximetry combined with frequent recordings of blood preassure and pulse provide additional safety. Patients should be allowed to recover for one hour with monitoring of vital signs after completion of the procedure.

Two basic techniques for performing falloposcopy have been described: a coaxial and linear everting catheter approach. The coaxial technique involves visualization of the uterotubal ostium (UTO) with a flexible hysteroscope during the follicular phase of the menstrual cycle after prophylactic antibiotic administration. Tubal access is achieved by cannulation of the UTO with a flexible guidewire (0.3-0.8 mm OD) and an over-the-wire soft Teflon-coated catheter (1.3 mm OD) introduced through the operating channel of the hysteroscope. The catheter and guidewire are advanced with a torque motion for a distance of 12 cm or until a point of resistance is met. The wire is then removed and a falloposcope with camera attachment is introduced through a Tuohy-Borst Y adaptor attached to the catheter and advanced under direct visualization until it reaches its distal end. Irrigation with Ringer's lacate solution employing a hand held syringe or infusion pump is used to achieve adequate visualization. The tubal lumen is viewed in a retrograde fashion. Dual video monitoring is employed to simultaneously appreciate images derived from the falloposcope and hysteroscope. This approach allows for simultaneous diagnosis and potential therapy of visualized lesions with the subsequent use of stiffer wires or balloon catheters [12]. The use of this technique in an office setting requires the infusion of minimal amounts of distending medium, and extremely gentle incremental movement of catheters and guidewires. This technique is summarized in Table 1.

An alternative approach involves the use of a linear everting catheter (LEC) (Imagyn, Laguna Niguel, CA) [17]. The LEC has an inner and outer body joined distally by a flexible balloon. When pressurized, the balloon is everted, as the inner body is advanced by slowly unrolling from the catheter tip. The UTO is visualized with the falloposcope placed through the central LEC lumen so that a hysteroscope is unnecessary. The LEC is incrementally everted to the desired distance and imaging performed in a retrograde fa-

Table 1. Coaxial falloposcopy: summary of technique

- Visualization of uterotubal ostium (UTO) with flexible hysteroscope
- Guidewire cannulation of UTO
- Over the wire catheter placement
- Removal of guide wire
- Introduction of falloposcope through catheter
- Retrograde visualization

shion (Fig. 2). This technique has been successfully used in an office based setting under local anesthesia by several investigative teams [14, 16, 18]. Dunphy and colleagues [19] reported that pain experienced during this procedure was no greater than that experienced during HSG.

## Findings and management

Kerin and coworkers [20] have developed a classification system to standardize and quantify findings at falloposcopy. Point scores are attributed for patency, dilation, vascular patterns, epithelial quality, and intralumenal adhesions (Fig. 3). Findings at falloposcopy have been shown to correlate poorly with findings at hysterosalpingography. In a large series of falloposcopies performed on 112 tubes in 75 women who had a presumptive diagnosis of proximal tubal occlusion based on laparoscopic or radiologic findings, no abnormalities were noted in 46 % [20]. Venezia and colleagues [15] noted that hysterosalpingography and LEC falloposcopy findings failed to correlate in 40% of tubes visualized. Grow et al. [21] reported that 9/12 tubes described as proximally

occluded by hysterosalpingogram were normal at falloposcopy. Surrey and coworkers [22] have recently reported that 40 % of visualized tubes in patients with otherwise unexplained infertility and normal HSG had abnormalities appreciated only at falloposcopy [22]. The likelihood of HSG or chromotubation depicting normal tubes when abnormalities were detected at falloposcopy was 22.7% in this study. Management changes were made in 52.4% of patients in this series as a result of falloposcopic findings. A clear correlation between falloposcopic findings and conception has been described [20, 23].

Patients with intralumenal mucous plugs or debris may best be managed with aquadissection techniques [24, 25]. Intralumenal endometriosis and endosalpingiosis may perhaps best be treated medically with a trial of gonadotropin releasing hormone agonist or danazol therapy, although minimal intralumenal adhesions may be more appropriately approached with gentle guide wire dissection. Denser adhesions or mild stenoses may also be approached employing balloon dilation techniques [12, 24, 25]. These procedures could possibly be performed in an office setting, once sufficient data addressing safety and patient tolerance has been reported. Increased analgesic require-

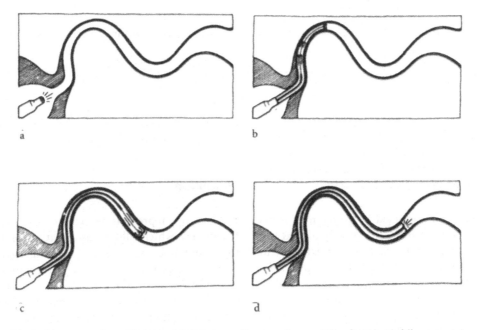

**Fig. 2.** Linear everting catheter and falloposcope (Imagyn, Laguna Niguel, CA). A) falloposcope is used to visualize utero-tubal ostium; B) LEC is everted into fallopian tube lumen; C) falloposcope is advanced through central lumen as LEC is everted; D) falloposcope is at tip of fully everted LEC and visualization performed in a retrograde fashion. (From [17] reprinted with permission)

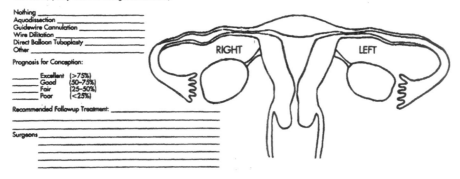

| SITE of DISEASE | RIGHT TUBE | | | | LEFT TUBE | | | |
|---|---|---|---|---|---|---|---|---|
| | INTRAMURAL | ISTHMIC | AMPULLARY | FIMBRIAL | INTRAMURAL | ISTHMIC | AMPULLARY | FIMBRIAL |
| **PATENCY** | | | | | | | | |
| Patency ____ 1 | | | | | | | | |
| Stenosis ____ 2 | | | | | | | | |
| Fibrotic obstruction ____ 3 | | | | | | | | |
| **EPITHELIUM** | | | | | | | | |
| Normal ____ 1 | | | | | | | | |
| Pale, Atropic ____ 2 | | | | | | | | |
| Flat, featureless ____ 3 | | | | | | | | |
| **VASCULARITY** | | | | | | | | |
| Normal ____ 1 | | | | | | | | |
| Intermediate ____ 2 | | | | | | | | |
| Poor pallor ____ 3 | | | | | | | | |
| **ADHESIONS** | | | | | | | | |
| None ____ 1 | | | | | | | | |
| Thin, weblike ____ 2 | | | | | | | | |
| Thick ____ 3 | | | | | | | | |
| **DILITATION** | | | | | | | | |
| None ____ 1 | | | | | | | | |
| Minimal ____ 2 | | | | | | | | |
| Hydrosalpinx ____ 3 | | | | | | | | |
| *OTHER ____ 2–3 | | | | | | | | |
| **CUMULATIVE SCORE** | | | | | | | | |

TOTAL SCORE    RIGHT TUBE =                    (NORMAL = 20)    LEFT TUBE =                    (NORMAL = 20)

A cumulative score for each tube of: 20 = Normal Tubal Lumen; >20 but <30 = Moderate Endotubal Disease; >30 = Severe Endotubal Disease.
* Mucus Plugs or Tubal Debris, Endotubal Polyps, Endometriosis, Salpingitis Isthmica Nodosa, Inflammatory, Infectious, Neoplastic
   conditions and absent tubal segments are each assigned a score of 2 to 3, depending on the significance of the lesion.

Treatment (Specify R & L Tube Surgical Procedures).

Nothing _____
Aquadissection _____
Guidewire Cannulation _____
Wire Dilitation _____
Direct Balloon Tuboplasty _____
Other _____

Prognosis for Conception:

____ Excellent    (>75%)
____ Good    (50–75%)
____ Fair    (25–50%)
____ Poor    (<25%)

Recommended Followup Treatment: _____
_____
_____

Surgeons _____
_____
_____
_____

**Fig. 3.** Classification system for falloposcopic findings. (From [20]; Fig. 1, reprinted with permission)

ments and inability to avoid tubal perforation by performing concomitant laparoscopy may prove to be limiting factors. Patients with dense fibrotic obstruction require tubal bypass with *in vitro* fertilization or resection and microsurgical anastomosis as appropriate.

The patient with suspected hydrosalpinges is managed in a different fashion. If a grossly dilated tube with no functional endothelial lining or extensive intralumenal adhesions is noted at falloposcopy, further surgical intervention may prove unnecessary. The patient should be referred directly for *in vitro* fertilization. If, however, the lining appears only minimally compromised, laparoscopic assessment of peritubal disease with the potential for neosalpingostomy should be performed. *In vitro* fertilization would be appropriate in the face of extensive peritubal disease

or more advanced maternal age. This management paradigm is summarized in Table 2.

## Conclusion

Falloposcopy represents an exciting new and evolving technology which allows visualization of the entire tubal lumen in a minimally invasive fashion. This procedure clearly lends itself to performance in an office setting with minimal anesthesia. As a result, management decisions can now be made based upon actual visualization of pathologic findings. A decision as to whether tubal endoscopy after selective salpingography should represent a standard part of the infertility evaluation shall come from the results of larger scale ongoing clinical trials.

**Table 2.** Management based upon findings at office fallo-poscopy

---

Normal lumen
- treat as unexplained infertility
- perform laparoscopy if indicated

Suspected proximal occlusion
- mucous plugs, debris: aquadissection
- endometriosis, endosalpingiosis: medical suppression
- nonobstructive adhesions: guide wire dissection
- moderate adhesions, stenosis: guide wire dissection or directed balloon tuboplasty
- dense obstruction: IVF/ET vs. resection and microsurgical anastomosis

Suspected distal occlusion
- severe disease: IYF/ET
- mild-moderate disease: IVF/ET vs. laparoscopy and possible distal neosalpingostomy

---

# References

1. Dor J, Homburg R, Rabau E (1977) An evaluation of etiologic factors and therapy in 665 infertile couples. Fertil Steril 28:718-722

2. Templeton AA, Penney GC (1982) The incidence, characteristics, and prognosis of patients whose infertility is unexplained. Fertil Steril 37:175-182

3. Cummings DC, Taylor PJ (1979) Historical predictability of abnormal laparoscopic findings in the infertile woman. J Reprod Med 23: 295-298

4. Gomel V, Taylor PJ (1995) Diagnostic laparoscopy in infertility. In: Keye WR Jr, Chang RJ, Rebar RW, Soules MR (eds) Infertility: Evaluation and Treatment. WB Saunders, Philadelphia, PA, pp 330-348

5. Sulak P, Letterie G, Coddington C et al (1991) Histology of proximal tubal obstruction. Fertil Steril 56:831-835

6. Surrey ES, Surrey MW, Kerin JF (1996) Salpingoscopy and falloposcopy. In: Adamson GD, Martin DC (eds). Endoscopic Management of Gynecologic Disease. Lippincott-Raven, Philadelphia, pp 345-358

7. Surrey ES, Surrey MW (1996) Correlation between salpingoscopic and laparoscopic staging the assessment of the distal fallopian tube. Fertil Steril 65:267-271

8. McComb PF, Fleige-Zahradka BG (1995) The Fallopian Tube: Pathophysiology. In: Keye WR Jr, Chang RJ, Rebar RW, Soules MR (eds). Infertility: Evaluation and Treatment. Saunders, Philadelphia, pp 444-473

9. Jansen RPS (1984) Endocrine response in the fallopian tube. Endo Rev 5:525-551

10. World Health Organization (1980) Comparative trial of tubal insufflation, hysterosalpingography, and laparoscopy with dye hydrotubation fo assessmant of tubal patency. Fertil Steril 46:1101-1107

11. Swart P, Mol BWJ, Van der Veen F, van Beurden M, Redekop WK, Bossuyt PMM (1995) The accuracy of hysterosalpingography in the diagnosis of tubal pathology: a meta-analysis. Fertil Steril 64:486-491

12. Kerin J, Daykhovsky L, Grundfest W, Surrey E (1990) Falloposcopy: a micro-endoscopic technique for diagnosting and treating endotubal disease incorporating guide wire cannulation and direct balloon turboplasty. J Reprod Med 35:606-612

13. Kerin J, Daykhovsky L, Segalowitz J, Surrey E et al (1990) Falloposcopy: a micro-endoscopic technique for yisual exploration of the human fallopian tube from the uterotubal ostium to the fimbria using a transvaginal approach. Fertil Steril 54:390-400

14. Scudamore IW, Dunphy BC, Cooke ID (1992) Outpatient falloposcopy: intra-lumenal imaging of the fallopian tube by trans-uterine fiber-optic endoscopy as an outpatient procedure. Br J Obstet Gynecol 99:829-835

15. Venezia R, Zangara C, Knight C, Cittadini E (1993) Initial experience of a new linear everting falloposcopy system in comparison with hysterosalpingography. Fertil Steril 60:771-775

16. Dunphy BC (1994) Office falloposcopy assessment in proximal tubal disease. Fertil Steril 61:168-70

17. Pearlstone AC, Surrey ES, Kerin JF (1992) The linear everting catheter: a nonhysteroscopic transvaginal technique for access and microendoscopy of the fallopian tube. Fertil Steril 58:854-857

18. Bauer O, Dietrich K, Bacich S, Knight C, Lowery G, van der Veen H et al (1992) Transcervical access and intra-lumenal imaging of the fallopian tube in the non-anesthetized patient: preliminary results using a new technique for fallopian access. Hum Reprod 7 [Suppl]: 7-11

19. Dunphy B, Tuwzer P, Bultz B et al (1994) A comparison of pain experienced during hysterosalpingography and in office falloposcopy. Fertil Steril 62:62-70

20. Kerin J, Williams D, San Roman G, Pearlstone AC, Grundfest W, Surrey E (1992) Falloposcopic classification and treatment of fallopian tube lumen disease. Fertil Steril 57:731-741

21. Grow DR, Coddington CC, Flood JF (1993) Proximal tubal occlusion by hysterosalpingogram: a role for falloposcopy. Fertil Steril 60:170-174

22. Surrey ES, Adamson GD, Surrey MW, Nagel T, Malo J, Jansen R, Molloy D (1997) Introduction of a new coaxial fallocopy system: a multicenter feasibility study. J Am Assoc Gynecol Lap 4:475-478

23. Dunphy B, Greene C (1995) Falloposcopic cannulation, oviductal appearances and prediction of treatment independent intrauterine pregnancy. Hum Reprod 10:3313-3316

24. Kerin JF, Surrey ES (1992) Tubal surgery from the inside out: falloposcopy and balloon tuboplasty. Clin Obstet Gynecol 35:299-312

25. Kerin J, Surrey E, Daykhovsky L, Grundfest W (1990) Development and application of a falloposcope for transvaginal endoscopy of the fallopian tube. J Laparoscopic Surg 1:47-56

# Traumatic complications

B. BLANC

## Cervical wounds

In case of cervical stenosis, forceful dilatation with bougies is necessary and traction on the tenaculum can cause lacerations of the paracervical fascia. Anatomic and physiologic conditions such as menopause, preoperative treatment by LH-RH agonists, cervical hypoplasia and the hysteroscopist's inexperience increase the risks of wounds.

Prevention includes gentle manipulation and progressive dilatation of the endocervical canal (dilating bougies of 0.5 mm). In certain cases (women who have never had children, postmenopausal women, or women treated by LH-RH analogs) synthetic laminaria which act quickly or antiprostaglandine medication should reduce their frequency. Surgical treatment of wide cervical wounds may be necessary and is realised with a 000 slow resorption thread set with a needle.

## Uterine perforations

Frequency varies according to the type of hysteroscopic procedure, with 1.2 °/00 of diagnostics hysteroscopics. During surgical hysteroscopic procedures, frequency is higher and certainly the number of perforations reported in the literature does not do justice to the facts, as many perforations go unsuspected. This frequency may be estimated at 1.77 to about 2%. (Table 1). March [5] reported 2 perforations out of 66 uterine synechiae.

Risks of perforation of surgical hysteroscopic procedures should be compared to other endouterine invasive methods [13-14] (Table 2).

Table 2.

| | |
|---|---|
| 0.02 to 1.5% | for curettages in first trimester abortions |
| 0.0 to 8.7% | for the placement of an IUD |
| 0.6 to 1.3% | during the sequence: dilatation, curettage (CDC) in menstruating women |
| 2.6% in menopausal women | |
| 5.1% in post-partum period | |

## Contributing factors [15]

1) special anatomic conditions;
2) some pathologies;
3) disregard of the rules of procedure;
4) some dangerous endoscopical procedures.

## Special anatomic conditions

Severe cervical atresia. The hysteroscope should never be introduced forcibly and without visual control. A diagnostic hysteroscopic procedure is necessary to evaluate the atresia and the lesion to be treated. Theuse of a hollow mandrin, into which the optical system of the diagnostic hysteroscope can be inserted, allows penetration under visual control. With ultrasonic control during penetration of the surgical hysteroscope, there should be no false passages.

Table 1. 1.2°/00 of diagnostic hysteroscopies

| Lindeman [1] | recorded | 6 perforations out of 5220 hysteroscopies |
|---|---|---|
| Hamou [2] | recorded | 1 perforation out of 1000 diagnostic hysteroscopies |
| Taylor [3] | recorded | 1 perforation out of 602 cases |
| Parent [4] | recorded | 3 perforations during diagnostic hysteroscopic procedures when assessing post menopausal metrorrhagia |

Menopausal uterus. Cervical atresia should be dilated by bougies as explained above, and prostaglandines prescribed except if there are contraindications.

## Special pathological states

Diffuse myomatosis: risks of uterine perforation are high when the uterine cavity is distorted by diffuse fibromatosis. The axis of the uterine cavity is displaced. Ultrasonographic control is necessary to avoid false passages.

Uterine hypoplasia and distilbene syndrome may be present, during the endocervical dilatation and surgical procedure, as well as endometrium carcinoma with risks of perforation due to myometrium infiltration and muscular changes.

## Disregard of the rules

The hysteroscope should always be inserted under visual control. The tip of the hysteroscope is bent at a variable angle. The 30° angle is the most common one. When the hysteroscope is inserted, a little experience is required to become accustomed to the "off-axis" view which should be taken into account to avoid false passages (Fig. 1). It is necessary to negotiate the cervico-isthmic passage dilated by the pocket of gas or of NACL. The crossing of the internal os needs some experience to avoid a false passage, for the zone under view is in fact 30° above the internal os.

The Foroblique lens allows the exploration of the entire uterine cavity by rotating the outside sheath of the hysteroscope to examine the two sides of the uterine cavity. Resection of a lesion (fibroid, polyp, endometrium) should always be performed under visual control. It should be done from back to front for a large lesion (fibroid or polyp), or from side to side for synechiae or uterine septa. Resection should be controlled by ultrasonography which gives better results than laparoscopy as regards resection of uterine septa, synechiae or integrity of the myometrium.

If the field of vision is obscured by bleeding, the bleeding vessel should be coagulated before going on with the surgery. If irrigation is poor, the resectoscope has to be moved inside the uterine cavity. The outside sheath, which has a number of orifices at its end to absorb the liquid, may be flattened against one wall of the uterus or the endocervical canal, thus preventing proper drainage of the intracavity liquid. If vision is still obscured, the procedure has to be stopped, the resectoscope withdrawn and gently cleaning of the blood clots that may have built up on the orifices of the outside sheath or between the two sheaths, has to be realized.

## Dangerous procedures

Complex uterine synechiae (5/187 reported by Valle) [10]. Ultrasonographic preoperative control is essential in the treatment of complex marginal synechiae.
Huge interstitial uterine fibroids with submucous jutting protusions. It is necessary to be very careful with the resecting loop particularly in the pericornua regions, as the myometrium is very thin.
Endometrectomy. During an endometrectomy, the periostial regions and the uterus fundus should be coagulated with the roller-ball so as to limit risks of uterine perforation.
Resection of uterine septa. It is necessary to associate hysteroscopic treatment with ultrasonic control so as to keep a security margin in the myometrium (8 to 10 mm in the uterus fundus).

Prevention of risks depends on meticulous attention to the rules of procedure, visual control of the resection of endouterine lesions and ultrasonic control when there are synechiae and uterine septa. Perforation often happens during resection of synechiae in complex synechiae. Per-operative ultrasonic control is not always sufficient to avoid them, as limits between the myometrium and the synechiae are not always clear-cut.

When resecting myoma or in case of endometrectomy, perforation most often occurs in the uterus fundus for it is more difficult to handle the resecting loop in the fundus and the pericornual region which are very thin (2 to 4 mm). To limit risks of perforation, the roller-ball should be used to realize coagulation in those areas.

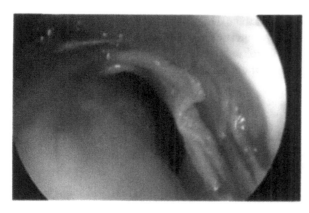

Fig 1. False passage with rigid hysteroscope

Table 3. Uterine perforations in the course of surgical hysteroscopy

| Authors | HSS | Nb of perf. | Comp | Therapeutic consequences |
|---|---|---|---|---|
| Hamou [6] | EUR | 2/96 (2%) | 1 bowelburn for endometrectomy | |
| Dargent [7] | EUR for benign intra cavitary lesions | 2/25 (8%) | 0 | 2 laparoscopies |
| Hallez [8] | EUR for fibroid | 1/92 (1%) | hemoperitoneum | hysterorrhaphy laparotomy |
| Goldrath [9] | Laser for endometrectomy | 2/22 (10%) | 0 | 0 |
| Valle [10] | Surgical HSS traumatic synechiae | 5/187 (2.7%) | 0 | 0 |
| Siegler [11] | Surgical HSS traumatic synechiae | 1/ ? | wound of the small intestine | laparotomy resection of the small intestine |
| Blanc/Boubli [12] | EUR | 7/400 (1.75%) | 0 | 1 laparoscopy |
| Blanc [16] | EUR | 8/506 (1.58%) | 0 | 1 laparoscopy |
| (Thesis Cravello) | fibroid, polyp endometrectomy | | | 1 laparoscopy with myomectomy |
| Loffer [17] | EUR | /43 (2.3%) | | |
| Corson [18] | EUR | 3/92 (3.3%) | | |
| Serden [19] | EUR | 1/216 (0.5%) | | |
| Hill [20] | EUR | 7/850 (0.8%) | | |
| Hucke [21] | EUR | 1/39 (2.6%) | | |
| Mergui [22] | EUR | 1/111 (0.96%) | | |
| Blanc [23] | EUR | 10/699 (1.4%) | | 1 laparoscopy 1 laparoscopy with myomectomy |

## Anatomic lesions

There are two kinds of uterine perforations: subperitoneal and intraperitoneal.

## Subperitoneal uterine perforations

They are most often due to false passages when the hysteroscope is pushed through the cervico-isthmic area. They occur either:

- *during dilatation of the cervical canal,* by forcibly inserting metallic bougies (Hegar bougies). They can be avoided by adapted measures;
- *during the endocervical penetration of the outside sheath of the resectoscope* containing the mandrin. This blind manoeuvre should be avoided; it is better to introduce the endoscope under visual control into the endocervical canal when dilatation has been reached. In certain cases (cervical stenosis, menopause or preoperative treatment by LH-RH agonist), the introduction of a hollow mandrin into which the optical system can be pla-

ced is necessary to achieve complete dilatation. Introduction is performed under visual control which lessens risks of perforation up to a certain point.

If the off-view axis is not taken into account, the bevelled end of the resectoscope can thus create a false passage. No treatment is necessary as there are no symptoms. The prognosis of subperitoneal perforations is usually excellent as they cause neither bleeding or infection, nor any gynecological or obstetrical problem. There is no need for hysterographic control. At least three ovulatory cycles should take place before a new endoscopical attempt.

## Intraperitoneal uterine perforations

Risks of intraperitoneal uterine perforations are increased with anteverted or retroverted uterus, complex synechiae or uterine hypoplasy. Disrespect of the basic rules or hysteroscopist's inexperience are other factors. Such perforation may be caused by:

- the tip of the hysterometer introduced at the beginning of the procedure to assess the limits of the uterine cavity;
- the tip of the mandrin forcibly and deeply introduced into the uterine cavity to obtain a sufficient cervico-isthmic dilatation. It is most often an anterior or posterior perforation;
- the tip of a pair of scissors to resect synechiae in the treatment of marginal complex synechiae or uterine septum;
- the resecting loop or the tip of the cutting loop during a resectoscopy (polyp, myoma or endometrectomy), or the resection of synechiae or uterine septum.

These perforations can have severe consequences because of the loss of myometrial substance and the risk of burns or resection of neighbouring organs (bowels, bladder, colon or sigmoid) if the perforation goes unnoticed during the procedure.

Perforations can and must be avoided by scrupulous attention to the rules of procedure. The rollerball loop or the tip of the knife must only be manipulated under visual control and from front to back toward the cervix for large lesions (polyps and fibroids) and from side to side for the section of a septum in an abnormal uterus. An ultrasonic control is essential during the procedure. If the vision is obscured by bleeding or poor irrigation, the procedure must be stopped and the cause of the problem evaluated and removed.

## Diagnostic and management of perforations

The following criteria have to be taken into consideration:
- the anatomic location: either sub or intraperitoneal perforations;
- the symptoms: bleeding, pains and shock.

The most important rule in all cases is to stop the procedure, withdraw the hysteroscope and evaluate the situations (type and means of perforation, anatomic lesions and clinical signs), and finally inform the patient or her family of the incident and its possible risks.

### Perforation during diagnostic hysteroscopy

If it is a subperitoneum perforation, the diagnosis is obvious (pains, bleeding, and the limits of the uterine cavity which are no longer visible). The procedure has to be stopped. No treatment is necessary, nor hospitalisation.

If the perforation is intraperitoneum, the diagnosis is usually easy because the hysteroscope "escapes" and if the procedure has been performed in the office without anesthesia, the patient complains of pains. Prognosis is good, for the mechanical perforation carries few risks for the neighbouring organs. An antibiotic therapy is not necessary nor is hospitalisation except if the patient is in pain or anxious. Day-time hospitalisation may be enough.

### Perforation during surgical hysteroscopy

It is a purely mechanical perforation caused by the tip of the mandrin of the hysteroscope or by scissors. It is a low-risk perforation as it is small and neighbouring organs are not hurt. A 24-hour hospitalisation is desirable for a careful assessment. An antibiotherapy should be administered.

It is an electrical perforation caused by the resecting loop and a high-risk complication since neighbouring organs may be hurt by the monophasic current. Laparotomy is indicated because of bleeding, shock or delay before a diagnosis is reached. It allows an objective assessment of the situation, such as location and dimension of the perforation and damage done to neighbouring organs (hemoperitoneum). In some cases, laparoscopy can be therapeutic and coagulation of the perforation zone can be achieved to reduce bleeding and avoid laparotomy. Hospitalisation is always necessary even if laparotomy is not indicated.

After an electric resection, an electrolytogram and protidemy tests should be carried out as soon as possible. Signs of a glycine resorption syndrome reveal a perforation. If the diagnosis of perforation is delayed, great quantities of liquid can pass into the peritoneal cavity. Ultrasonography will help to discover an important effusion in the Douglas. In such a case, it is preferable to puncture around the Douglas'pouch to decrease the risks of vascular passage of glycine. Antibiotherapy is necessary. In a young woman of child-bearing age, a hysterographic control three to six months after the perforation will allow the evaluation of the scars.

## References

1. Lindeman HJ (1975) Komplicationen bei der CO2 hysteroskopie. Arch Gynakol 219-257
2. Hamou JE (1981) Hysteroscopy and microcolpohysteroscopy. Text and Atlas. Appleton Lange Norwalk, p 52

3. Taylor PJ, Leade RA, Georgere (1983) Combined laparoscopy and hysteroscopy in the investigation of infertility. In: Siegler AM, Lindeman HJ (eds) Hysteroscopy, Principles and Practices. Lippincot, p 207

4. Parent B, Gued JH, Barbot J, Nodarian P (1985) Hystéroscopie panoramique. Maloine ed, Paris, p 113

5. March, C, Israel, R, March AD (1978) Hysteroscopic management of uterine synechiae. Am J Obstet Gynecol 130:653-657

6. Hamou JS, Alatbaroux J (1988) Hystéroscopie et microhystéroscopie opératoire. Mise à jour en gynécologie-obstétrique. Collège National des Gynécologues-Obstétriciens. Vigot Diffusion, Paris, pp 111-197

7. Dargent TD, Mellier G, Jacquot F (1988) Electro-résection endo-utérin: une série préliminaire de 25 cas. J Gynecol Obstet Biol Reproduc 17(7):940

8. Hallez JP, Neter A, Cartier R (1987) Methodical intrauterine resection. Am J Obstet Gynecol 156(5):1080-1084

9. Goldrath M, Fuller T, Segal S (1981) Laser photovaporization of endometrium for the treatment of menorrhagia. Am J Ostet Gynecol 140:14-19

10. Valla RF, Sciarra JJ (1988) Intra-uterine synechiae, hysteroscopic diagnosis, classification, treatment and reproductive outcome. Am J Obstet Gynecol 158:14-59

11. Siegler A, Valler F (1988) Therapeutic hystereoscopic procedures. Fertil Steril 50(5):685-701

12. Blanc B, Boubli L (1991) Manuel d'hystéroscopie opératoire. Vigot ed, Paris, pp 107-109

13. Stirk GJ (1993) Uterine perforation- endoscopic treatment and complication. In: Corfman RS, Diamond M, Decherney A (eds) Complications of laparoscopy and hysteroscopy. Blackwell Scientific Publ, p 192

14. Benbaruc HG, Menczer J, Shale VJ et al (1980) Uterine perforation rates and post-perforation management. ISRJ Med SC 16:821-824

15. Valler F (1993) Cervical and uterine complications during insertion of the hysteroscope. In: (as in ref. 13)) Complications of laparoscopy and hysteroscopy. Blackwell Scientific Publ, pp 167-176

16. Cravello L (1994) Le traitement hystéroscopique des lésions endoutérines bénignes (à partir d'une série de 506 résections). Thèse médecine, Marseille

17. Loffer FD (1990) Removal of large intra uterine growths by the hysteroscopic resectoscope. Obstet Gynecol 76: 836-840

18. Corson SL, Broks PG (1991) Resectoscopic myomectomy. Fertil Steril 55:1041-1044

19. Serdens P, Brooks PG (1991) Treatment of abnormal uterine bleeding with the gynecologic resectoscope. J Reprod Med 36:697-699

20. Hild, Mher P, Wood C, Lawrence A, Downing B, Lolatgis N (1992) Complications of operative hysteroscopy. Gynaecological Endoscopy 1:185-189

21. Huck EJ, Campor L, Debruyme F, Freikha A (1992) Hysteroscopic resection of submucous myoma. Geburtshilfe Frauenheilkd, 51:214-218

22. Mergui JL, Renolleau C, Salat-Baroux J (1993) Hystéroscopie opératoire et fibromes. Gynecol, 1:325-337

23. Cravello L, d'Ercole C, Boubli L, Blanc B (1995) Les complications des résections hystéroscopiques. Contracept Fertil Sexual

# Infectious complications

B. Blanc, R. de Montgolfier

Infections complications are rare and may be caused by the endoscopic procedure. Contamination may occur during the cervical passage from contact with some infected discharge. Risks are theoretically higher with liquid distending media, which easily carry germs whereas possibility of contamination is lower with gas. Latent endometritis or unknown salpingitis can be exacerbated by any endouterine manipulation including hysteroscopic procedures. Rupture of a hydrosalpinx may theoretically occur during gaseous distension. Siegler [1] reported such a case during a diagnostic hysteroscopy. It is, however, exceptional.

In case of infection, the patient runs a temperature (above 38° C) or complains of pains in the pelvic abdomen. In a series of 1000 hysteroscopical examinations, Hamou noted one case of severe infection and seven cases of mild infection [2]. In a personal series of 1000 diagnostic examinations performed in the same conditions, we noted one severe case of infection which was favorably resolved with antibiotherapy and hospitalisation [3].

Salat-Baroux and Hamou [4] studied the bacteriologic effects of the routine use of a microhysteroscope. Bacteriologic investigations of the optical system and the cervix were carried out before and after the examination. No germs were found on the endoscope. Saprophyte germs such as enterococci and *Escherichia coli* were found on the cervix. No germs were transferred from one patient to another. No infection was observed after surgical hysteroscopies. Darabi found 0.7% cases of endometritis out of a series of 773 hysteroscopic examinations with tubal sterilisation [5]. Valle and Sciarra reported seven genital infections after 4000 hysteroscopic examinations [6]. Preventive antibiotic therapy does not seem necessary as the risks of infection are so low. Their frequency varies between 0.5 and 3.5% but the different series in the literature have little in common.

We do not advise preventive antibiotherapy after endouterine resections.

We carried out a prospective study to investigate:
- risks of contamination of the endometrium in case of vaginal contamination;
- risks of clinical endometritis;
- risks according to the type of procedure, either diagnostic or therapeutic hysteroscopy.

This study was realised between February and October 1993 on 81 hysteroscopies (34 diagnostic and 47 surgical hysteroscopies). Vaginal samples were taken before the hysteroscopic procedure, and endouterine samples after the procedure [7].

According to our findings:
- risks of high genital infection after hysteroscopy are low compared to risks after hysterosalpingography (from 0.3 to 1.3 according to the series);
- risks of endouterine contamination are real and differ according to the degree of infection in the vagina (3.4 if the sample is sterile and 56.5% if the sample is infected);
- the hysteroscopical examination may reveal an infection even if there is no infected discharge when the prescribed conditions of asepsis are not respected. Risks of iatrogenous contamination by hepatitis B virus, VIH or papilloma virus are similar;
- vaginal disinfection is of utmost importance to diminish the risks of infections before any kind of endoscopical examination, either diagnostic or therapeutic.

## References

1. Siegler AM, Kemman E (1975) Hysteroscopy. Obstet Gynecol Survey, 30(5): 67
2. Hamou J, Salat-Baroux J (1987) Hystéroscopie et microhystéroscopie. Atlas et Traité, Masson, Paris, pp 83-84
3. Blanc B, Boubli L (1992) HSS Opératoire. Vigot, Paris, p 108
4. Hamou J (1999) Hysteroscopy. Masson, Paris-New-York, p 51
5. Daraki KF, Richart RM (1977) Collaborative study on Hysteroscopic Sterilisation Procedures. Obstet Gynecol 49:48-54
6. Valle R, Sciarra JJ (1979) Current status of hysteroscopy in gynecologic practice. Fertil-Steril 32:619-632 (Livre complications ref 28 p 202)
7. Boubli L, Porcu G, Gantois SM, d'Ercole C, Blanc B (1997) Risques infectieux de l'hystéroscopie. J Gynecol Obstet Biol Reprod 26:250-255

# Hemorrhagic complications

B. BLANC

Postoperative hemorrhage is rare and the need for a blood transfusion exceptional. Bleeding may be caused by vascular injury of intralesional blood vessels in uterine fibroids, fibro-muscular synechiae or intramyometrial vessels during the resection of interstitial myoma or endometrectomy. The best preventive measure and specific treatment are to carry out all resections under strict visual control [1].

Prevention of hemorrhages is essential. The first step before an endoscopic resection is to examine the lesion and perform preventive coagulation on visible vessels. In case of vascularized fibro-muscular synechiae, coagulation of the vessels comes first, before resection of the synechiae. This precaution is unnecessary for uterine septum as it is avascular.

Hemorrhages have to be carefully controlled. Every vascular perforation has to be electrically coagulated with the resection loop or the tip of the knife. Pumps which deliver fluids under permanent pressure control afford an elective treatment of vascular effraction [2]. In case of severe bleeding and when no irrigation pumps are available, and in any case at the end of the procedure, the glycine flow should be stopped for a few moments while keeping some liquid in the uterine cavity. Barohemostasis being thus suppressed, it is possible to visualise the vascular effraction and treat them accordingly. If bleeding comes from the vascular bed, the resection loop is used with little successive touches. The high frequency knife is most useful in these cases (see Table).

Corson and Brooks [3] recommend preventive recourse to vasopressive medication. Decherney [4, 5] controlled postoperative bleeding by placing a Foley catheter balloon similar to the one used by urologists in the surgical treatment of prostate adenoma. It was left in place for a few hours (1 to 4, exceptionally 24 hours). Loffer [6] used it three times out of 55 endocavitary myomectomies.

In our experience, out of more than 1500 resectoscopies we used a Foley catheter only in one case for an hemorrhage which was finally favorably resolved without any other treatment (Table 1). We never used preventive oxytocic substances in the postoperative phase as some have done [7, 8].

## References

1. Blanc B, Boubli L (1991) Manuel d'hystéroscopie opératoire. Vigot, Paris, pp 109-110
2. Hamou J, Salat-Baroux J (1988) Hystéroscopie et microhystéroscopie opératoire. Mise à jour en Gyncol

Table 1. Hemorrhagic complications after endouterine resection

| Authors | No. of cases | Treatment |
|---|---|---|
| De Cherney [5] | 1 | Foley catheter |
| Loffer [6] | 3 | Foley catheter |
| Corson [3] | 1 | Foley catheter |
| Serden [9] | 4 | Foley catheter |
| Istre [10] | 1 | Hysterectomy at day 1 |
| Hill [11] | 5 | Foley catheter |
| | 1 | Progestatives |
| | 1 | Hysterectomy at day 21 |
| Blanc [12] | 2 | Foley catheter |

Obstet Collège National des Gynécologues Obstétriciens. Vigot Diffusion, Paris, pp 111-197

3.  Corson SL, Brooks PG (1991) Resectoscopic myomectomy. Fertil Steril 55:1041-1044

4.  Cooerman AB, Decherney A (1993) Hysteroscopic resection of uterine leiomyomas and post-operative metrorrhagy in complications of laparoscopy and hysteroscopy. In: Corfman RS, Diamond MP, Decherney A (eds) Blackwell Scientific Publications 76:836-840

5.  De Cherney, Polan ML (1983) Hysteroscopic management of intra-uterine lesions and intractable uterine bleeding. Obstet Gynecol 61:392-397

6.  Loffer FD (1990) Removal of large symptomatic intra-uterine growths by the hysteroscopic resectoscope. Obstet Gynecol 76:836-840

7.  Magos A, Bauman R, Turnbull A (1989) Transcervical resection of endometrium in women with menorrhagia. Br Med J 298:1209-1212

8.  Neuwirth R (1983) Hysteroscopic management of symptomatic submucous fibroids. Obstet Gynecol 62(4):509

9.  Serden SP, Brooks PG (1991) Treatment of abnormal uterine bleeding with the gynecologic resectoscope. J Reprod Med 36: 697-699

10.  Istre O, Schiotz H, Sadik L, et al (1991) Transcervical resection of endometrium and fibroids: initial complications. Acta Obstet Gynecol Scand 70:363-366

11.  Hill D, Maher P, Wood G, et al (1992) Complications of operative hysteroscopy. Gynaecol Endosc 16: 781-785

12.  Cravello L, D'Ercole C, Boubli L, Blanc B (1995) Les complications des résections hystéroscopiques. Contracep Fertil Sexual 23(5):335-340

# Complications linked to gaseous distension media

B. Blanc, R. de Montgolfier

$CO_2$ is widely used as a distension medium for diagnostic hysteroscopies (HSS) as it allows an excellent vision of the uterine cavity. Risks can and must be avoided by using machines which automatically control gas flow and pressure. $CO_2$ is easily miscible with blood. At body temperature and atmospheric pressure, 54.1 ml of $CO_2$ can be absorbed per 100 ml of blood. The risks of gaseous embolism are low if pressure is kept under 100 mmHg.

Experimenting on animals, Lindeman [1] reported no changes in blood PH, $PCO_2$, bicarbonates or electrocardiogram when the $CO_2$ flow rate is under 100 ml/min. Accidents occur when $CO_2$ flow rate is higher than 350 ml/min. Toxic signs such as tachycardia and arrhythmia always appear first. Risks of gaseous embolism are thus limited but should not be disregarded though $CO_2$ blood solubility limits the formation of bubbles [2]. Gomar [3] and more recently Mac Grath [4] reported cases of embolism which could not be formally attributed to $CO_2$. Cases of gaseous embolism were described during hysteroscopic procedures using liquid distension media [5]. Though there may have been bubbles in the solute, yet it seems more likely that embolism was due to $CO_2$ produced by electroresection or by laser photovaporization of tissues.

A prodromic phase with arrhythmia and respiratory disorders is observed prior to gaseous embolism and then the procedure has to be stopped immediately, assisted ventilation installed, blood gases drawn from a central catheter and hyperbaric oxygenotherapy started immediately [6].

Pierre [7] researched 18 departments of hyperbaric oxygen therapy and carried out a prospective enquiry about all the hysteroscopic procedures performed in 84 public departments of gynecology over a two-year period. He reported 11 cases of gaseous embolism but out of 5140 patients who had undergone exploratory hysteroscopic procedures, he noted only 3 cases of embolism (one resulting in death), that is a 0.58%. Close analysis of the data showed there are no risks of gaseous embolism in ambulatory procedures. Accidents happen with general anesthesia when there are bleeding problems often linked with cervical dilation and long procedures.

Prevention of complications is essential. All severe accidents reported in the literature occurred when the $CO_2$ flow and pressure were not duly controlled. In 1972, Porto [8] reviewed the literature and reported six fatal cases. In all the accidents gas flow exceeded 350 ml/min. Thus control of volume and pressure is essential.

There are three types of insufflating apparatus:
- the Wisap insufflator with preset pressure at 100 mmHg. Gas flow varies from 0 to 80 ml/min until pre-set pressure is reached;
- the Hysteroflator (Storz) insufflator with constant flow set at 40 ml/min. Pressure rises from 0 to 180 mm/Hg when flow is turned off;
- Hamou microhysteroflator-Storz insufflator with variable flow and pressure. There is a constant balance between flow and pressure which cannot increase beyond 180 mmHg without turning off the gas flow.

In fact, a diagnostic hysteroscopic procedure should be performed in the office without anesthesia or with a local anesthetic or analgesia. General anesthesia is a contraindication. Gas flow should never exceed 80 ml and pressure 100 mmHg. No cases of gaseous embolism have ever been reported when those conditions are applied.

## References

1. Lindeman HJ, Siegler AM, Mohr J (1976) The Hysteroflator 1000 S. J Reprod Med 11(6):145
2. Etches RC (1990) Hyperbaric oxygen and $CO_2$ embolism. Can J Anesth 37:270, 271
3. Gomar C, Fernandez C, Villalonova et al (1985) Carbon dioxide embolism during laparoscopy and hysteroscopy. Ann Fr Anesth Reanim 4:380-382
4. MacGrath RJ, Zimmermann JE, William JF et al (1989) Carbon dioxide embolism treated with hyperbaric oxygen. Can J Anaesth 36:586-589
5. Perry PM, Baughlman VL (1990) A complication of hysteroscopy: air embolism. Anestesiol 73:546-547
6. Turkaspa H (1990) Hyperbaric oxygen therapy for air embolism complicating operative hysteroscopy. Am J Obstet Gynecol 163:680-688
7. Pierre F, Lansac J, Soutoul JH (1995) Embolie gazeuse et hystéroscopie exploratoire. Mythe ou réalité. J Gynecol Obtest Biol Reprod 1:19-23
8. Porto R, Gaujoux J (1972) Une nouvelle méthode d'hystéroscopie: Instrumentation et technique. J Gynecol Obstet Biol Reprod 1:691

# Complications linked to use of glycine in hysteroscopic surgery

L. Boubli

Glycine solution is very often used for hysteroscopic surgery. This fluid has interesting properties like excellent optical quality and poor miscibility with blood and mucus.

The biochemical composition does not include glucose or natrium and allows the electrosurgery.

The urologist surgeons have a long experience with that fluid. However, some complications have been described.

The rate of those is very low, and if the common rules of hysteroscopic surgery are respected, the severe complications can be easily avoided.

## Glycine

Glycine is an aminoacid, used in a dilution of 1,5%. Its metabolism is linked with many others among which several are potentially toxic (Fig. 1).

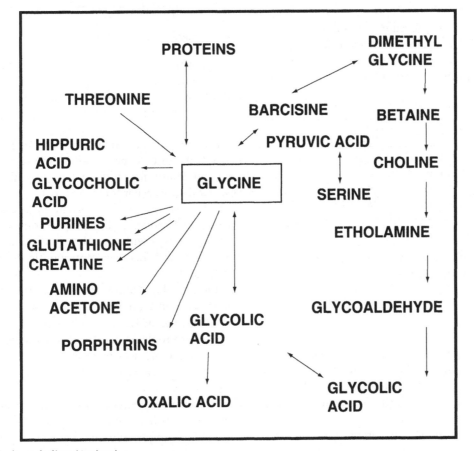

**Fig. 1.** Glycins' metabolism (Arvieux)

## Biological modifications during hysteroscopic surgery

### Surgery using glycine

Hysteroscopic surgery needs the transformation of the virtual uterine cavity into a real cavity; this is made by carrying out a liquid irrigation with inflow and outflow of glycin solution.

In order to know the biological modifications associated with that irrigation, we fixed some plasmatic rates before the surgery, immediately after the surgical procedure and two hours later.

|         | Before surgery | After surgery |         |
| ------- | -------------- | ------------- | ------- |
| Creat   | 70,5 ± 2,4     | 70,9 ± 2      | NS      |
| Urea    | 4,46 ± 0,18    | 4,25 ± 0,14   | NS      |
| Protid  | 67,7 ± 1       | 63,8 ± 0,9    | < 0,01  |
| Glycine | 330 ± 42       | 1074 ± 25     | < 0,005 |
| Natrium | 140,05 ± 02    | 136,2 ± 1,2   | < 0,005 |
| Haemat  | 38,2 ± 0,5     | 36,2 ± 0,9    | < 0,005 |

At the end of the procedure, several modifications are statistically significant but in a normal range.

Thus, even without complication, the values of natrium and haematocrit indicate a tendency to hemodilution.

|         | Before surgery | 2h later    |         |
| ------- | -------------- | ----------- | ------- |
| Protid. | 67,7 ± 1       | 66,4 ± 0,9  | < 0,02  |
| Glycin  | 330 ± 42       | 519 ± 46    | < 0,005 |
| Natrium | 140,05 ± 02    | 135,8 ± 0,6 | NS      |
| Haemat  | 38,2 ± 0,5     | 36,7 ± 4,9  | NS      |

Two hours after surgery, quite all the value return to the initial rate, but the glycine remains increased.

### Complications

Complications have been described by urologist surgeons as "transuretral resection syndrome", which asociate several signs. Neurological and ophthalmic are the first to appear; the other are pulmonary, cardiovascular and nephrologic.

Classically, the immediate complications are related to a direct toxicity of glycine.

The delayed complications are the consequences of the overload.

The threshold of biological values indicatig a complication was 5% for natrium and haematocrit.

|                  | < 5%        | > 5%        |          |
| ---------------- | ----------- | ----------- | -------- |
| Diameter of myoma | 2,21 ± 0,2 | 2,82 ± 0,37 | NS       |
| Duration         | 29,7 ± 3,02 | 45 ± 8,37   | < 0,05   |
| Hte              | 97,6 ± 0,38 | 90,1 ± 3,76 | < 0,005  |
| Glycine          | 2,59 ± 0,35 | 10,1 ± 3,7  | < 0,0005 |

If we consider that threshold for the natrium, the variations are significantly linked to duration of the procedure, variation of haematocrit and glycine.

The rate of metabolic complications is discussed.

It's difficult to know the rate of biological and clinical forms. Therefore, the rate is low.

| Studies        | NB HSS | Biological complications |
| -------------- | ------ | ------------------------ |
| Magos          | 250    | 2                        |
| Scottish study | 978    | 0,1                      |
| Osei           | 90     | 3,33                     |
| AAGL (1988)    | 7293   | 0,34                     |
| AAGL (1991)    | 17298  | 0,14                     |
| Personal data  | 699    | 1,14                     |

The consequences of the overload are not really severe if the discrepancy is low (1 l for a healthy patient and 750 ml for an old patient or with a cardiovascular disease, according to Magos)

If the discrepancy is important, in default of correction, the hyponatremia may have some neurological consequences with a cerebral oedema and, in the most important forms, a centropontic demyelinization (Fig. 2).

However, the relation between hyponatremia and demyelinization is not very clear; a hypercorrection of the biologic perturbation would increase the risk.

Another problem concerns a potential direct toxicity of the glycine, which seems to get an important affinity for the gabaergic receptors and can act like benzodiazepin.

The terminal consequence of the neurological toxicity is a biochemical pontomesencephalic section. This kind of complication may happen only in case of quick and important overload.

In surgical terms it may be observed in case of prolongation of the procedure, with a very high intrauterine pressure and/or perforation.

The variations of glycine are directly linked to discrepancy between inflow and outflow, but intrauterine high pressure and perforation provoke a very rapid variation (Fig. 3).

## Modifications of glycin plasmatic rates

The variation of glycine is directly linked to the intrauterine pressure. The main variation is observed in case of perforation (Fig. 3).

## Prevention

The conditions of high risk of biological complications are easy to avoid. The intrauterine fluid pressure must be low, less than 100 mm of water. It is important to realize a permanent monitoring of outflow and inflow.

In case of perforation, but also of suspicion of perforation, the procedure must be immediately stopped. The first signs are neurological and ophthalmic; so the presence of nausea or amaurosis yields to increase the clinical monitoring and to perform biological samplings, essentially ionogram and haematocrit.

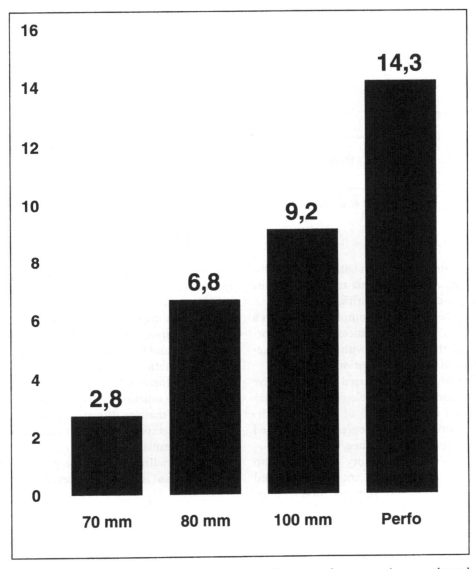

Fig 2. In the additional case of perforation, two hours after surgery the rate remains at an elevated level with a potential risk of neurological complication

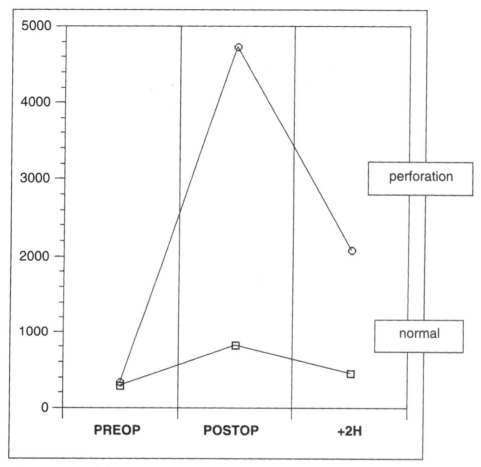

**Fig 3.** Variations of glycine rates after perforation

## Treatment

In case of moderate complication with only some discrete clinical signs, if the natremia returns to a quite normal value, the clinical monitoring is efficient.

The management of severe complications needs a real resuscitation. The circumstances are an important duration of the procedure with a major discrepancy especially in case of perforation.

The patient must be transferred to an intensive care unit. The correction of biological disease may need a parenteral administration of a loop diuretic, but the correction must be progressive, the speed being diversely appreciated (0,5 meq/h - 2meq/h).

The management of circulatory overload is also necessary by increasing inspired concentrations and improving cardiac function (nitrates, dobutamine, dopamine).

## Conclusion

The metabolic complications of glycine use during hysteroscopic surgery are rare if the safety conditions are respected.

The most important is to avoid high intrauterine pressure, to have a permanent monitoring of inflow and outflow and to stop immediately the procedure in case of perforation or suspicion of perforation.

The treatment of the severe complications needs a transfer to an intensive care unit. The biological treatment must manage the overload and its consequences: direct toxicity of glycin and indirect effect by the hyponatremia.

The normalization must be progressive, but the most important is always the prevention.

# References

1. Bauman et al (1990) Absorption of glycine irrigating fluid during transcervical resection of the endometrium. Br Med J 300-305

2. Boubli L et al (1990) Le risque métabolique de l'hystéroscopie opératoire. J Gyn Obst Biol Repr 19:217-222

3. Byers G et al (1993) Fluid absorption during transcervical resection of the endometrium. Gynaecol Endoscopy 2:21-24

4. Hill D et al (1992) Complications of operative hysteroscopy. Gynaecol Endoscopy 1-4:185-190

5. Lewis BV, Magos A Endometrial ablation.

6. Sterns RH et al (1986) Osmotic demyelinization syndrome following correction of hyponatremia. N Engl J Med 314:1535-1542

Lightning Source UK Ltd.
Milton Keynes UK
UKOW07f1225141116

287614UK00001B/7/P